Perinatal and Postpartum Mood Disorders

Susan Dowd Stone, MSW, LCSW, was president of Postpartum Support International (2006–2008), the organization's vice-president and conference chair (2005–2006), and currently chairs PSI's President's Advisory Council (2008–2010). She is a NJHSS Certified Perinatal Mood Disorders Instructor and Adjunct Lecturer in the MSW program at the Silver School of Social Work, New York University, where she presents on Cognitive Behavior Therapy. Ms. Stone received her clinical social work education at New York University where she received a President's Service Award and has been the recipient of numerous other awards for community service including the development of facility based programs supportive to mental health. Intensively trained in Dialectical Behavior Therapy while working in the Department of Psychiatry at Hackensack University Medical Center, she helped form and facilitate the Postpartum Psychotherapy Program which helped identify women at high risk for perinatal mood disorders. She also offered socialization groups for new mothers and their babies, as well as individual and group therapy specifically designed to support recovery from perinatal mood disorders.

Ms. Stone was a contributor to the NJ Governor's Task Force Educational Webinar on postpartum depression and is a frequent author and cited resource on the topic of perinatal mental health; recent writings include an article in the NJ Psychological Association journal *Empowering PPD with Dialectical Behavior Therapy* and a chapter on the treatment of perinatal mood disorders in a graduate textbook entitled *Cognitive Behavior Therapy in Clinical Social Work Practice,* the first text of its kind for social workers with foreword by Aaron Beck (Ronen & Freeman, Springer, 2006). Her PowerPoint presentation, "Telling the Birth Story," has been widely resourced around the world by health care facilities, agencies and mental health professionals as a guide for those interested in implementing PPD programs. She regularly presents on women's reproductive mental health issues at educational conferences, seminars and in the media; national television appearances have included the CBS Early Show, ABC News, NJN News, NBC News, The New Morning Show (Hallmark), A Place of Our Own (PBS), The Morning Show (Fox), and many others.

At the invitation of Congressional Leaders, Ms. Stone has presented at Capitol Hill press conferences and briefings on perinatal legislation and is frequently invited to contribute viewpoint or review pending legislation, media content, or commentary relevant to PPD issues and emerging research. She is a nationally recognized advocate for the promotion of evidenced based clinical programs contributing to the perinatal wellness of women and their infants. She maintains a private practice in Englewood Cliffs, NJ, specializing in women's reproductive mental health in both group and individual format. She can be reached at susanstonelcsw@aol.com.

Alexis E. Menken, PhD, is a Clinical Psychologist licensed in New York, New Jersey and Connecticut. She developed her career at Columbia Presbyterian Medical Center where she worked for approximately 10 years as a staff psychologist in Community Psychiatry conducting women's groups and training psychology interns. Dr. Menken developed a specialty in Maternal Mental Health and is the co-founder of the Pregnancy and Postpartum Resource Center at Columbia Presbyterian Medical Center in the Department of Behavioral Medicine. She has served as a Board Member for Depression After Delivery and as a Board Member and Public Relations

Chairperson for Postpartum Support International. Dr. Menken was invited by Governor Codey to represent women's mental health at his first state-of-the-state address when he announced his groundbreaking initiative for postpartum depression. Dr. Menken was also a member of Governor Codey's Postpartum Depression Task Force where she worked on the professional education subcommittee. In this capacity she helped write the training program and Webinar titled "Perinatal Mood Disorders: Psychiatric Illnesses During Pregnancy and Postpartum."

Dr. Menken is currently an instructor in Clinical Psychology in the Department of Psychiatry at Columbia University and an Assistant Professional Psychologist at Columbia Presbyterian Medical Center. She serves on the Maternal Mortality Review Committee for Governor Corzine. She also serves as both the NJ Coordinator and is a Presidential Advisory Council Member for Postpartum Support International. Through PSI, Dr. Menken currently writes the "Expert Advice" section for DestinationMaternity.com, answering all questions related to postpartum depression. She teaches a Mind/Body course for infertility patients at the Institute for Reproductive Medicine & Science at St. Barnabas Hospital in Livingston, NJ. Dr. Menken has a private practice in Montclair, NJ where she offers psychological testing for ovum donors and gestational carriers, and provides psychotherapy for women with disorders related to reproductive mental health.

Perinatal and Postpartum Mood Disorders

Perspectives and Treatment Guide for the Health Care Practitioner

SUSAN DOWD STONE, MSW, LCSW

ALEXIS E. MENKEN, PhD

Editors

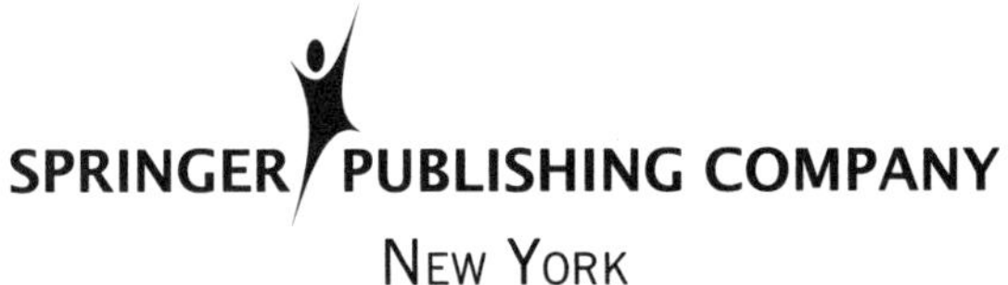

Springer Publishing Company, LLC
11 West 42nd Street
New York, NY 10036
www.springerpub.com

Acquisitions Editor: Sheri W. Sussman
Production Editor: Julia Rosen
Cover design: Joanne E. Honigman
Composition: Apex Publishing, LLC

07 08 09 10/ 5 4 3 2 1

Library of Congress Cataloging-in-Publication Data

Perinatal and postpartum mood disorders : perspectives and treatment guide for the healthcare practitioner / Susan Dowd Stone, Alexis E. Menken [editors].
p. cm.
Includes bibliographical references and index.
ISBN 978-0-8261-0116-7 (alk. paper)
1. Postpartum depression. 2. Postpartum psychiatric disorders. 3. Pregnant women—Mental health. I. Stone, Susan Dowd. II. Menken, Alexis E.
RG852.P438 2008
618.7'6—dc22 2008005869

Printed in the United States of America by Bang Printing.

Contents

Contributors

Cheryl Tatano Beck, DNSc, CNM, FAAN, is a Board of Trustees Distinguished Professor at the University of Connecticut School of Nursing and a fellow in the American Academy of Nursing. She has developed the Postpartum Depression Screening Scale (PDSS), published by Western Psychological Services. She is a prolific writer who has published over 125 journal articles on topics such as postpartum depression, birth trauma, and PTSD due to childbirth. She co-authored with Dr. Jeanne Driscoll *Postpartum Mood and Anxiety Disorders: A Clinician's Guide* which received the 2006 American Journal Nursing Book of the Year Award.

Kristin Bergman, PhD, has a first degree in psychology and has just completed her PhD at Imperial College, London investigating the effects of prenatal stress on child development. Dr. Bergman has studied women recruited at amniocentecis to show a relationship between both the maternal prenatal stress and the in utero hormone environment with child cognitive and emotional outcomes.

Lisa Bernstein is the Executive Director of The What To Expect Foundation in NYC, a non-profit that provides the Baby Basics Prenatal Health Literacy Program for underserved expecting and new families nationwide. Ms. Bernstein is a former commercial book publishing executive who founded the organization with Heidi Murkoff, the author of the bestselling *What To Expect When You're Expecting*. She has lectured nationally and internationally on strengthening health education and communication skills in order to break cycles of poverty and illiteracy.

Catherine A. Birndorf, MD, is Assistant Professor of Psychiatry and Obstetrics & Gynecology at The New York Presbyterian Hospital–Weill Cornell Medical College. She is Program Director of the Payne Whitney Women's Program, a program designed to evaluate and treat women with emotional distress and psychiatric illness throughout the life cycle. Dr. Birndorf has expertise in reproductive psychiatry, treating women before, during, and after pregnancy as well as at other times of hormonal changes in the life course. Board-certified in Psychiatry and Psychosomatic Medicine, Dr. Birndorf, a Smith College graduate, received her medical degree from Brown University and completed her psychiatry residency at New York Presbyterian Hospital/Payne Whitney Clinic.

Andrea Mechanick Braverman, PhD, is the Director of Psychological and Complementary Care at the Reproductive Medicine Associates of New Jersey. She has lectured internationally and published widely in the area of infertility and particularly in third party reproduction.

Julia Chase-Brand, MD, PhD, is currently the Medical Director of Outpatient Psychiatry at Lawrence & Memorial Hospital in New London, CT. Prior to completing her MD at Albert Einstein College of Medicine, Dr. Chase-Brand was a biologist who taught at Barnard College as a Professor of Physiology. She developed a specialty in child psychiatry while on staff at several facilities, including Montefiore Medical Center and Hackensack University Medical Center. She presents nationally and internationally on the effects of maternal stress on infant and child development and is also a recognized expert in animal behavior.

Ian Brockington, PhD, FRCPsych, has a distinguished career in maternal mental health that has spanned decades and has mightily contributed to our body of knowledge in this field. He was a Professor of Psychiatry, University of Birmingham (1983–2001, now emeritus), a Visiting Professor at The University of Chicago (1980–1981), Washington University in St. Louis (1981), Nagoya University (2002), and Kumamoto University (2003). Dr. Brockington is the Founder and First President of the Marcé Society. He was also the Founder and 1st Chairman, Section on Women's Mental Health, World Psychiatric Association. Dr. Brockington has written extensively on the subject. Notable contributions include "Motherhood and Mental Health" (1996) and "Eileithyia's Mischief: the Organic Psychoses of Pregnancy, Parturition and the Puerperium" (2006).

Vivette Glover, PhD, DSc, is currently Professor of Perinatal Psychobiology at Imperial College, London. She was trained as a biochemist at Oxford and did her PhD in neurochemistry at University College, London. Recent projects include studies characterizing the stress responses of the fetus and the first trial of analgesia in the fetus; studies showing that maternal antenatal stress or anxiety increases the risk for a range of emotional, behavioral and cognitive adverse outcomes for the child; and studies showing possible mechanisms by which maternal stress or anxiety may affect the development of the fetus. This work shows the importance of the fetal period and the emotional state of the mother during pregnancy for the later neurodevelopment of the child. She has published over 400 papers.

Jane Israel Honikman, MS, co-founded Postpartum Education for Parents (PEP) in 1977 and became the Executive Director of the Santa Barbara Birth Resource Center in 1984. She founded Postpartum Support International in 1987 and was elected as PSI's first president in 1989. She has authored many articles and educational materials on postpartum depression, including her books "Step by Step" (2000) and "I'm listening" (2002). She lectures extensively on the role of social support and the emotional health of families during the perinatal period.

Karen Joe, BSc Honours, is a research coordinator for the Reproductive Mental Health Program, an outpatient tertiary care clinic located out of BC Women's and St. Paul's Hospitals in Vancouver, Canada. Karen has a BSc in Biology and has recently completed a study examining antidepressant usage during pregnancy. She has also contributed manuscripts to peer-reviewed journals and presented posters at large scale conferences outlining recent research topics in the area of perinatal depression and anxiety disorders.

Sandra Jolley, PhD, ARNP, is an Assistant Professor in Family and Child Nursing at the University of Washington, Seattle. She has worked as pediatric Nurse Practitioner and Lactation Consultant for decades, where she developed her interest in Postpartum Depression and doctoral study. She focuses her research on the psychobiology of PPD, particularly the stress system (relationships between ACTH and cortisol). She has been involved with Washington State PPD organizations for the last 10 years, and is currently a PSI board member.

Kathleen Kendall-Tackett, PhD, IBCLC, is a Health Psychologist, international board certified Lactation Consultant, and research associate specializing in women's health at the Family Research Lab, University of New Hampshire. Dr. Kendall-Tackett is a Fellow of the American Psychological Association in both health and trauma psychology. She has a long-standing interest in maternal depression, perinatal health, and family violence, and is the author of 17 books and 175 articles on depression and related topics including *Depression in New Mothers, The Hidden Feelings of Motherhood* and *Handbook of Women, Stress, and Trauma.* Her latest book is *Non-Pharmacologic Treatments for Depression in New Mothers* (2008).

Linda G. Klempner, PhD, Clinical Psychologist and certified Psychoanalyst, began Women's Health Counseling & Psychotherapy 25 years ago in Teaneck, NJ to address psychological difficulties related to reproductive health issues. She is currently a board member of Postpartum Support International and on the Nothern New Jersey Maternal Health & Child Consortium PPD taskforce. Dr. Klempner is on the faculty of the Contemporary Center for Advanced Psychoanlytic Studies at Fairleigh Dickinson University in Madison, NJ. She has written, taught, and appeared on television regarding reproductive and emotional health.

Mary Ann LoFrumento, MD, FAAP, attended Barnard College and the University of Pennsylvania where she received her medical degree. After her pediatric residency at Babies Hospital, Columbia Presbyterian, she started Franklin Pediatrics, where for 17 years she was a managing partner with one of the largest pediatric groups in New Jersey. She is currently an Attending Physician at the Goryeb Children's Hospital in Morristown, NJ and Clinical Assistant Professor of Pediatrics at the Mt. Sinai School of Medicine. She is the author and producer of the *Simply Parenting* series of childcare books and DVDs and a regular contributor for parenting magazines, radio, and cable television networks.

Shaila Misri, MD, FRCPC, is a reproductive psychiatrist with longstanding research interests in psychopharmacology related to pregnancy and the postpartum, with special interest in secretion of medications in the breast milk and developmental effects on the baby. In the past 15 years she has developed interests in understanding and improving how maternal mental health and exposure to medications affect the growing fetus/child. She is the medical director of the Provincial Reproductive

Mental Health Program in Vancouver, Canada as well as a Clinical Professor of both OB/GYN and Psychiatry at the University of British Columbia.

Thomas G. O'Connor, PhD, is Associate Professor of Psychiatry and of Psychology and Director of the Laboratory for Mental Disorders at the University of Rochester Medical Center. He has directed and collaborated on many studies tackling a wide array of questions in development and psychopathology. His work in these areas has been supported by research grants in the US, UK, and Canada. He has also received distinguished awards for his research, including the Boyd McCanless Award from the American Psychological Association (2001) and the American Psychological Association Distinguished Scientific Award for Early Career Contribution to Psychology (2004).

George Parnham, JD, has practiced law for 37 years in Houston, Texas, specializing in criminal defense. He is a nationally and internationally recognized expert on the defense of individuals with mental illness and a passionate advocate for legal reform of their treatment in the criminal justice system. He represented Andrea Pia Yates who was found not guilty by reason of insanity in July of 2006 in the drowning deaths of her five children and is an internationally sought-after speaker, writer, and consultant on legal issues associated with perinatal mental health. Mr. Parnham is on the President's Advisory Council of Postpartum Support International and founded, with his wife Mary, The Yates Children Memorial Fund in coordination with the Mental Health Association of Houston.

Alexandra Sacks, BA, is completing medical school at Mount Sinai School of Medicine via its Humanities and Medicine program. She will grade with a Medical Degree in May 2008 and is headed to a clinical residency in Psychiatry. Her clinical and research interests include women's mental health and psycho-oncology; she has co-authored several publications in these subspecialties. Alexandra graduated Phi Beta Kappa in English from Amherst College in 2003.

Tricia Spach, MN, ARNP, is a psychiatric nurse practitioner with a private practice specializing in the care and treatment of women with perinatal mood disorders. She works as an inpatient ARNP providing care to acutely ill psychiatric patients, including women with postpartum psychosis. In addition, she works at a non-profit clinic that provides care to the uninsured, both for general psychiatric care and for women with perinatal mood disorders. She has been the Director of the Washington State PPD warm line. In addition, she served as a PSI board member and is speaker for the program for Early Parent Support.

Alexandra C. Spadola, MD, received her medical degree in 1999 at the Mayo Medical School in Rochester, MN. She completed her residency in Obstetrics and Gynecology at New York Presbyterian Hospital, Sloane Hospital for Women. Dr. Spadola also completed a fellowship in Maternal and Fetal Medicine at New York Presbyterian Hospital, Sloane Hospital for Women. Dr. Spadola is currently an Assistant Professor of Obstetrics and Gynecology with a clinical specialty in Maternal and Fetal Medicine at SUNY Upstate Medical University, Syracuse, NY.

Margaret Spinelli, MD, is an Associate Professor of Clinical Psychiatry at Columbia University College of Physicians and Surgeons and the founder and the Director of the Women's Program in Psychiatry at Columbia University. She has been the recipient of research awards from the National Institutes of Mental Health to study depression and pregnancy. Dr. Spinelli received her medical degree from the Cornell University Medical College after a 15-year career in obstetrical nursing. During medical school, she received additional training in the United Kingdom on the Mother-Baby Postpartum Unit of the Maudsley and Royal Bethlem Hospital in London. Dr. Spinelli's clinical, teaching, and research activities as well as publications have focused on psychiatric disorders during pregnancy and the postpartum periods. Her book *Infanticide: Psychosocial and Legal Perspectives on Mothers Who Kill* (2002) was recognized when Dr. Spinelli was awarded the prestigious Manfred S. Guttmacher Book Award for "outstanding literary contribution to psychiatry and the forensic sciences" in 2004 from the American Psychiatric Association and the American Association of Psychiatry and the Law.

Eve Weiss, MS, is a consultant/writer for The What To Expect Foundation, which provides prenatal and pediatric health information, materials, and education to low-income families. Her professional background includes health policy analysis, scientific writing, journalism, and philanthropic work. Her career has focused on fostering access to quality health services among vulnerable populations and understanding the barriers that prevent equal access. In addition to The What To Expect Foundation, Ms. Weiss works with other nonprofit and academic institutions, including the University of Pennsylvania's Health of Philadelphia Photo-documentation Project. She earned a BA in anthropology at the University of California at Berkeley and an MS in health policy and management at the Harvard School of Public Health.

Foreword

Motherhood is skilled, emotionally demanding, and exhausting work. In most families, the mother is the main source of comfort, care, and counsel: all members benefit from her devotion, enthusiasm, and resourcefulness, and all—especially the children—suffer from her discouragement. Every effort we make to improve mothers' well-being and morale is a contribution to family life, and the health of the next generation. Helping mothers is the responsibility of many professionals and professions—clinical and scientific psychology, psychiatry, social work, midwifery, academic nursing, general medical practice, obstetrics, pediatrics, pharmacology, pathology, and law. In addition, laity in many countries have organized their own networks of support, which play a vital role.

Our knowledge of the mental disorders that afflict mothers has made strides in recent times, with a deluge of publications from all over the world. In my book, *Motherhood and Mental Health* (1996), I reviewed about 4,000 works that had appeared up to that time, dating back to Hippocrates. Much of the best literature was German, French, and Scandinavian, with, of course, contributions from other Western European nations and North America. But since then—within 12 years—at least as many more papers have been published, with many other nations contributing—Chile, Hong Kong, India, Japan, Nigeria, Singapore, and Turkey, to name a few. These countries represent those parts of our world where most of the infants are born, so it is appropriate that we are now hearing how their women experience motherhood.

The science of maternal mental illness has become more detailed. When I entered this field of clinical work and science in 1975, it was usual to speak of three postpartum psychiatric entities—the maternity blues, postpartum psychosis, and postnatal depression. The *blues* (strictly defined) is a transient, subclinical disturbance, and concern has been displaced to more severe and persistent disorders. Postpartum psychoses, we now know, are of many distinct kinds. At least a dozen forms of organic (neuropsychiatric) psychoses can complicate pregnancy, parturition, or the puerperium; these are now rare, but they used to account for at least one-quarter of cases, and certain forms (eclamptic psychosis, infective delirium, Wernicke-Korsakov psychosis, and cerebral venous thrombosis) may still be prevalent in the Third World. That form of psychosis that is still relatively common in Europe and North America (rather less than 1/1,000 births) is considered to be a variant of bipolar (manic depressive) disorder, but sometimes the illness is atypical, with *cycloid* or *acute polymorphic* features. (These terms are not used in the United States, where *schizophreniform* is perhaps equivalent.) As for *postnatal depression,* this is also heterogeneous. In some mothers, the main disorder is not depression, but anxiety. There are anxious themes specific to pregnancy—for example, *tocophobia* (the fear of delivery). In the puerperium, the main themes are infant-focused anxiety, which can reach the severity of a phobia, or agonizing foreboding about the child's health and safety, especially the fear of crib death (SIDS). In addition, a particular variant of obsessive compulsive disorder—obsessions of infanticide—is quite common. In other mothers, depression is a mask for a completely different disorder. A large modern literature has been concerned with the consequences of severe or traumatic labor, which can be followed by persistent stress symptoms or pathological complaining. Unwanted pregnancy is another source of extreme stress. It is still common in nations with ready access to termination, and surely much more common in those that forbid or strongly discourage abortion: it carries an increased risk of several forms of psychopathology. It may lead to denial of pregnancy (conscious or hysterical), which has obstetric risks and occasionally ends in neonaticide (the killing of the newborn). Another disorder, described and explored by American academic nurses, is a disturbance of the mother-fetus relationship (affiliation), which in extreme degree can lead to fetal abuse. After delivery, severe disorders of the mother-infant relationship are seen; often these are combined with depression, but not always. Thus we now confront an array of different pre- and postpartum disorders that challenge the diagnostic skills of mental health professionals, but also lead in to an arsenal of specific therapies.

The present compendium is focused on perinatal mood disorders. Appropriately, the authors come from many professions, including social work, psychology, law, psychiatry, nursing, health education, neurobiology, pediatrics, and obstetrics. Lay organizations are represented by both the founder and current president of Postpartum Support International and the What to Expect Foundation. The purpose is education, targeted at health care professionals of all kinds, and students in all those professions. The importance of recognizing, assessing, and treating perinatal mood disorders cannot be too strongly emphasized. This volume will summarize what is now known and serve as a primer for clinical reference. It will broadcast an optimistic message. Ignorance and pessimism are no longer justified. We are in a much stronger position to understand what is wrong with these troubled mothers and to intervene effectively. A great deal can now be done to restore mothers to full mental health.

Ian Brockington, PhD, FRCPsych
Professor Emeritus
University of Birmingham
Birmingham, United Kingdom

Acknowledgments

With great appreciation, I would like to acknowledge the following individuals whose vision, passion, and dedication have inspired my pursuit of remedial social and health care action on this issue. Thank you to Former New Jersey First Lady Mary Jo Codey, Sylvia Lasalandra, Carol Blocker, Joan Mudd, Valerie Plame Wilson, Gena Zaks, Katherine Stone, and Kimberly Wong for turning agony into advocacy and daring to share your stories with a nation of women closeted in shame.

Thank you to the army of courageous men who stand beside us, soldiers who have lent their power and initiated action responsive to this critical issue; these include U.S. State Senate President and former New Jersey Governor Richard J. Codey, U.S. Senator Robert Menendez, Congressman Bobby L. Rush, attorney George Parnham, Matthew Margo, Laurence Kruckman, PhD, Tom Davis, Brian Shanahan, David Klinker, Merrill Sparango, MD, Chris Armstrong, Dr. Manny Alvarez, and my husband, Stephen Stone, who provides an unwavering foundation of love, belief, and encouragement.

Thanks to many mentors, colleagues, and advocates whose guidance and wisdom have led to great clinical and social gains for our nation's women, including Shari Lusskin, MD; Sarah Schleifer, LCSW; Katherine Wisner, MD; Frances Smith, LCSW; Dora Pierakkos, MD; Shoshana Bennett, PhD, Diana Lynn Barnes, PsyD, Erin Jameson, LSSW; Emma Palmer; Aysha Moshi, Thyatiria Towns, Haydee Mato, and Dr. Robert and Mary Ellen Logan. Many thanks to our editor, Sheri W. Sussman, for her professional and personal belief and support of this project; Alexis Menken for her assistance as co-editor, and Katherine Tengco, whose invaluable and patient orchestration of this compilation sustained its progress.

Greatly shaping my career are those whose past lives of service modeled social awareness, compassion, and the need for vigorous response to injustice; they are Frederick Rish, MD; John Francis Dowd; Dickens

Stone; Nancy Dowd Raife; and Finvola Drury. Thanks to the board members, coordinators, and supporters of Postpartum Support International whose volunteer spirit reaches out on a daily basis around the world to end the ignorance and suffering associated with perinatal mood disorders (www.postpartum.net). Thank you to my clients, whose extension of trust in treatment brings constant lessons of survival and renewal.

Finally, my love, pride, and admiration are endlessly extended to my precious daughter, Julia Michelle Rish, whose ever-watchful curiosity and support of her mother's journey brings joy at every turn. This is for you Julia, and beloved children everywhere who have endured with their mothers and found the loving strength to understand. By your sound rejection of stigma and ignorance, you offer hope to future generations of mother and child and bear witness to triumph over tragedy.

Susan Dowd Stone

Having immersed myself in the world of maternal mental health for the past 15 years, I have found the opportunity to think deeply about the meaning of motherhood, with all its challenges, risks, demands, and rewards, to be tremendously valuable. Many thanks to our editor, Sheri W. Sussman, for her faith in this book and Katherine Tengco for her tireless editorial assistance. The development of my career path has been deeply influenced by Mary D'Alton, MD; Catherine Monk, PhD; and Governor Richard Codey and Mary Jo Codey. I am fortunate to be surrounded by a wonderful study group, and teachers such as Gary Kose, PhD; Ivan Bresgi, PhD; Dorothy Cantor, PsyD; and others too numerous to mention. My greatest teachers have been my parents, Drs. Etta and Milton Ehrlich, both of whom are psychologists and have generously shared their wisdom. More important, both have taught me mindful and nurturing mothering. I am grateful to my brothers, Dimitri and Gregor Ehrlich, for their vast compassion and endless humor. My life and work has been deeply influenced by Virginia Brown and Melissa Neubauer, dear friends who have taught me so much about the meaning of motherhood by surviving extraordinary and unspeakable loss. There is no greater model for maternal love than the following friends, all of whom have shown me that they know how to live with profound intention and kindness: Lisa Tuttle, Mark Burrell, Karen D'Avanzo, Cynthia Green, Michelle Phillips, Melissa Katz, and, of course, my much-loved Mariana Castaneda. I am especially grateful to Peg Rosen for her lucid thinking and bottomless friendship. I am indebted to Bruce Menken, love of my life and fearless voice to the voiceless. It is with unending gratitude that I thank Max, Oliver, and Sonia for filling my heart and soul with joy and providing me with the chance to be a mother. Last but not least, I have learned so much from my patients who have shown enormous bravery in examining their innermost worlds with me, and without whose trust this work would not be possible.

Alexis E. Menken

Introduction

Our nation is finally awakening to acknowledge the full spectrum of maternal experience. Medical, neurobiological, and psychiatric research are merging and sharing their growing knowledge base with clinical, social, and legislative communities. Some states, such as New Jersey and Illinois, already have laws encouraging screening, detection, treatment delivery, and additional research for the long-ignored public health crisis of perinatal mood disorders. As we have become better equipped and more motivated to carefully assess the mental health of childbearing mothers, the incidence of such illnesses has appeared to increase, but perhaps we are simply illuminating long existent facts.

One major task of this growing interdisciplinary initiative is the education of our health care providers. As professional caregivers from many disciplines provide services to women anticipating pregnancy, who are currently pregnant, or who are in the postpartum, the need for consistent evaluative awareness to the full spectrum of perinatal mental health outcomes requires organization and attention.

Perinatal and Postpartum Mood Disorders: Perspectives and Treatment Guide for the Health Care Practitioner is meant to offer an overview and classic text responsive to the need for multidisciplinary education specific to the perinatal period. Such disciplines include obstetrics, gynecology, psychiatry, medicine, social work, psychology, nursing, social support, law, and literacy, professions that acknowledge and accept their responsibility to attend to the full spectrum of maternal experience, including mental health. While ambitious in reach, the authors who contributed time and thought to this project are well recognized leaders, thinkers, clinicians, and advocates within this practice specialty. We, therefore, wish to begin this introduction by offering our respectful appreciation of each contributing author who has honored this text and its readers with his or her considerable knowledge. Please take a moment to read of their significant contributions to the issue and this text. Many authors have additional and more extensive writings also worthy of your pursuit. We hope this overview will encourage further in-depth exploration of the subject matter.

The enormous impact of compromised maternal mental health on child development, social stability, and family health has offered indisputable evidence demanding less vertical and broader, more inclusive research and study. This text is an effort to bring perspective to the issue and help practice evolve toward current dictates of evidence-based science and research in perinatal mental health.

The textbook begins by establishing the importance of maternal mental health. Vivette Glover, Kristin Bergman, and Thomas G. O'Connor have written a chapter on groundbreaking research explaining the effects of maternal stress, anxiety, and depression during pregnancy on the neurodevelopment of the child. These authors present compelling evidence for the importance of assessing and treating maternal anxiety and stress during pregnancy to prevent neurodevelopmental sequalea in the fetus.

Ian Brockington, who has studied maternal child attachments across the decades and has researched the topic for major studies and diagnostic evaluations, shares his wisdom and current view of the diagnostic spectrum of attachment disorders. Julia Chase-Brand, a psychiatrist with a background in biology, brings both disciplines to bear in evaluation of maternal mental illness as it affects children and adolescents. Her work with this population brings rich perspective to her findings and evaluative overview.

Shaila Misri and Karen Joe's chapter offering an in-depth exploration of diagnostic etiology and should be required reading for many professionals developing perinatal specialties. Dr. Misri's prolific written and research contributions to our current body of knowledge offer readers further opportunities for learning.

The second part of this textbook addresses different perspectives on risk factors, screening, and diagnosis. Linda Klempner has written a summary overview of the history of postpartum depression and how screening tools have been developed. Dr. Klempner's chapter will provide the reader with necessary tools to begin screening patients. Kathleen Kendall-Tackett is a health psychologist and researcher who presents the reader with an overview of alternative treatments. As many women make inquiries about alternate roads to recovery, this chapter will help prepare the clinician for those questions.

Sandra N. Jolley and Tricia Spach have provided health care professionals with psychobiological underpinning to understand Perinatal Mood Disorders. While many clinicians feel that there is a biological basis for perinatal mood disorders, Jolley and Spach elucidate brain physiology and how this contributes to the perinatal period. Andrea Braverman gives voice to the role of assisted reproductive technology in perinatal mood disorders. Dr. Braverman's chapter is one of the first published works to tackle this severely neglected area.

The third part of this text addresses perinatal mood disorders from the perspective of four different professionals. Alexandra Spadola speaks to the experience of the obstetrician. She acknowledges the special role that an obstetrician can play in the life of the patient and how this relationship can be pivotal to helping women get the treatment they need. Mary Ann LoFrumento provides the pediatrician's perspective with an all-inclusive guideline for pediatric practice. Dr. LoFrumento's chapter should serve as a template for pediatric practice guidelines for helping with perinatal mood disorders. Cheryl T. Beck describes the nurses' vantage point. Dr. Beck provides concrete and manageable steps, not only for nurses, but for all professionals working with new mothers. George Parnham is our nation's foremost leading legal expert on the evolution of appropriate recourse and defense for the small percentage of women whose undetected, untreated, and severe maternal mental illness has led them into the justice system. Mr. Parnham challenges our nation's response to such cases, and offers current status and perspective on the insanity defense as applied to this population.

The fourth section of this volume offers an overview of various treatment options. Catherine Birndorf and Alexandra Sacks grapple with the complicated decision-making process that couples must face when considering psychotropic medication during pregnancy and lactation. This is never a simple evaluative process and the authors provide a meticulous explanation of how to explore the decision tree with your patient. This is not a one-size-fits-all approach, and they clarify essential issues that must be explored when helping couples make these difficult decisions. Co-editor Susan Dowd Stone emphasizes the need for research and treatment that includes focus on common comorbidities presenting across the perinatal period, suggesting this could lead to better treatment outcomes. Dowd Stone also proposes consideration of Dialectical Behavior Therapy for treatment of complex cases as its theory appears to be well aligned with the presumed etiology of perinatal mood disorders. Margaret Spinelli makes the case for Interpersonal Psychotherapy as an efficacious treatment for perinatal depression. IPT has consistently demonstrated reduction in depressive symptoms, attends to the profound role changes of parenthood, helps with grief responses, and targets more skillful management of interpersonal transactions. Co-editor Alexis Menken has written about the psychodynamic approach to working with postpartum depression. Her focus is on the development of maternal identity and the dynamics that need to be addressed to help a woman find her own voice as a mother. Lisa Bernstein, Executive Director of the What to Expect Foundation, addresses, with Eve Weiss, the issues of literacy and effective disbursements of needed information to often-underserved populations. Finally, Jane Honikman, founder of Postpartum Support International, the world's leading network devoted to perinatal mental health, gives us a history of grassroots efforts to connect women to appropriate services, and, most important, to each other.

The Importance of Maternal Mental Health

PART I

1 The Effects of Maternal Stress, Anxiety, and Depression During Pregnancy on the Neurodevelopment of the Child

VIVETTE GLOVER, KRISTIN BERGMAN, AND THOMAS G. O'CONNOR

Symptoms of anxiety and depression are frequent during pregnancy. Indeed, they are more common in late pregnancy than in the postpartum period (Heron, O'Connor, Evans, Golding, & Glover, 2004). Pregnancy is also a period in which major life events cluster, as women, and their partners, begin to adjust to a major life transition. Several studies show that domestic violence in pregnancy is common (Chhabra, 2007; Macy, Martin, Kupper, Casanueva, & Guo, 2007). It is now apparent that it is important to recognize and reduce all this, both for the woman herself, and also for the sake of her future child. There is evidence that maternal anxiety and stress during pregnancy can affect the neurodevelopment of the fetus.

It is a commonly held belief in many societies that the mood of a mother during pregnancy can affect the development of the child she is bearing. In 400 B.C., Hippocrates was already aware of the importance of emotional attitudes for the outcome of pregnancy. In China, more than a thousand years ago, recognition of the importance of prenatal attitudes led to the institution of the first antenatal clinic (Ferreira, 1965). However, it is only recently that this idea has been investigated scientifically in both animal and human research.

Note: The authors' work was supported by NIH grant R01MH073842.

There is very strong evidence from animal studies that maternal stress in pregnancy has a long-term effect on the behavior of the offspring (Weinstock, 2001). With animals, it is possible to cross foster the prenatally stressed pups to control mothers after birth, and thus clarify the timing of the exposure. Prenatal stress in animal models has been linked with a wide range of outcomes, including altered cerebral laterality and abnormal sexual behavior. However, the most widely reproduced effects are on cognition, including reduced memory and attention, and increased anxiety and emotional dysregulation. Work with nonhuman primates has identified some brain bases of the prenatal stress effects. For example, Coe et al. have shown that exposure to unpredictable noise, either early or late in pregnancy, resulted in reduced volume of the hippocampus in the offspring (Coe et al., 2003). This is a part of the brain that is important for memory. The responsiveness of the hypothalamic-pituitary-adrenal axis (HPA), which produces the stress hormone called cortisol, was also increased in the offspring. Other experiments have shown the effects of prenatal stress may be moderated and even reversed by positive postnatal rearing, suggesting that, although there may be persisting effects of prenatal stress, it is not inevitable (Maccari et al., 1995).

STUDIES SHOWING A LINK BETWEEN ANTENATAL STRESS AND ANXIETY AND THE NEURODEVELOPMENT OF THE CHILD

There is now good evidence in humans also that if a mother is stressed or anxious while pregnant, her child is substantially more likely to have emotional or cognitive problems, including an increased risk of symptoms of attention deficit/hyperactivity, anxiety, or language delay (for reviews, see Talge, Neal, & Glover, 2007; Van den Bergh, Mulder, Mennes, & Glover, 2005). These findings are independent of effects due to maternal postnatal depression and anxiety.

A pioneering study linking antenatal stress with effects on the child was published by D. H. Stott in 1973 (Stott, 1973). Information was collected from 200 women in Scotland in 1965–1966, at the end of their pregnancy. The questions asked of the mother concerned her physical and mental health, the course of the pregnancy, and her social circumstances. The health, development, and behavior of the child were followed for the next 4 years. Stott's major conclusion was that stresses during pregnancy involving severe and continuing personal tensions, in particular marital discord, were closely associated with child morbidity in the form of ill health, neurological dysfunction, developmental delays, and behavior disturbance.

In a study carried out in Washington, D.C., with predominantly primiparous African American women, it was found that several psychosocial variables, including stress, anxiety, and partner interaction, were associated with reduced behavioral scores on the Brazelton Neonatal Behavior Assessment Scale (NBAS) when the newborns were 2 days of age (Oyemade et al., 1994). An Israeli study examined the outcome for two cohorts of boys, one group consisting of those born in the year of the Six-Day War and a second group born 2 years later. The children from the "war exposed pregnancies" had significant developmental delays and evinced regressive behavior (Meijer, 1985), although antenatal and postnatal stress effects were not distinguished in the analyses. A retrospective study by McIntosh et al. (McIntosh, Mulkins, & Dean, 1995) showed that if the mother experienced moderate emotional stress, or smoked cigarettes during pregnancy, her child was more likely to be diagnosed with an attention deficit disorder. These studies laid the important groundwork and provided a springboard for the better-controlled more recent studies described below.

The Effects on the Child

There is now good evidence from many independent prospective studies that antenatal stress predicts adverse social/emotional and cognitive outcomes during childhood. In the last 5 years several prospective studies have been published. Even though these studies used a wide range of different methods, both for measuring antenatal stress or anxiety and for assessing the child, they all found links in a way that revealed an effect on the development of the fetal brain. These studies are mainly European with two conducted in North America (Field et al., 2003; Laplante et al., 2004); none are from developing countries or countries at war, where one might predict that the effects would be even more marked.

It is clear that a wide range of different outcomes can be affected by prenatal stress. One set of studies shows an effect of prenatal stress or anxiety on the cognitive development of the child as assessed by scores on the Bayley Mental Developmental Index (MDI) (Bergman, Sarkar, O'Connor, Modi, & Glover, 2007; Huizink, Robles de Medina, Mulder, Visser, & Buitelaar, 2003) or language development (Laplante et al.,

2004). The MDI is a widely used standardized tool for the assessment of cognitive development in infants and young children. Other studies have shown links between antenatal stress/anxiety and behavioral/emotional problems in the child. The most consistent adverse outcome is in symptoms of Attention Deficit Hyperactivity Disorder (ADHD) (O'Connor, Heron, Golding, Beveridge, & Glover, 2002; Rodriguez & Bohlin, 2005; Van den Bergh & Marcoen, 2004). However, other effects have been observed also, such as an increase in anxiety (O'Connor et al., 2002; Van den Bergh & Marcoen, 2004) and in externalizing problems (Van den Bergh & Marcoen, 2004). It is likely that the particular outcome affected depends on the specific genetic vulnerabilities of the child. There is now good evidence for gene/environment interactions with respect to the postnatal development of psychopatholgy (Caspi et al., 2003); it is probable that the same occurs prenatally.

The studies have examined children at a wide range of ages, from the newborn to 17 years, and it is clear that the effects of prenatal stress can be long lasting. Two studies found impairment in the newborn using the Brazelton NBAS (Brouwers, van Baar, & Pop, 2001; Field et al., 2002) and one study used the Prechtl neurological assessment (Lou et al., 1994). Field et al. (2003) reported that the newborns of mothers with high anxiety had greater relative right frontal brain activation (as measured by EEG) and lower vagal tone. The babies also spent more time in deep sleep and less time in quiet and active alert states, and showed more state changes and less optimal performance on the NBAS (motor maturity, autonomic stability, and withdrawal). Lou et al. (1994) proposed that there may be a "fetal stress syndrome" analogous to the "fetal alcohol syndrome," on the basis of their study showing that antenatal life events resulted in a smaller head circumference, lower birthweight, and lower neurological scores on the Prechtl scale.

O'Connor, Heron, Golding, and Glover (2003) showed a continuity of effects from 4 to 7 years old and Van den Bergh and colleagues have found links between antenatal anxiety and child depression in adolescence (Van den Bergh, Van Calster, Smits, Van Huffel, & Lagae, 2007).

Another effect of prenatal stress appears to be on laterality. Glover, O'Connor, Heron, and Golding (2004) used the large community ALSPAC cohort to test the hypothesis that antenatal maternal anxiety is associated with altered lateralization in humans, as demonstrated by mixed handedness. Maternal anxiety at 18 weeks of pregnancy predicted an increased likelihood of mixed handedness in the child, independent of parental handedness, obstetrical and other antenatal risks, and postnatal anxiety. For this outcome measure, unlike with late ADHD symptoms or anxiety, there was no link with anxiety at 32 weeks. Obel, Hedegaard, Henriksen, Secher, and Olsen (2003) have also shown that antenatal life events are associated with a higher prevalence of mixed handedness in the child. Both studies found that this effect was stronger with antenatal anxiety/stress than with antenatal depression.

Atypical laterality has been found in children with autism, learning disabilities, and other psychiatric conditions, including problems with attention as well as in adult schizophrenia (Glover et al., 2004). There is anecdotal evidence for a link between antenatal maternal stress and both autism and dyslexia, in addition to the evidence discussed already for ADHD. It is an interesting possibility that many of these symptoms or disorders, which are associated with mixed handedness, share some neurodevelopmental components in common, which may be exacerbated by antenatal maternal stress or anxiety.

More needs to be understood about the exact period of gestation that is most important for all the effects described here. Different studies have found different periods of vulnerability. What is clear is that the effects are not confined to the first trimester. Although the basic body structures are formed early, the brain continues to develop, with neurons making new connections, throughout gestation. In the study of O'Connor et al. (2002) anxiety was measured only at 18 and 32 weeks gestation, and the associations were stronger with the latter time point. It remains possible that the effects were actually maximal at midgestation, for example, about 24 weeks. It is also likely that the gestational age of sensitivity is different for different outcomes. Brain systems underlying different aspects of cognition or behavior mature at different stages.

What Causes Risk to the Child?

The evidence shows that the effect is not specific to one type of stress or anxiety. It also seems that many neurodevelopmental effects can be observed with relatively low levels of anxiety or stress (O'Connor, Heron, & Glover, 2002). Most of the studies have used maternal self-rating questionnaires, some used anxiety questionnaires, and others measures of stress (O'Connor et al., 2002; Van den Bergh & Marcoen, 2004). Some studies assessed daily hassles (Huizink et al., 2003), whereas others focused on life events (Bergman et al., 2007; Lou et al., 1994), perceived stress (Rodriguez & Bohlin, 2005), or pregnancy specific worries. Others have used exposure to an external trauma, such as a severe Canadian ice storm (Laplante et al., 2004) or the Chernobyl disaster.

However, it is also of interest that one study has found, in a cohort of financially and emotionally stable women, that there was a small but significant positive association between antenatal stress and both the mental and physical development of the child (DiPietro, Novak, Costigan, Atella, & Reusing, 2006). The authors suggest that a small to medium amount of antenatal stress may actually be helpful for the development of the child, although this remains to be confirmed.

None of the published studies have used clinical interviews, and, consequently, none can demonstrate if there are differences among these disorders with respect to the effect on the fetus and child. Many subtypes of anxiety disorder are recognized, including generalized anxiety, panic, specific phobia, posttraumatic stress, acute stress, and obsessive-compulsive disorders. These disorders may involve quite different physiological processes (Tsigos & Chrousos, 2002). It is interesting that the actual life events found in one study to be most linked with both low scores on the Bayley Mental Developmental Index and increased fear reactivity were "separation/divorce" and "cruelty by the partner" (Bergman et al., 2007). This finding is similar to the conclusion by Stott (1973) that continuing personal tensions (in particular, marital discord) were a particular risk factor for later "neurological dysfunction, developmental delays and behavior disturbance in the child" (p. 785).

The high co-occurrence of symptoms of anxiety and depression raises questions about the specific predictions from maternal anxiety. However, there is some evidence that the effect on the child derives more from prenatal anxiety rather than depression. O'Connor et al. (2002) found that, although antenatal depression was associated with child behavioral problems in a similar way to prenatal anxiety, the effect was smaller; furthermore, when prenatal anxiety was covaried, the association with depression was not significant. In contrast, the prediction from prenatal anxiety to child behavioral problems was substantial and not reduced when prenatal depression was covaried. The authors also found that the link between antenatal anxiety and child behavioral problems was separate and additive to the effects of postnatal depression (O'Connor, Heron, & Glover, 2002).

There have been no studies that have addressed the important question of whether stress due to the mother working during pregnancy has adverse effects on neurodevelopment of the child. There have been several such studies in relation to preterm delivery and these suggest that work per se is not damaging; it only becomes harmful when the woman is working when she does not want to, or feels out of control (Homer, James, & Siegel, 1990).

In summary, there is growing evidence that the risk most closely linked with adverse child outcomes is maternal anxiety/stress. There is also evidence that the effects on the child are not restricted to extreme anxiety or stress in the mother, but can occur across quite a wide range (O'Connor et al., 2002). On the other hand, more research is needed into what types of anxiety/stress are most predictive of later developmental and health problems. The consistent findings across studies, despite different measures of anxiety and stress, may indicate that the risk derives from a broad range of negative emotions that occur in stressed and anxious individuals.

Magnitude of Effect

The size of the effects found in many of these studies is considerable, although it is important to emphasize that most children are not affected. In the general population study of O'Connor et al. (2002), it was found that women in the top 15% for symptoms of anxiety at 32 weeks gestation had double the risk of having children with behavioral problems at 4 and 7 years of age, even after allowing for multiple covariates. It raised the risk for a child of this group of women having symptoms of ADHD, anxiety or depression, or conduct disorder, from 5% to 10%. Thus 90% were not affected. However these results imply that the attributable load in behavioral problems due to antenatal anxiety is of the order of 15%.

Van den Bergh and Marcoen (2004) found that maternal anxiety during pregnancy accounted for 22% of the variance in symptoms of ADHD in 8–9-year-old children. LaPlante et al. (2004) showed that the level of prenatal stress exposure accounted for 11.4% and 12.1% of the variance in the toddlers' Bayley MDI and productive language abilities, respectively, and accounted for 17.3% of the variance of their receptive language abilities. Bergman et al. (2007) also observed an effect of antenatal life events at 18 months of age, accounting for 22% of the variance in Bayley's MDI scores.

Most of these are substantial effects, but there remains considerable variation across children. Bergman et al. (2007), for example, have found that, although antenatal maternal stress increases the risk for both cognitive delay and raised anxiety, these do not necessarily occur in the same children.

Possible Mechanisms

The mechanisms underlying the effects of prenatal stress in women on the development of the fetus and child are far from clear. In animal models, the central role of the stress hormone cortisol in mediating prenatal stress effects in both mother and offspring is well established (Schneider, Moore, Kraemer, Roberts, & DeJesus, 2002; Weinstock, 2001), although many other systems, such as those involving dopamine and serotonin have also been shown to be involved.

In humans, presumably stress or anxiety changes the maternal physiology, including her hormonal levels, and these in turn affect the development of the fetus. Stress and anxiety are generally associated with elevated activity in both the HPA axis and the sympathetic system, although the relationships are complex. However, the maternal HPA axis becomes desensitized to stress during pregnancy, as gestation increases (Kammerer, Adams, Castelberg Bv, & Glover, 2002; Sarkar, Bergman, Fisk, & Glover, 2006). Even though we know that there is a strong correlation between maternal and fetal levels of cortisol (Sarkar, Bergman, Fisk, O'Connor, & Glover, 2007), and that this correlation is increased with higher maternal anxiety (unpublished observations), suggesting that the placenta becomes more permeable to cortisol with increased stressor anxiety, much remains to be understood.

Maternal anxiety during pregnancy has also been associated with reduced blood flow to the baby through the uterine arteries (Teixeira, Fisk, & Glover, 1999), but we do not know whether this is of clinical significance.

CLINICAL IMPLICATIONS AND OPPORTUNITY FOR INTERVENTIONS

The implications of the research described above is that anxiety and stress during pregnancy should receive more attention, both for the sake of the woman herself and for the development of her future child.

Effective interventions to reduce maternal stress and/or anxiety during pregnancy should help to decrease the incidence of cognitive and behavioral problems in children. The evidence suggests that it is not only extreme levels of stress and anxiety that need attention, but possibly, the most affected 15% of the population. Also, it is not only clinically diagnosed mental illness that is important here, but stress due to other factors too, especially the relationship with the partner.

However, there have been few studies that have directly evaluated nonpharmacological, psychological, or social support interventions in pregnancy, and only one research program that has followed up with the child. This is the program that has been conducted by Olds and coworkers over many years, the nurse family partnership (Olds, 2002; Olds et al., 2002; Olds et al., 2004). Although this program was not specifically targeted to help the mental health or emotional state of the mother, it provides considerable social support to vulnerable mothers, starting in pregnancy. The subjects were asked about, and helped with, both support networks and domestic violence. The participants were especially deprived groups of mostly teenage, first-time mothers. Specially trained nurses completed an average of 6.5 home visits during pregnancy and 21 visits from birth to the children's second birthdays, with a focus on health care, development and education of the mother, and teaching parenting skills. The outcomes were compared with standard care. The nurse visitations produced significant effects on a wide range of maternal and child outcomes. Nurse-visited mothers and children interacted with one another more responsively, and 6-month-old infants were less likely to exhibit emotional distress in response to fear stimuli. At 21 months, nurse-visited children born to women with low psychological resources were less likely to exhibit language delays, and, at 24 months, they exhibited superior mental development on the MDI. The children have been followed up for 15 years, and findings include fewer long-term behavioral problems and fewer convictions (Olds et al., 1998). There is no direct evidence that a reduction of maternal stress during pregnancy contributed to the positive gains in the intervention group, but that is a very plausible hypothesis. It is well established that lack of social support or confiding relationships are strong risk factors for antenatal mood disturbance (Bowen & Muhajarine, 2006). Additional studies to evaluate the efficacy of similar types of interventions starting during pregnancy, with a special focus on mental illness, social support, and help with partner relationships, should be part of the agenda for new public health research.

One small randomized, controlled trial of 16 sessions of interpersonal psychotherapy for antenatal depression has been conducted (Spinelli & Endicott, 2003). It was found to be effective in reducing the depression, and the authors recommend it as a first line of antidepressant treatment during pregnancy. There has been a meta-analysis of treatments for depression in both pregnancy and postpartum (Bledsoe & Grote, 2006). The authors conclude that a range of treatments have been found to be effective, with cognitive behavioral therapy producing the largest effect sizes.

Teixeira, Martin, Prendiville, and Glover (2005) assessed whether a short period of directed or passive relaxation would reduce maternal self-rated anxiety, heart rate, plasma catecholamines, cortisol and uterine artery blood flow in pregnant women. Both methods reduced maternal state anxiety and heart rate, the directed therapy more so. Passive relaxation while sitting on a chair had a greater effect in reducing cortisol and norepinephrine. There was a striking lack of correlation between the psychological effects and all the biological indices measured. We have to be aware that it is possible that in order to reduce the physiological effects of anxiety during pregnancy, different methods may be needed from those that are effective at ameliorating subjective anxiety.

CONCLUSION

There is now good evidence that maternal anxiety and stress during pregnancy substantially increase the risk for adverse long-term effects on the neurodevelopment of her child, even though most children are not affected. These effects are not limited to mothers experiencing extreme distress, but occur across the range. Neither are they limited to mothers suffering from a diagnosed mental illness. Relationship strain with the partner is a strong risk factor for adverse child outcome. Different children can be affected in different ways, probably depending on their genetic vulnerabilities and timing of the exposure. We do not know the critical gestational ages of sensitivity, and they are likely to vary for different outcomes. Independent studies have found effects from early to late gestation, suggesting that it is important to recognize and treat emotional problems from early in pregnancy, but that it is not too late to provide benefit later on. There have been few studies that have studied psychological interventions during pregnancy, and only one support study that has subsequently followed up with the child. However, it is reasonable to assume that interventions for which there is evidence of efficacy outside pregnancy, to treat anxiety, depression, or partner relationship problems, will be of benefit to the mother, and that they should be tailored to meet each woman's particular problems. They may well be of benefit to her child also.

REFERENCES

Bergman, K., Sarkar, P., O'Connor, T., Modi, N., & Glover, V. (2007). Maternal stress during pregnancy predicts cognitive ability and fearfulness in infancy. *Journal of the American Academy of Child and Adolescent Psychiatry, 46,* 1454–1463.

Bledsoe, S. E., & Grote, N. K. (2006). Treating depression during pregnancy and the postpartum: A preliminary analysis. *Research on Social Work Practice, 16,* 109–120.

Bowen, A., & Muhajarine, N. (2006). Antenatal depression. *Can Nurse, 102*(9), 26–30.

Brouwers, E., van Baar, A., & Pop, V. (2001). Maternal anxiety during pregnancy and subsequent infant development. *Infant Behavior and Development, 24,* 95–106.

Caspi, A., Sugden, K., Moffitt, T. E., Taylor, A., Craig, I. W., Harrington, H., et al. (2003). Influence of life stress on depression: Moderation by a polymorphism in the 5-HTT gene. *Science, 301*(5631), 386–389.

Chhabra, S. (2007). Physical violence during pregnancy. *Journal of Obstetrics and Gynaecology, 27*(5), 460–463.

Coe, C. L., Kramer, M., Czeh, B., Gould, E., Reeves, A. J., Kirschbaum, C., et al. (2003). Prenatal stress diminishes neurogenesis in the dentate gyrus of juvenile rhesus monkeys. *Biological Psychiatry, 54*(10), 1025–1034.

DiPietro, J. A., Novak, M. F., Costigan, K. A., Atella, L. D., & Reusing, S. P. (2006). Maternal psychological distress during pregnancy in relation to child development at age two. *Child Development, 77*(3), 573–587.

Ferreira, A. J. (1965). Emotional factors in prenatal environment. *Journal of Nervous and Mental Disease, 141,* 108–118.

Field, T., Diego, M., Hernandez-Reif, M., Salman, F., Schanberg, S., Kuhn, C., et al. (2002). Prenatal anger effects on the fetus and neonate. *Journal of Obstetrics and Gynaecology, 22*(3), 260–266.

Field, T., Diego, M., Hernandez-Reif, M., Schanberg, S., Kuhn, C., Yando, R., et al. (2003). Pregnancy anxiety and comorbid depression and anger: Effects on the fetus and neonate. *Depress Anxiety, 17*(3), 140–151.

Glover, V., O'Connor, T. G., Heron, J., & Golding, J. (2004). Antenatal maternal anxiety is linked with atypical handedness in the child. *Early Human Development, 79*(2), 107–118.

Heron, J., O'Connor, T. G., Evans, J., Golding, J., & Glover, V. (2004). The course of anxiety and depression through pregnancy and the postpartum in a community sample. *Journal of Affected Disorder, 80*(1), 65–73.

Homer, C. J., James, S. A., & Siegel, E. (1990). Work-related psychosocial stress and risk of preterm, low birthweight delivery. *American Journal of Public Health, 80*(2), 173–177.

Huizink, A. C., Robles de Medina, P. G., Mulder, E. J., Visser, G. H., & Buitelaar, J. K. (2003). Stress during pregnancy is associated with developmental outcome in infancy. *Journal of Child Psychology and Psychiatry, 44*(6), 810–818.

Kammerer, M., Adams, D., Castelberg Bv, B., & Glover, V. (2002). Pregnant women become insensitive to cold stress. *BMC Pregnancy Childbirth, 2*(1), 8.

Laplante, D. P., Barr, R. G., Brunet, A., Galbaud du Fort, G., Meaney, M. L., Saucier, J. F., et al. (2004). Stress during pregnancy affects general intellectual and language functioning in human toddlers. *Pediatric Research, 56*(3), 400–410.

Lou, H. C., Hansen, D., Nordenfoft, M., Pyrds, O., Jensen, F., Nim, J., et al. (1994). Prenatal stressors of human life affect fetal brain development. *Developmental Medicine and Child Neurology, 36,* 826–832.

Maccari, S., Piazza, P. V., Kabbaj, M., Barbazanges, A., Simon, H., & Le Moal, M. (1995). Adoption reverses the long-term impairment in glucocorticoid feedback induced by prenatal stress. *Journal of Neuroscience, 15*(1 Pt 1), 110–116.

Macy, R. J., Martin, S. L., Kupper, L. L., Casanueva, C., & Guo, S. (2007). Partner violence among women before, during, and after pregnancy: multiple opportunities for intervention. *Women's Health Issues, 17*(5), 290–299.

McIntosh, D. E., Mulkins, R. S., & Dean, R. S. (1995). Utilization of maternal perinatal risk indicators in the differential diagnosis of ADHD and UADD children. *Journal of Neuroscience, 81*(1–2), 35–46.

Meijer, A. (1985). Child psychiatric sequelae of maternal war stress. *Acta Psychiatr Scand, 72*(6), 505–511.

Obel, C., Hedegaard, M., Henriksen, T. B., Secher, N. J., & Olsen, J. (2003). Psychological factors in pregnancy and mixed-handedness in the offspring. *Dev Med Child Neurol, 45*(8), 557–561.

O'Connor, T. G., Heron, J., & Glover, V. (2002). Antenatal anxiety predicts child behavioral/emotional problems independently of postnatal depression. *J Am Acad Child Adolesc Psychiatry, 41*(12), 1470–1477.

O'Connor, T. G., Heron, J., Golding, J., Beveridge, M., & Glover, V. (2002). Maternal antenatal anxiety and children's behavioral/emotional problems at 4 years. Report from the Avon Longitudinal Study of Parents and Children. *Br J Psychiatry, 180,* 502–508.

O'Connor, T. G., Heron, J., Golding, J., & Glover, V. (2003). Maternal antenatal anxiety and behavioral/emotional problems in children: A test of a programming hypothesis. *J Child Psychol Psychiatry, 44*(7), 1025–1036.

Olds, D. L. (2002). Prenatal and infancy home visiting by nurses: From randomized trials to community replication. *Prev Sci, 3*(3), 153–172.

Olds, D., Henderson, C. R., Jr., Cole, R., Eckenrode, J., Kitzman, H., Luckey, D., et al. (1998). Long-term effects of nurse home visitation on children's criminal and antisocial behavior: 15-year follow-up of a randomized controlled trial. *Jama, 280*(14), 1238–1244.

Olds, D. L., Kitzman, H., Cole, R., Robinson, J., Sidora, K., Luckey, D. W., et al. (2004). Effects of nurse home-visiting on maternal life course and child development: Age 6 follow-up results of a randomized trial. *Pediatrics, 114*(6), 1550–1559.

Olds, D. L., Robinson, J., O'Brien, R., Luckey, D. W., Pettitt, L. M., Henderson, C. R., Jr., et al. (2002). Home visiting by paraprofessionals and by nurses: A randomized, controlled trial. *Pediatrics, 110*(3), 486–496.

Oyemade, U., Cole, O., Johnson, A., Knight, E., Westney, O., Laryea, H., et al. (1994). Prenatal predictors of performance on the Brazelton Neonatal Behavioral Assessment Scale. *J Nutr., 124*(Suppl. 6), 1000S–1005S.

Rodriguez, A., & Bohlin, G. (2005). Are maternal smoking and stress during pregnancy related to ADHD symptoms in children? *J Child Psychol Psychiatry, 46*(3), 246–254.

Sarkar, P., Bergman, K., Fisk, N. M., & Glover, V. (2006). Maternal anxiety at amniocentesis and plasma cortisol. *Prenat Diagn, 26*(6), 505–509.

Sarkar, P., Bergman, K., Fisk, N. M., O'Connor, T. G., & Glover, V. (2007). Ontogeny of foetal exposure to maternal cortisol using midtrimester amniotic fluid as a biomarker. *Clin Endocrinol (Oxf), 66*(5), 636–640.

Schneider, M. L., Moore, C. F., Kraemer, G. W., Roberts, A. D., & DeJesus, O. T. (2002). The impact of prenatal stress, fetal alcohol exposure, or both on development: Perspectives from a primate model. *Psychoneuroendocrinology, 27*(1–2), 285–298.

Spinelli, M. G., & Endicott, J. (2003). Controlled clinical trial of interpersonal psychotherapy versus parenting education program for depressed pregnant women. *Am J Psychiatry, 160*(3), 555–562.

Stott, D. H. (1973). Follow-up study from birth of the effects of prenatal stresses. *Develop Med Child Neurol, 15,* 770–787.

Talge, N. M., Neal, C., & Glover, V. (2007). Antenatal maternal stress and long-term effects on child neurodevelopment: How and why? *J Child Psychol Psychiatry, 48* (3–4), 245–261.

Teixeira, J. M., Fisk, N. M., & Glover, V. (1999). Association between maternal anxiety in pregnancy and increased uterine artery resistance index: Cohort based study. *Bmj, 318*(7177), 153–157.

Teixeira, J., Martin, D., Prendiville, O., & Glover, V. (2005). The effects of acute relaxation on indices of anxiety during pregnancy. *J Psychosom Obstet Gynaecol, 26*(4), 271–276.

Tsigos, C., & Chrousos, G. P. (2002). Hypothalamic-pituitary-adrenal axis, neuroendocrine factors and stress. *J Psychosom Res, 53*(4), 865–871.

Van den Bergh, B. R., & Marcoen, A. (2004). High antenatal maternal anxiety is related to ADHD symptoms, externalizing problems, and anxiety in 8- and 9-year-olds. *Child Dev, 75*(4), 1085–1097.

Van den Bergh, B. R., Mulder, E. J., Mennes, M., & Glover, V. (2005). Antenatal maternal anxiety and stress and the neurobehavioral development of the fetus and child: Links and possible mechanisms. A review. *Neurosci Biobehav Rev, 29*(2), 237–258.

Van den Bergh, B. R., Van Calster, B., Smits, T., Van Huffel, S., & Lagae, L. (2007). Antenatal maternal anxiety is related to HPA-axis dysregulation and self-reported depressive symptoms in adolescence: A prospective study on the fetal origins of depressed mood. *Neuropsychopharmacology, 33*(3), 536–545.

Weinstock, M. (2001). Alterations induced by gestational stress in brain morphology and behavior of the offspring. *Prog Neurobiol, 65*(5), 427–451.

2 Maternal Attachment and Bonding Disorders

IAN BROCKINGTON

Just as the emerging relationship with the fetus is important during pregnancy, so the growth of the mother-infant relationship is the key psychological process in the puerperium. *Bonding* is a popular lay term. Some professionals prefer the synonym *attachment*, but one must not confuse this with infant-mother attachment, which develops more slowly over the first 6–9 months of the baby's life. The mother-infant relationship consists essentially of ideas and emotions aroused by the infant, which find their expression in affectionate and protective behavior. Its power is revealed in self-sacrifice, and the pains of separation. Its inner presence is betrayed by external signs—touching and fondling, kissing, cuddling and comforting, prolonged gazing and smiling, baby talk, recognizing signals, tolerating demands, and resisting separation; but it is hard to select a single activity that lies at the core. Particular behaviors wax and wane, but the relationship endures, even when the child is absent, even when it is gone forever. This emotional response enables the mother to maintain the never-ending vigilance and endure the exhausting toil of the nurture of the newborn.

The relationship begins during pregnancy. The mother "bonds" or "affiliates" to the unborn child in a way analogous to the formation of postpartum attachment. Prepartum bonding is promoted by quickening and probably by ultrasound examination. The mother begins to have fantasies about the baby and talks affectionately to it. She may engage the husband and other children in "playing" with the baby. At the same time she prepares for the birth and motherhood ("nesting behavior"). There is pathology to the affiliative stage. About half of all pregnancies are unplanned, and a proportion of unplanned pregnancies are not welcomed. Sometimes pregnancy is denied, or rejected. Not surprisingly, attachment may be minimal in these unwanted pregnancies. The fetus is viewed as an intrusion, whose movements annoy the mother and disturb her sleep. When a mother deeply resents her pregnancy, she may try to harm the fetus. This occurs, with determined intent, in self-induced abortion. It may also occur as a manifestation of rage against the baby: a pregnant woman may pound on her abdomen, even to the point of causing bruising. A poor mother-fetus relationship is one of the predictors of impaired mother-infant bonding.

After the birth, there is no so-called critical period in the development of the maternal response. Proximity from the start ("rooming-in") gives confidence in mothering skills, and breast-feeding may help. The infant plays an important part. At an early stage, it can discriminate speech, and reacts preferentially to the human face and voice. Eye-to-eye contact mediates the interaction, and gazing becomes an absorbing activity on both sides. The baby's smile is another catalyst. Videotape studies have shown the infant contributing to a dialogue with its caregiver. Sometimes the maternal response is immediate, primed by affiliation to the fetus, but sometimes there is a worrying delay. For the first 3 to 4 weeks many mothers feel bruised, tired, and insecure, and their babies may seem strange and distanced. As the baby begins to respond socially, a normal relationship develops rapidly.

When an impaired response progresses to persistent negative feelings, it is appropriate to recognize a mother-infant relationship (or *bonding*) disorder. This concept covers a spectrum of clinical states, which has two main dimensions:

- A negative emotional response, amounting, in severe cases, to hatred of the baby and rejection of it.
- Pathological anger. The infant's demands provoke aggressive impulses, which may lead to shouting, cursing, screaming, abusive assaults, and, in extreme instances, infanticide.

REVIEW OF THE LITERATURE

History

The first indications that there was a psychological process to be recognized—a process, which could fail, with dire consequences—were in European medico-legal reports. In 1845, a forensic pathologist in Fulda (Germany) described this case:

> A child died at six months. His mother was dominant, and completely lacked human sympathy or motherly feelings; the children were just a burden to her. She threatened to kill her eldest son (who was reared by his grandparents) because he surreptitiously tried to feed his baby brother some milk. The corpse weighed 6 ½ lb. There was no trace of fat and the gut was completely empty. It was rumored that earlier children had died the same way. (Rothamel, 1845)

This is not extremely rare. I have seen a case in which a 9-month-old child weighed 7 pounds at his death. Trube-Becker (1968) described 13 cases seen in Düsseldorf. Such extreme neglect testifies to profound rejection of the infant—there seems no other plausible explanation. Not long after Rothamel's case report, Tardieu (1860)—the *doyen* of French forensic medicine—described 24 cases of deliberate injury of children by their parents, including five infants young enough to be breast-fed and one baby only 15 days old. These cases of child abuse testify to maternal rage and loss of control.

The term *misopédie* (hatred of children) was introduced at this time (Boileau de Castélnau, 1861); Oppenheim (1919) used the same term in one of his cases:

> A 36 years old woman with tocophobia (fear of childbirth) married on condition she would never become pregnant. She was bitterly angry when she conceived. After the birth, she was cold & indifferent, and unable to cuddle or kiss her daughter, who seemed like a foreign being. Her husband had to employ another woman to care for her.

Child psychiatrists (e.g., Newell, 1934) have long been familiar with the problem of rejected children; but the recognition of the early stages came later. Luft (1964) reported on 40 cases of "postpartum depression": in the overwhelming majority the pregnancy was planned and welcomed, and not a single birth was out of wedlock. Despite that, there was estrangement from the newborn. "The essence of this syndrome is a disturbance of the instinctive bond between mother and child—a perversion of the maternal instinct."

Robson (1967) pioneered the close study of early maternal behavior. He spent 400 hours observing 30 mothers and infants. Mothers started playing with their babies at about 4 weeks, when they began to look at each other *en face.* Visual contact gave them a feeling of recognition in a personal and intimate way. Gazing—the core of the dyadic relationship—became a mutually absorbing activity. Since then, there has been a spate of sophisticated studies of the normal mother-infant relationship, using ethological techniques and videotape analysis.

In 1970 Robson and Moss reported 54 interviews with American mothers 3 months after birth. Most felt tired and distanced from their babies for 3–4 weeks. At 4–6 weeks the baby "became a person" and recognized its mother. Feelings grew steadily until, at 3 months, the mother felt a pang on leaving the infant. Seven mothers had an accelerated maternal response, but in nine it was delayed or absent; they included six with unwanted pregnancies. This was an early quantification of the prevalence of pathological maternal responses.

From 1975, American academic nurses began to focus on the relationship between a pregnant woman and the fetus. Observation of deviant behavior at this stage was noted by Cohen (1966 and 1988) and Leifer (1977). Several self-rating scales were introduced (Arbeit, 1975; Cranley, 1981; LoBiondo-Wood & Vito-O'Rourke, 1990; Müller, 1993; Nagata et al., 2000). In Adelaide, Condon (1986) described fetal abuse.

It is difficult to say when it became generally recognized that severe disorders of the mother-infant relationship were a major clinical problem and a scientific challenge. I reviewed these disorders in chapter 6 of *Motherhood and Mental Health* (Brockington, 1996), with 140 references, but they have still not achieved general acceptance. There is no mention of them in the 10th edition of the *International Classification of Mental and Behavioural Diseases* (World Health Organization, 1992), and hardly any mention in the 4th revision of the *Diagnostic and Statistical Manual of Mental Disorders* (APA, 1994). But, in spite of a lack of funding, a fair volume of research has been published in the last 10 years.

Symptoms

Symptoms can be placed in five groups:

- In rejection of the baby, the core of the disorder is the pathological affective response—its mildest degree is disappointment over the lack of feeling, followed by dislike, hostility, and hatred. The intensity of this aversion is shown in illustrative case no. 1.
- Resulting from this emotional response, there is a lack of interaction—no talking, playing, or cuddling. This may extend to a lack of eye contact, as shown in illustrative case no. 2.
- These mothers regret the pregnancy and feel trapped, so it is not surprising that they seek a way of escape from infant care. Some (illustrated by case no. 3) run away from home. Others try to persuade their own mother or another relative to take over. If this is not possible, the idea of fostering or adoption is considered, first privately, then publicly.
- The most poignant manifestation is a secret wish that the baby "disappear"—be stolen, or die (illustrated by case no. 4).
- In pathological anger, the degree of the mother's irritation with the baby's demands varies from occasional shouting, swearing, or screaming to various forms of rough treatment. At first these impulses are resisted, but later self-control gives way.

Before diagnosing a mother-infant relationship disorder, certain other disorders must be considered. The most important differential diagnosis for rejection is child-centered anxiety. These mothers love their infants, but feel so anxious in their presence that they develop a phobia for it (De Armond, 1954; Sved-Williams, 1992).

In pathological anger, the main differential diagnosis is obsessions of infanticide, of which there are American descriptive studies (Chapman, 1959). These gentle, devoted women have extraordinary fantasies of destroying their infants—for example, by decapitation or throwing them into the fire. It is vital to distinguish this symptom from anger-based impulses to "batter" the child.

Assessment

There are now several questionnaires that can be used for early detection of disturbed bonding (Brockington et al., 2001; Brockington, Fraser, &

Wilson, 2006; Nagata et al., 2000; Taylor, Atkins, Kumar, Adams, & Glover, 2005). These are useful for screening, but are insufficient for diagnosis. The main clinical resource is an interview exploring the mother's emotional response and behavior; this should include:

- Her account of the pregnancy
- Her feelings about the infant
- Any morbid ideas and aggressive impulses
- The severity of depression or other comorbid symptoms.

In many cases, such an interview provides a good basis for diagnosis and the planning of treatment. But in severe, intractable cases, further assessment is necessary. The most intensive assessment can be made by conjoint (mother and baby) in-patient admission. This allows 24-hour observation by a multidisciplinary team, each member contributing to the overall picture. The psychiatrist monitors the mother's mental state, the social worker assesses family and network support, a psychologist can perform specialized assessments, and pediatric nurses assess the baby; but the crucial observations on maternal behavior are made by psychiatric nurses, who keep a shift-by-shift record of salient incidents, reporting the mother's statements about the baby, her competence and skill, affectionate behavior and her response to crisis. Scales can be used (Hipwell & Kumar, 1996; Salariya & Cater, 1984), but a narrative record gives sufficient information. In severe cases and in research, the gold standard is direct observation. In the study of normal mother-infant relationships, 5-minute videotaped observations of mothers playing with their infants have often been used, but it has not yet been demonstrated that such brief observations are sufficient to diagnose severe disorders, nor that these disturbed mothers can tolerate such intrusions. It seems best that observations are made over a substantial length of time.

Frequency

There are at present few data on the frequency of these disorders in the general community. At the level of "threatened rejection," when the mother has an aversion to her child and seeks temporary escape from child care, this is probably about 1%. It is much higher in mothers who seek help for "postnatal depression." In a study of more than 200 mothers referred to specialist services in Birmingham (United Kingdom) and Christchurch (New Zealand), we made consensus diagnoses, based on a

Table 2.1

ANGLO-NEW ZEALAND STUDY: FREQUENCIES OF MOTHER-INFANT RELATIONSHIP DISORDERS

DIAGNOSIS	FREQUENCY AMONG 205 PATIENTS
Rejection (threatened or established)	52 (27%)
Pathological anger at least moderate (i.e., impulses to child harm)	42 (20%)
Infant-focused anxiety	38 (19%)
Threatened rejection (i.e., a mother with aversion to her infant seeks temporary transfer of care)	30 (15%)
Established rejection (mother seeks permanent placement of child, or expresses hatred or wish for crib death)	22 (11%)
Severe anger (frank abuse)	17 (8%)
Phobia for the infant	14 (7%)

2-hour structured interview (Brockington, Aucamp, & Fraser, 2006) and the case records: they showed the following frequencies (see Table 2.1) (Brockington, Aucamp, & Fraser, 2006).

Therapy

Treatment can sometimes begin during pregnancy. If a mother's attitude to the pregnancy is obstinately rejecting, therapists can direct her attention to the child within. Stroking the abdomen and identifying fetal body parts, or telling stories about the baby's future life, have been suggested (Jernberg, 1988).

If, after childbirth, the maternal emotional response is delayed, and a mother so distressed by her lack of affection for her baby that she seeks professional help, the first step is explanation: such delays are common, and usually brief; a full relationship will develop as the mother recovers from delivery, and the baby responds with smiling, laughter, and babbling.

Indeed, as the first illustrative case shows, a mother may even recover spontaneously from established rejection.

For those who suffer prolonged and increasingly severe negative feelings for their infants, or who have difficulty in controlling their irritation at its demands, reassurance is insufficient. The threshold for active intervention is pathological anger or threatened rejection—when the mother begins to seek temporary respite or separation from the baby.

In the treatment of these severe cases, there have been no randomized, controlled double-blind trials. This is partly because the recognition of these disorders is in its early stages, and funding has been unobtainable. But, with full funding, the matching of patients and controls will be difficult, given differences in severity and duration, and the presence of comorbid postpartum psychopathology. There will be large placebo effects, due to spontaneous recovery and response to antidepressive treatment. At this stage, therefore, therapy is still at the stage of heuristic ideas and single case studies. From my clinical experience, I recommend that management proceeds in these stages:

1. The primary decision is whether to attempt treatment. The mother must be given freedom of choice; it is dangerous for her to feel trapped in unwelcome motherhood. At the same time, the father has his rights. The option of relinquishing the infant must be openly acknowledged, and fully discussed with both parents. Provided the infant is safe, this stage should not be rushed. In the short term it is often easy to arrange alternative baby care. Illustrative case no. 5 shows how long-term alternative care can be perfectly satisfactory. Every case is different, and a cautious but optimistic approach should be taken.
2. If it is decided to embark on treatment (as in most cases), depression should be treated, with psychotherapy, drugs, or (occasionally) electroconvulsive therapy. There is much evidence that, in some cases, depression, or even a bipolar disorder, is an important etiological factor. Since depression can be occult, it is sensible always to deal with it thoroughly in all cases.
3. In other cases (such as illustrative case no. 6) prolonged and intensive antidepressive treatment is of no avail. Progress, therefore, depends on specific psychological treatment. Treatment focused on the mother alone (such as analytic psychotherapy) is inappropriate. It is necessary to work on the dyadic relationship. This relationship, like others, grows through shared pleasure.

The baby alone has the power to awaken its mother's feelings, so the aim is to create circumstances in which mother and child can enjoy each other. Various techniques can be used to facilitate this

- Play therapy with participant modeling
- Baby massage (Onazawa, Glover, Adams, Modi, & Kumar, 2001)
- Singing lullabies
- Mother and infant bathing together

In Heidelberg, videotape feedback has been used, with success.

It is a mistake to separate the mother and baby completely. It merely compounds the problem by adding an element of avoidance. But, if there is any hint of abuse or aggressive impulses, the mother must never be left alone with her infant. She must be relieved of all irksome burdens of infant care. When mother and baby are calm, she is encouraged and helped to interact with him or her—to cuddle, talk, play, and bring out the child's smile and laughter.

Treatment can take place in various settings. Home treatment can be successful, provided there is enough support to relieve the mother of night care and stressful duties: the maternal grandmother, an understanding husband, or a family group can sometimes achieve this. Day-hospital treatment provides individual support and group discussion, as well as specific therapies. In the most severe and refractory cases, the proper setting is an inpatient mother-and-baby unit, where an experienced team of psychiatric and nursery nurses, available 24 hours a day and 7 days a week, can provide full support. Even in the most severe cases, one can feel optimistic about a successful outcome.

Prevention

In Brazil, Wendland-Carro, Piccinini, and Stuart Millar (1999) conducted a randomized controlled trial in 37 mothers: one-half received videotaped instruction on interaction with their babies, and the other received lectures on care-giving skills. One month later, home observations showed increased sensitive responsiveness in mothers instructed about interaction. In South Africa, Cooper et al. (2002) studied Xhosa women living in poverty: one group received 20 visits by unqualified community workers and the control group received routine care. The study showed that those given additional support had better mother-infant interaction, and the children gained more height and weight.

Long-Term Effects

Since the mother is the child's primary environment, one would expect her persistent hostility to have serious and long-term effects. A number of studies have confirmed this:

- Children whose mothers showed (in videotaped play) poor parenting had insecure attachment at 18 months (Tomlinson, Cooper, & Murray, 2005).
- Because of the reduction in verbal interaction, the children show deficits in learning. Although most studies of the effects of postnatal depression on the child have not assessed the early mother-infant relationship, the one study that did so showed that interactions (videotaped at 2 months), and not depression, predicted cognitive functioning at 5 years ($r = .29$, $p = <.05$) (Murray, Hipwell, & Hooper, 1996).
- In Sweden, Finland, the Czech Republic, Denmark, Germany, and Australia, there have been a number of long-term follow-through studies of unwanted pregnancy (see Table 2.2); refused abortion has been one of the main indicators. This is not an ideal predictor because some mothers, whose pregnancy is unwelcome, make a satisfactory adjustment during pregnancy, and others have a normal reaction to the newborn; so the sample will be diluted by many mothers with normal emotional responses. The results are not completely consistent, and not dramatic; moreover, two studies have shown a lessening of disadvantage after the age of 30—when, presumably the "changes and chances of this mortal life" have drowned out adversity in early childhood. But on the whole, they show deficits in education and relationships.
- Child abuse, child neglect, and abusive filicide are all increased when a mother has a severe mother-infant relationship disorder. This has not yet been confirmed by cohort studies, but many rejecting mothers, presenting in the clinic, have already acted out their hostility and perpetrated frank abuse.

Causes

These disorders are not confined to White mothers living in isolated nuclear families. They have been observed in Pakistani and Sikh mothers (living with their extended families), in Afro-Caribbean women, Maoris, and the Japanese.

Table 2.2

LONG-TERM FOLLOW-UP OF UNWANTED PREGNANCY

FIRST AUTHOR	SUBJECTS	FOLLOW-UP	MAIN FINDINGS
Forssman & Thuwe (1966, 1981)	Controlled study of 120 children of Swedish mothers who refused abortion.	35 years	At 21, fewer children attended higher education, and more had psychiatric care, social assistance, and criminal records. These differences were less marked at 35.
Matejcek et al. (1978), Kubicka et al. (1995), and David (2006), who summarized the whole series	220 children born in Prague after abortion was twice refused.	35 years	In school the children obtained lower grades in Czech, had fewer friends, and higher maladaptation scores. They more often dropped out of education, and had conflict at work, or with friends. They were more often imprisoned, unmarried or divorced, or in psychiatric treatment. These differences narrowed after the age of 30.
Blomberg (1980) summarized by Höök	A cohort of unwanted Swedish children collected by Hultin and Ottoson (1971).	15 years	School performance was worse in unwanted children, especially in Swedish and mathematics. More had psychiatric care and social assistance.
Rantakallio & Myhrman (1980), Myhrman (1988) and Myhrman et al. (1996)	Controlled study of 284 unwanted Finnish children from 12,068 pregnancies in Oulu and Lapland in 1966.	28 years	Primary school performance was worse, especially writing skills. There was no difference in emotional development. At 16, there were no differences in boys, but girls had poorer relationships with their fathers and with peers, and more often left school early. At 28 the incidence of schizophrenia was doubled.

(*continued*)

Table 2.2

LONG-TERM FOLLOW-UP OF UNWANTED PREGNANCY (CONTINUED)

FIRST AUTHOR	SUBJECTS	FOLLOW-UP	MAIN FINDINGS
Netter (1982)	3 year follow-up of 6,117 German pregnancies, of which 28.8% were "unambiguously unwanted."	3 years	The infants showed more aggressive or regressive tendencies.
Raine et al. (1994)	Male infants from 4,269 pregnancies in Copenhagen, 1959–1961. Of these, 447 were rejected, that is, an attempt was made to abort an unwanted pregnancy, or the child was in institutional care for 4 months in its first year.	19 years	Criminal violence in adolescence was *not* associated with rejection or birth complications alone, but was strongly associated with a combination of these two factors.
Bor et al. (2003)	An Australian cohort of 7,000 mothers. At 6 months, the mother's attitude was assessed by a 6-item scale. Mothers who scored in the lowest 10th percentile were considered to have a negative attitude.	5 years	The children had more childhood behavior problems.

In spite of the dearth of research, we can be fairly certain that the following factors have a part in their causation:

- Unwanted pregnancy. This emerged from the very first study of Robson and Moss (1970). It has been confirmed by the Anglo-New Zealand study (Brockington, Aucamp, & Fraser, 2006): when mothers with rejection (threatened or established) were compared with the other mothers, the relative risks of predictor varibles were:
    - 4.2 Negative reaction to the newborn
    - 3.9 Termination of pregnancy considered
    - 3.0 Fetal abuse
    - 2.3 Lack of interaction with the fetus
    - 2.0 Negative attitude to the pregnancy.
- "Negative reaction to the newborn" may be the early stages of a pathological response; the other four items reflect unwanted pregnancy or disturbance of affiliation with the fetus. The association of prepartum and postpartum bonding has also been demonstrated by Damato (2004) in her study of 139 mothers of twins in Indiana: mothers completed self-rating questionnaires before and after delivery, and there was a significant correlation between the two ($r = .38$, $p < .001$). Siddiqui and Hägglöf (2000) demonstrated that various subscales of the Prenatal Attachment Inventory (Müller, 1993) predicted maternal involvement, measured from videotapes made at home, when the infant was 12 weeks old.
- Depression. In clinical practice, most mothers with bonding disorders are depressed to a greater or lesser extent. Berkson bias will have exaggerated this association. Berkson showed that the concurrence of diseases must be exaggerated in clinics, because patients with two diseases have two "tickets of admission." Nevertheless, there are strong clinical reasons for regarding depression as a causal factor:
    - Mothers sometimes lose an established bond when they become depressed.
    - Some mothers show a dramatic improvement when treated with ECT.
    - Some mothers later show evidence of bipolar disorder (as in illustrative case no. 2).
- The follow-through study of Murata and colleagues (n.d.) found evidence that prepartum depression was a factor.

- Infant temperament. Clinical experience suggests that difficult babies—those that cry excessively, sleep poorly, or are cranky eaters—can disturb the bonding process. Sick infants and those with delayed social responses may also be at risk. A difficult temperament may be more strongly associated with a mother's pathological anger than with rejection.
- Unfortunate events at the time of childbirth, such as desertion by the infant's father, death of a twin, or an unusually painful delivery may play a part, although the evidence is anecdotal.
- One would expect that poor parenting by the mother's own mother would be important. Kumar's (1997) postal study of 800 mothers with postnatal depression put a ceiling on this, by showing that 7 of 29 multiparous mothers who failed to love their babies had a normal response to their first child.

Status of the Concept

Those who oppose the concept of mother-infant relationship disorders believe they are merely a manifestation of "postnatal depression." There is every reason to expect such an association: a failure to love one's child is depressing, and depression is probably a causal factor in such disturbances. But there are many reasons to reject the alternative concept of "postpartum depression with impaired mother-infant interaction":

1. A disturbed relationship is different from a mood disorder.
2. Impaired interaction, although it can be recorded and measured, is not the essence of the phenomenon, but merely its behavioral manifestation.
3. Impaired interaction has other causes, especially infant-centered anxiety and obsessions of infanticide.
4. When depression is associated with phobias, obsessions, or deviant behavior, these comorbid phenomena are still considered worthy of study and treatment in their own right.
5. When depression and "bonding disorders" coexist, their severity and course often differ:
   a. The disturbed relationship sometimes precedes the depression.
   b. Depression sometimes seems mild, relative to the gravity of the relationship disorder.

  c. The mother feels better when she is separated from her infant.
  d. Psychological treatment of the relationship disorder sometimes cures the depression.
  e. Pharmaceutical or electrical treatment of depression sometimes has no effect on the relationship with the child.
6. Some of these mothers are not depressed. This is based not only on clinical observations, but also on community studies: Righetti-Veltema, Conne-Perréard, Bousquet, & Manzano (2002) followed a cohort of 570 normal Swiss women from pregnancy, assessing postpartum depression and the mother-infant relationship. Inadequate holding, gazing and talking, lack of pleasure and awkwardness were found in 11%–31% of depressed and 3%–24% of nondepressed women; 22% of depressed and 11% nondepressed mothers had pathological interaction scores. Bernazzani et al. (2005) used the Contextual Assessment of Maternity Experience (CAME) in 85 women with a history of depression: they found no correlation between postpartum depression and negative feelings about the child.
7. Only a minority of depressed mothers have this problem. It is important to select them for treatment and not to stigmatize the others.
8. The risks—including child abuse and neglect—are higher. It is these disorders, rather than uncomplicated depression, that have serious and long-term effects on the child's development. These mothers are a high-risk group that can contribute to the vital task of preventing child abuse and neglect.
9. The treatment is different and specific. Assessment and treatment of this relationship forms an important part of the work of mother-infant mental health teams.
10. Management must be made aware of the need for training and service provision.
11. The etiology is different, with more emphasis on unwanted pregnancy and challenging infant behavior.

Psychiatrists sometimes get entangled in disputes about "disease entities." Whether maternal attachment disorders are diseases depends on the definition of *disease;* in psychiatry, this is seldom related to bodily function and sometimes has a social component. *Bonding disorders* are emotional and behavioral phenomena and deserve the universal scientific response—definition, measurement, and the search for causes, effects, intervention, and prevention. These disorders are a *syndrome*—that is, a group of symptoms and behaviors that concur, and follow the same course over time. They are *disorders,* because they cannot, in any sense of the word, be regarded as "normal"; they are even abnormal in the biological sense of threatening the survival of the newborn. Hatred of an infant, unlike hatred of a rival, is squarely in the clinical domain, because mothers seek help, and treatment is available and often given with full success. Helping professions like medicine, nursing, clinical psychology, and social work cannot refuse treatment and must find concepts that channel patients toward effective interventions. For all these reasons, these disorders should find a place in the *Diagnostic and Statistical Manual of Mental Disorders*, so that practitioners become fully aware of them, know how to make the diagnosis, and deploy therapy.

Research is in its early stages. There is a wealth of studies of the normal mother-infant relationship, using rigorous measurements. But in the future, it will be necessary to focus on clinical disorders. For this, we need robust methods of studying disturbed *bonding* in oversensitive mothers with infants of any age, from a few days to a year or more. All follow-through studies of *postnatal depression* should include measures of bonding. Once the problems of measurement and matching have been solved, we need to study the active components of intervention. In the search for causes and effects, cohort studies starting with high-risk groups will be informative: unwanted pregnancy could be the starting point, using prepartum and postpartum interviews and self-rating questionnaires, and (at follow-up) observations of mother-infant interaction; large samples, for example, 1,000 mothers, will be necessary to explore infrequent effects such as child abuse and neglect.

Recently, a promising new validator has become available—functional magnetic resonance imaging (fNMR). This can be used to study regional brain blood flow, and locate the cerebral basis of emotional phenomena. When the brain areas are known, normal and pathological responses can be distinguished, and their strength measured. Lorberbaum et al. (2002) studied healthy, breast-feeding first-time mothers with 4–8-week-old babies as they listened to infant cries (not their own infants): the areas associated with infant crying were the medial thalamus, medial prefrontal and right orbitofrontal cortices, midbrain, hypothalamus, dorsal and ventral striatum and lateral septal region. Squire and Stein (2003), in an editorial, suggested that visual, olfactory, or tactual images of the infant could be used; the areas important in the processing of salient emotions included amygdala, hippocampus, anterior cingulated gyrus and insula. This method has already been used to study bonding. An unpublished Manchester study compared *schizophrenic* mothers with normals. Nitschke et al. (2004) studied 6 normal mothers viewing photographs of their infants, and of unfamiliar infants: there was bilateral activation of the orbitofrontal cortex when they viewed their own infants. What is needed now is to apply this method to the study of rejecting or angry mothers, before and after treatment. Perhaps one day such techniques will become as mundane as chest radiographs, and will be used to confirm diagnoses and measure severity.

ILLUSTRATIVE CASES

In the *first case*, the description of maternal emotions before and after the illness is taken from the mother's handwritten personal account. This 32-year-old nurse was referred 2 years after the birth of her first child. After 2 years of happy marriage, she achieved a planned pregnancy. Prepartum bonding was normal. Labor was prolonged, with inadequate pain control. In the early puerperium, she found that she did not want her baby Sam and had thoughts of throwing him out of the window.

> I remember the total helplessness of not being able to care for him properly . . . my Mum and [my sister] Eileen passed him from one to another . . . with me sitting in the back room pretending he didn't exist. I am left with a terrible feeling of guilt about the deep hate I had for Sam. I feel . . . so dreadfully ashamed to admit it, but I absolutely hated him, wishing to God he'd never been born, wishing terrible things would happen—cot death [crib death]—how on earth could I have thought it? . . . What kind of person am I? . . . How on earth could I have felt such terrible hate towards such a beautiful little boy? [Even now] I can't bear to see tiny babies and my friends happy with them. Every time I watch newborn babies on the television, I cry because of the way I felt towards Sam. I want to move house to leave all these memories behind. I am frightened he might know how I felt towards him when he grows up, and I don't want more children because I must make it up to Sam.

She also suffered from suicidal depression, losing 35 pounds in weight:

> I was in a hopeless state of deep deep despair . . . Those terrible nights of being awake for hours . . . I knew I would have to die to be rid of him . . .

> I lay in the bath for 2½ hours planning what to do, thinking how to put the pipe in the car.

She sought, and received, no help, but spontaneously recovered. Her weeks of suffering in the puerperium left a "deep scar," and she was still trying to come to terms with it.

> No-one suspected anything . . . I was probably just tired or had the baby blues. Why didn't anybody guess something could be wrong? I can't really believe that I finally saw a light at the end of such a long tunnel . . . One day [3–4 months later] I was getting Sam dressed, looking straight at him (which I'd never seemed to do), and suddenly I loved him—he was mine and I absolutely loved him. I don't know where those feelings come from. It seemed unbelievable. I never even dreamed I could ever feel like that. I absolutely adored him. [Now] he is the most precious thing in the world. I can't bear to share him—I want him all to myself. He is my life, my whole life.

The *second case* history illustrates the striking symptom of gaze avoidance.

A 33-year-old doctor's wife, herself employed by the Health Authority, gave birth to her second child. She was referred because she had not bonded and was tearful and withdrawn, especially in the morning. At the clinic she said:

> It is like he isn't my baby. I feel quite cold and empty towards him—he is just a baby that needs looking after. I am starting to resent him. I don't think of him as a person. I don't like to look at him if he looks at me. It's his eyes. I can't look at him. I don't know why.

She felt like running away, or leaving him in the park, where someone would remove him. She sometimes got angry with him—"It's his fault. He did it to annoy me." She sometimes had an impulse to put a hand over his mouth or shake him. Outpatient treatment with oral antidepressive agents had a slight effect on depression, but she still had difficulty looking at him, and, during massage therapy, was unable to touch him or stroke his hand. After 9 weeks, there was no change in her scores on a self-rated bonding questionnaire. She was admitted to the Mother and Baby unit, where, within a few days, she started to bond; swimming therapy seemed to be the most effective form of play therapy for her. After 4 weeks, antidepressants were stopped because of retention of urine, and her depression returned. But her relationship with her baby maintained its improvement. There was evidence of a mood disorder related to menstruation, and brief menstrual hypomanic phases.

The *third case* illustrates the mother's attempts to escape, which can be a clue to the diagnosis, when she is too ashamed to describe her feelings:

> A mother became depressed after the birth of her third baby, and was "unable to cope." She took a train to London for no known reason. She was admitted to the hospital *without her baby* for 3 weeks, and investigated in the usual way. She seemed quite well, and was discharged without the relationship disorder being suspected. After returning home, she ran away twice, and made a suicide attempt. She could not tolerate the presence of her infant. She was reluctantly persuaded to accept admission to a mother and baby unit, and rapidly responded to treatment. (This mother's history is briefly summarized in Brockington, Aucamp, & Fraser, 2006: she had a bonding disorder after three of her four pregnancies.)

The *fourth case* illustrates the most poignant symptom—wish for the death of the infant:

> A mother looked forward to "a beautiful baby tucked up in bed, or going for walks, proudly pushing a pram." But he went only one hour between feeds, and cried unless held. One night he screamed for 5 hours. In the pram he would scream constantly, and strangers would stop to tell her what was wrong. After 10 days she was exhausted—"It was the biggest mistake of my life." She considered having him adopted, and moving house to start again. Later she shared her feelings with her husband—"We were surprised to learn that we *both* thought a cot death would be a welcome release."

The *fifth case* illustrates the successful decision not to engage in active therapy:

> A 35-year-old mother presented after her 4th (unwanted) pregnancy. She "did not take to the baby," who was looked after by her own mother, with whom she lived. When offered day hospital treatment, she panicked. Her mother intervened to explain that the patient was "not maternal" and had delegated care of all four children. Management consisted of reassuring her that it was perfectly satisfactory for the grandmother to provide baby care. After 3 years, the toddler wheedled her way into her mother's affections, and she formed a good relationship.

The *sixth case* illustrates the power of play therapy after all other treatments failed:

> A newlywed looked forward to her first baby—a boy. She developed postpartum depression and rejected him. "I can't bear him. I don't want to know him." The child was taken over by her mother-in-law, amidst severe family friction. There were suicidal attempts and homicidal threats against her husband, who obstinately refused to give up his baby or his marriage. She failed to respond (as in-patient or day patient), to several courses of antidepressant drugs, 3 courses of ECT, psychotherapy by two gifted therapists, and marital therapy. After 3 years, a clinical psychologist intervened, and with four sessions of participant play therapy, established a normal bond. The intractable depression evaporated (Brockington & Brierley, 1984).

SUMMARY

This chapter reviews severe disorders of the mother-infant relationship, which are seen in a substantial proportion of mothers seeking help for postpartum mood disorders. These disorders involve rejection of the infants and/or pathological anger. In all these mothers, the relationship with the infant should be thoroughly explored, starting with the circumstances of pregnancy and attitudes to the unborn child, and continuing with emotional responses to the newborn and the child as it matures. Infants, whose mothers suffer from these disorders and who do not spontaneously recover or receive therapy, may suffer far-ranging and long-term disadvantages, especially during their education. Treatment, which includes various forms of play therapy, is often effective. Although research is in its early stages, the causation probably includes unwanted pregnancy, depression, and challenging infant behavior. These disorders are risk factors for child abuse and neglect. They should be more widely recognized, and changes in the *Diagnostic and Statistical Manual of Mental Disorders* would help.

REFERENCES

American Psychiatric Association. (1994). *Diagnostic and statistical manual of mental disorders* (4th ed.). Washington, DC: Author.

Arbeit, S. A. (1975). *A study of women during their first pregnancy.* Unpublished doctoral dissertation, Yale University, New Haven, CT.

Bernazzani, O., Marks, M. N., Bifulco, A., Siddle, K., Asten, P., & Conroy, S. (2005). Assessing psychosocial risk in pregnant/postpartum women using the Contextual Assessment of Maternity Experience (CAME). *Social Psychiatry and Psychiatric Epidemiology, 40,* 497–508.

Boileau de Castélnau, P. (1861). Misopédie ou lésion de l'amour de la progéniture. *Annales Médico-psychologiques, 3rd series, 7,* 553–568.

Bor, W., Brennan, P. A., Williams, G. M., Najman, J. M., & O'Callaghan, M. (2003). A mother's attitude towards her infant and child behaviour five years later. *Australian & New Zealand Journal of Psychiatry, 37,* 748–755.

Brockington, I. F. (1996). *Motherhood and mental health.* Oxford, England: Oxford University Press.

Brockington, I. F., Aucamp, H. M., & Fraser, C. (2006). Severe disorders of the mother-infant relationship: Definitions and frequency. *Archives of Women's Mental Health, 9,* 243–251.

Brockington, I. F., & Brierley, E. (1984). Rejection of a child by its mother successfully treated after 3 years. *British Journal of Psychiatry, 145,* 316–318.

Brockington, I. F., Fraser, C., & Wilson, D. (2006). The postpartum bonding questionnaire: A validation. *Archives of Women's Mental Health, 9,* 233–242.

Brockington, I. F., et al. (2001). A screening questionnaire for mother-infant bonding disorders. *Archives of Women's Mental Health, 3,* 133–140.

Brockington, I. F., et al. (2006). *The Birmingham Interview for Maternal Mental Health.* Bredenbury, England: Eyry Press.

Chapman, A. H. (1959). Obsessions of infanticide. *Archives of General Psychiatry, 1,* 12–16.

Cohen, R. L. (1966). Some maladaptive syndromes of pregnancy and the puerperium. *Obstetrics & Gynecology, 27,* 562–570.

Cohen, R. L. (1988). *Psychiatric consultation in childbirth settings.* Plenum, New York.

Condon, J. T. (1986). The battered fetus syndrome. *Journal of Nervous and Mental Disease, 175,* 722–725.

Cooper, P. J., Landman, M., Tomlinson, M., Molteno, C., Swartz, L., & Murray, L. (2002). Impact of a mother-infant intervention in an indigent peri-urban South African context. *British Journal of Psychiatry, 180,* 76–80.

Cranley, M. S., (1981). Development of a tool for the measurement of maternal attachment during pregnancy. *Nursing Research, 30,* 281–284.

Damato, E. G. (2004). Prenatal attachment and other correlates of postnatal maternal attachment to twins. *Advances in Neonatal Care, 4,* 274–291.

David, H. P. (2006). Born unwanted, 35 years later: The Prague study. *Reproductive Health Matters, 14,* 181–190.

De Armond, M. (1954). A type of post partum anxiety reaction. *Diseases of the Nervous System, 15,* 26–29.

Forssman, H., & Thuwe, I. (1966). One hundred and twenty children born after application for therapeutic abortion refused. *Acta Psychiatrica Scandinavica, 42,* 71–88.

Forssman, H., & Thuwe, I. (1981). Continued follow-up study of 120 persons born after refusal of application for therapeutic abortion. *Acta Psychiatrica Scandinavica, 64,* 142–149.

Hipwell, A. E., & Kumar, R. (1996). Maternal psychopathology and prediction of outcome based on mother-infant interaction ratings. *British Journal of Psychiatry, 169,* 655–661.

Höök, K. (uncertain date). *Psychic insufficiency reactions in pregnancy—effects on mother and child. A long-term follow-up study.* Unpublished manuscript.

Jernberg, A. M. (1988). Untersuchung und Therapie der pränatalen Mutter-Kind-Beziehung. *Praxis der Kinderpsychologie und Kinderpsychiatrie, 37,* 161–167.

Kubicka, L., Matejcek, Z., David, H. P., Dytrych, Z., Miller, W. B., & Roth, Z. (1995). Children from unwanted pregnancies in Prague, Czech Republic, revisited at age thirty. *Acta Psychiatrica Scandinavica, 91,* 361–369.

Kumar, R. (1997). Anybody's child: Severe disorders of mother-to-infant bonding. *British Journal of Psychiatry, 171,* 175–181.

Leifer, M. (1977). Psychological changes accompanying pregnancy and motherhood. *Genetic Psychology Monographs, 95,* 55–96.

LoBiondo-Wood, G., & Vito-O'Rourke, K. (1990). The Prenatal Maternal Attachment Scale: A methodological study. Cited by Beck, C. T. (1999). Available instruments for research on prenatal attachment and adaptation to pregnancy. *Maternal Child Nursing Journal, 24,* 25–32.

Lorberbaum, J. P., et al. (2002). A potential role for thalamocingulate circuitry in human maternal behaviour. *Biological Psychiatry, 51,* 431–445.

Luft, H. (1964). Die Wochenbettdepression: Klinik und pathogenetische Factoren. *Nervenarzt, 35,* 185–194.

Matejcek, Z., Dytrych, Z., & Schüller, V. (1978). Children from unwanted pregnancies. *Acta Psychiatrica Scandinavica, 57,* 67–90.

Müller, M. I. (1993). Development of the Prenatal Attachment Inventory. *Western Journal of Nursing Research, 15,* 199–215.

Murata, H., Kaneko, H., Hashimoto, O., Honjo, S., & Ozaki N. (n.d.). *A longitudinal study of maternal depression and its correlates from later pregnancy to 6 months postpartum.* Unpublished manuscript.

Murray, L., Hipwell, A., & Hooper, R. (1996). The cognitive development of 5-year-old children of postnatally depressed mothers. *Journal of Child Psychology and Psychiatry, 37,* 927–935.

Myhrman, A. (1988). Family relation and social competence of children unwanted at birth. *Acta Psychiatrica Scandinavica, 77,* 181–187.

Myhrman, A., Rantakallio, P., Isohanni, M., Jones, P., & Partanen, U. (1996). Unwantedness of a pregnancy and schizophrenia in the child. *British Journal of Psychiatry, 169,* 637–640.

Nagata, M., Nagai, Y., Sobajima, H., Ando, T., Nishide, Y., & Honjo, S. (2000). Maternity blues and attachment to children in mothers of full-term normal infants. *Acta Psychiatrica Scandinavica, 101,* 209–217.

Netter, P. (1982). Unerwünschte Schwangerschaft als Ursache für kindliche Entwicklungsstörungen. *Zeitschrift für Geburtshilfe und Perinatologie, 186,* 256–262.

Newell, H. W. (1934). The psychodynamics of maternal rejection. *American Journal of Orthopsychiatry, 4,* 387–401.

Nitschke, J. B., Nelson, E. E., Rusch, B. D., Fox, A. S., Oakes, T. R., & Davidson, R. J. (2004). Orbitofrontal cortex tracks positive mood in mothers viewing pictures of their newborn infants. *Neuroimage, 21,* 583–592.

Onazawa, K., Glover, V., Adams, D., Modi, N., & Kumar, R. (2001). Infant massage improves mother-infant interaction for mothers with postnatal depression. *Journal of Affective Disorders, 63,* 201–207.

Oppenheim, H. (1919). Über Misopädie. *Zeitschrift für die gesamte Neurologie und Psychiatrie, 45,* 1–18.

Raine, A., Brennan, P., & Mednick, S. A. (1994). Birth complications combined with early maternal rejection at age 1 year predispose to violent crime at 18 years. *Archives of General Psychiatry, 51,* 984–988.

Rantakallio, P., & Myhrman, A. (1980). The child and family eight years after undesired conception. *Scandinavian Journal of Social Medicine, 8,* 81–87.

Righetti-Veltema, M., Conne-Perréard, E., Bousquet, A., & Manzano, J. (2002). Postpartum depression and mother-infant relationship at 3 months. *Journal of Affective Disorders, 70,* 291–306.

Robson, K. S. (1967). The role of eye-to-eye contact in maternal-fetal attachment. *Journal of Child Psychology & Psychiatry, 8,* 13–25.

Robson, K. S., & Moss, H. A. (1970). Patterns and determinants of maternal attachment. *Journal of Pediatrics, 77,* 976–985.

Rothamel, G.C.F. (1845). Eine Mutter führt durch allmähliger Entziehung der Nahrungsmittel den Tod ehres ehelichen Kindes herbei. *Henke's Zeitschrift für den Staatsarzneikunde, 50,* 139–155.

Salariya, E. M., & Cater, J. I. (1984). Mother-child relationship: FIRST score. *Journal of Advanced Nursing, 9,* 589–595.

Siddiqui, A., & Hägglöf, B. (2000). Does maternal prenatal attachment predict postnatal mother-infant interaction? *Early Human Development, 59,* 13–25.

Squire, S., & Stein, A. (2003). Functional MRI and parental responsiveness: A new avenue into parental psychopathology and early parent-child interactions. *British Journal of Psychiatry, 183,* 481–483.

Sved-Williams, A. E. (1992). Phobic reactions of mothers to their own babies. *Australian and New Zealand Journal of Psychiatry, 26,* 631–638.

Tardieu, A. (1860). Étude medico-légale sur les sévices et mauvais traitements exercés sur des enfants. *Annales d'Hygiène, 15,* 361–398.

Taylor, A., Atkins, R., Kumar, R., Adams, D., & Glover, V. (2005). A new mother-to-infant bonding scale: Links with early maternal mood. *Archives of Women's Mental Health, 8,* 45–51.

Tomlinson, M., Cooper, P., & Murray, L., (2005). The mother-infant relationship and infant attachment in a South African peri-urban settlement. *Child Development, 76,* 1044–1054.

Trube-Becker, E. (1968). Zur Tötung von Kleinkindern durch Nahrungsentzug. *Deutsche Zeitschrift für gerichtliche Medizin, 64,* 93–101.

Wendland-Carro, J., Piccinini, A., & Stuart Millar, W. (1999). The role of early intervention on enhancing the quality of mother-infant interaction. *Child Development, 70,* 713–721.

World Health Organization. (1992). *International classification of mental and behavioural disorders* (10th ed.). Geneva: Author.

3

Effects of Maternal Postpartum Depression on the Infant and Older Siblings

JULIA CHASE-BRAND

In the normal course of events, the birth of a new child brings joy to a family but also presents stressful challenges. Toddlers and older children are expected to adjust to a crying baby, frequent interruptions in daily routines, and the relative unavailability of the mother who is recovering from childbirth and who usually is the infant's primary caretaker. Dynamically, everyone's role shifts. The father may have to get the children off to school in the morning and supervise homework at night. The youngest sib may feel displaced by the new arrival and react with anger, sadness, or jealousy. Older children may be drafted into more parentified roles, getting food on the table, pulling on mittens, and supervising younger sibs. When these challenges are successfully met, they cement the sense of the family as a cooperative unit that can lovingly rise to the challenge and provide mutual support.

However, the birth of a new child may also overwhelm the family system. This is especially true if the mother experiences postpartum depression, anxiety, or psychosis. Unlike the mild, transient depressive symptoms ("baby blues") that occur in approximately one- to two-thirds of new mothers, 10%–15% of mothers will experience significant

Acknowledgments: I wish to thank Dr. Eleanor Burlingham, Dr. Hugh Bases, Dr. Punam Kashyap, Gretchen Ross, Jonathan Brand, and Ryan Uhlich for help in the preparation of this manuscript.

postpartum depression that, left untreated, will be felt throughout the family system. Recent studies have shown that 10% of fathers also become depressed in the postpartum period (Edhborg, Lundh, Seimyr, & Widstrom, 2003; Paulson, Dauber, & Leiferman, 2006), further reducing family resilience.

The effects of maternal depression on an individual child will depend on the child's age and developmental stage, his or her temperament, the family dynamics, and such variables as financial security and the availability of external supports. The newborn, whose early socialization, cognitive development, and speech acquisition are largely in the mother's hands, is at greatest risk. The following chapter reviews the literature on the effects of maternal postpartum depression on the mental health of children at different developmental stages. It also considers the long-term outcome for such children and suggests measures for identifying and effectively intervening on behalf of children and their parents.

EFFECTS OF MATERNAL DEPRESSION ON THE INFANT

Normal Attachment Formation in the Mother-Infant Dyad

Human infants are programmed to attend from birth to maternal stimuli. An hour-old baby can discriminate a face from a nonface, shows a preference for a face that makes eye contact, and will follow a moving face with both its head and eyes (Farroni, Menon, & Johnson, 2006; Goren, Sarty, & Wu, 1975). Newborns who are only a few hours old will respond selectively to their mother's voice, which they have heard *in utero,* in preference to the speech of strangers (DeCasper & Fifer, 1980), and within hours of birth, infants orient preferentially to their own mother's breast odors and amniotic fluid, distinguishing these from the odors of other new mothers (Porter & Winberg, 1999). Human mothers are likewise programmed to attend to their newborn offspring and as in other primates, they vocalize, touch, cuddle, nurse, groom, soothe, and look intently at their newborn. A human mother exposed to her newborn for as little as 10 minutes can discriminate and identify the odor of her own child from that of other newborns (Kaitz, Good, Rekem, & Eidelman, 1987) and mothers of day-old infants can identify their offspring in a photograph (Porter, Cernoch, & Balogh, 1984).

Thus primed, mother and infant engage in reciprocal behaviors from the first day of life. The mother looks at the baby and the baby looks back, the baby cries and the mother soothes it, the mother vocalizes and the baby gurgles back. This alternation of maternal and infant responses or reciprocal "turn-taking" is characteristic of the healthy mother-infant dyad. Other markers of a secure relationship are the amount of eye contact and the presence of positive affect (e.g., smiling), vocalizing, and play. Mothers in healthy dyads are responsive to distress vocalizations from the infant and react to the child's discomfort by feeding, cuddling, rocking, and other measures. Infants in turn respond to cuddling by quieting down and "molding" into their mother's embrace.

The Effects of Postpartum Depression on Attachment Formation

The first four months of life appear to be the "sensitive period" for establishing a secure attachment (Moehler, Brunner, Wiebel, Reck, & Resch, 2006). Bonding requires active participation of both mother and child and the depressed mother is less able to maintain her side of this developmental duet. Severely depressed mothers may become apathetic, emotionally withdrawn, and unresponsive to their offspring, and even mild depression can leave a mother sad, irritable, and fatigued. Feelings of guilt or a sense of inadequacy and worthlessness often accompany the depression. Anxiety symptoms are even more common in the postpartum than depressive symptoms and also interfere with the relaxed flow of mother-child interaction that underlies healthy infant bonding (Ross & McLean, 2006; Wenzel, Haugen, Jackson, & Brendle, 2005). Finally, severe postpartum depression or mania can precipitate psychosis, and, with it, an increased risk of neglect, abuse, infanticide, and suicide in the postpartum.

Research over the past decades has documented the abnormal behavior of depressed mothers. Women with postpartum depression (PPD) smile less and make less eye contact with their infants, and the infants in turn mirror this with gaze avoidance and a low level of positive affect (Field et al., 1988; Reck et al., 2004). Depressed mothers talk less to their infants, and their vocal patterns differ from those of nondepressed mothers (Reissland, Shepard, & Herrera, 2003). Researchers note a marked reduction in maternal touch and cuddling when the mother is depressed, and infants of depressed mothers are noted to spend more time "self-touching" in what is thought to be compensatory behavior (Herrera, Reissland, & Shepard, 2004). Finally, depressed mothers are found to be less affectionate and more anxious. Their children play less and show less reciprocity or "turn-taking" in speech, affect, and behavior (Righetti-Veltema, Bousquet, & Manzano, 2003). The cumulative effect is a "depressed dyad" and impaired mother-infant bonding.

Reactive Attachment Disorder

The *DSM–IV* recognizes the most severe form of insecure attachment under the diagnosis of Reactive Attachment Disorder. Children with severe disruption of the primary bond, whether due to maternal depression, neglect, abuse, or institutionalization, show markedly abnormal styles of relatedness. Some show indiscriminant friendliness toward acquaintances and strangers alike (the "disinhibited" form), while others present as negative and withdrawn from social contact (the "inhibited" form). In a study of children in Romanian orphanages, it was found that individual children often vacillated between these two symptom sets, but it was also found that their function improved markedly if the number of caregivers was reduced so that selective bonding was possible (Smyke, Dumitrescu, & Zeanah, 2002; see also Minnis, Marwick, Arthur, & McLaughlin, 2006).

Anaclitic Depression

Rene Spitz described infantile depression in 1946, based on observations of 6- to 11-month-old children, who had formed a secure attachment in their first half-year, but who were then separated from their primary caretaker, for example, due to hospitalization. Such children soon became apprehensive and tearful. If the separation continued, they began to shut down. Babbling quieted, their interest in food diminished, and motor activity slowed. Increasingly, such children became unresponsive to social contact, and, in the worst cases, these children essentially turned their face to the wall and died (Spitz & Wolf, 1946).

Since PPD strikes some women fully half a year after childbirth when mother-infant attachment has already taken place, the children of these "late-onset" depressed mothers are also at risk for infantile depression despite a secure initial bond. Like the children in Spitz's studies, these infants face the devastating loss of their attachment figure as the mother withdraws into the shadows of depression. If substitute attachment figures are not readily available, these infants, like those in Spitz's studies, begin to withdraw from social interaction. Appetite and activity levels may drop, vocalization, eye contact, and positive affect all decline, and these youngsters show little of the positive mood and animated social give-and-take that are characteristic of the secure older infant.

Failure to Thrive

The pediatric term *failure to thrive* is used for infants, toddlers, and preschool children who fall below the 5th percentile on the growth curves whether this is the result of medical illness (e.g., infection or inborn metabolic disease) or emotional deprivation, but in the latter case, it is termed *non organic failure to thrive* (NOFTT). The pediatric classification NOFTT partially overlaps the psychiatric designation of anaclitic depression, but it is applied to a wider age range and is defined by growth parameters rather than by behavior. Not surprisingly, however, studies of children with NOFTT describe a similar behavioral profile to that seen for children with anaclitic depression. Children with NOFTT show more negative affect, less vocalization, and more gaze aversion. Their mothers are less involved and their environment is often more chaotic (Steward, 2001). Infants with NOFTT vocalize less and their mothers are less responsive to their infant's vocalizations and touch their youngsters less (Berkowitz & Senter, 1987). As one might expect, the literature reports that mothers of children with NOFTT are frequently found to be depressed (Feldman, Keren, Gross-Rozval, & Tyano 2004; Polan & Ward, 1994). In a nationwide pediatric study of 5,089 American families, maternal depression was significantly correlated with less healthy feeding and sleep practices in infants (Paulson et al., 2006), and, in a totally different study population, rural Pakistan, maternal postpartum depression was correlated with a 4-fold rate of infants being undernourished and stunted (Rahman, Iqbal, Bunn, Lovel, & Harrington, 2004).

Neglect, Child Abuse, and Infanticide

Killing of a newborn (*neonaticide*) is associated with maternal denial of pregnancy (Spinelli, 2001). Child neglect, child abuse, and child murder in the postpartum and beyond are both associated with parental psychopathology, most commonly, depression, mania, psychosis, and personality disorders (Milne & Milne, 2002). An analysis of mothers who killed their children but were considered "not guilty by reason of insanity" reported that half of the mothers were depressed at the time that they killed their children and two-thirds were experiencing auditory command hallucinations (Friedman, Hrouda, Holden, Noffsinger, & Resnick, 2005).

The magnitude of the child abuse and filicide problem is summarized in the public health record. In 1995, for example, there were a million substantiated cases of child abuse and 1,000 fatalities from abuse and neglect, of which three-quarters were of children age 3 or younger (Milne & Milne, 2002; U.S. Department of Health and Human Services, 1997).

Other Medical and Safety Issues for Infants of Depressed Mothers

The National Evaluation of Healthy Steps for Young Children analyzed parenting practices of more than 5,000 mother-infant dyads during the children's first 3 years. The evaluations occurred when the infants were 2–4 months of age and again at 30–33 months of age. Mothers with depression, by self-report, were less likely to talk or play with their children, to show them books, keep them on a daily routine, or limit TV time. Depressed mothers were also more likely to use harsh punishments such as slapping an infant and were, on average, less likely to observe fundamental infant safety precautions such as using car seats, safety latches, and electrical outlet covers. Additionally, young children of depressed mothers were less likely to be up-to-date with their immunizations, were more likely to have missed well-baby appointments, and were more likely to have had emergency room visits (McLearn, Minkovitz, Strobino, Marks, & Hou, 2006a, 2006b; Minkowitz et al., 2005).

Babies of depressed mothers are more prone to colic (Akman et al., 2006; Milgrom, Westley, & McCloud, 1995; Miller, Barr, & Eaton, 1993) and chronic infant crying, in turn, may aggravate the mother's depressed mood and is sometimes cited as the proximate trigger for abuse. Babies at risk for asthma whose mothers are depressed are significantly more likely to have developed asthma by age 6 to 8 than the children of nondepressed mothers (Klinnert et al., 2001). Similarly, infants of depressed mothers are reported to have increased frequency of diarrhea in the first year (Rahman et al., 2004).

Exposure to Maternal Depression During Infancy: Long-Term Effects

Without intervention, children whose mothers were depressed during their infancy continue to show insecure attachments as toddlers and are less interested in other toddlers and adults than are their securely attached peers (Cicchetti, Rogosch, & Toth, 1998; Easterbrooks & Lamb, 1979). They also display diminished language skills and cognitive development (Sohr-Preston & Scaramella, 2006). By age 3, boys with insecure attachments in infancy showed more behavioral problems than 3-year-olds who were rated as securely attached in infancy (Shaw & Vondra, 1995).

These infantile deficits can persist into middle childhood and beyond. In a longitudinal study of children of depressed mothers, 83% of 7-year-olds identified by their teachers as "highly externalizing" had been classified as having "highly disorganized" attachments in infancy, and children classified as having an "avoidant" attachment in infancy were more likely to show internalizing symptoms by age 7 (Lyons-Ruth, Easterbrooks, & Cibelli, 1997). Eight- and nine-year-olds born to depressed mothers show, on average, less social competence (Luoma et al., 2001), and teens whose mothers experienced PPD during their infancy are more prone to acting-out behavior (Pilowsky et al., 2006) and anxiety (Halligan, Murray, Martins, & Cooper, 2007).

EFFECTS OF POSTPARTUM DEPRESSION ON THE OLDER CHILDREN

Preschool Children

The birth of a new baby can have an unsettling effect on the older children, even when there is no postpartum depression. The most vulnerable child is usually the youngest child who has just been displaced as "the baby of the family." In a study of firstborn preschool children, whose nondepressed mothers had given birth to a second child, there was a measurable disruption of the mother-firstborn attachment in the first months as measured by the Ainsworth Strange Situation test. At 4 months, there was still some residual anxiety, but by 8–12 months the preschoolers with nondepressed mothers generally showed normalization of their attachment (Touris, Kromelow, & Harding, 1995). However, if the mother became depressed in the postpartum period, the firstborn's security of attachment following the birth of a second child was markedly worse (Teti, Sakin, Kucera, Corns, & Eiden, 1996).

Common behavioral responses of preschoolers to the birth of a younger sib include regressive behaviors (e.g., resumption of thumb sucking or enuresis), imitation of infantile behaviors (e.g., trying to nurse), and anxiety (e.g., new onset of fear of the dark or strangers). Some preschoolers may attempt aggressive confrontations with the mother-infant pair or engage in attention-seeking behaviors (Sawicki, 1997), while others show depressive symptoms and become withdrawn, quiet, or tearful. In well-functioning households, these symptoms are temporary. Parents deal with these changes by providing the older child emotional support and intervening during outbursts as needed. However, if the parents are unable to support and intervene appropriately with the older sib because of their own emotional issues, the child's anxieties, depression, and/or acting-out behaviors are likely to persist or worsen.

School-Aged Children and Teens

For school-aged children and teens, it is also common to feel stressed after the birth of a new sib even if mother and infant are doing well. School-aged children may show a mix of anxious, depressive, and externalizing symptoms, and, again, these tend to wane within months in healthy families, but are more intense and persistent when the mother experiences depression in the postpartum (Luoma et al., 2001).

There is an extensive literature on the pathological effects of maternal depression on children in early, middle, and late childhood that is applicable here, though most of these studies consider the effects of all forms of maternal depression, not just postpartum depression. In one such study, 34% of children aged 7–17 whose mothers had moderate to severe depression were found to have a diagnosable psychiatric disorder. Disruptive behavior disorder accounted for 22% of the diagnoses, 16% were diagnosed with anxiety, and 10% with depression. If past episodes of psychiatric diagnoses in these offspring were included in the analysis, nearly half (45%) of the children of depressed mothers had had a psychiatric disorder at some point during the mother's depression (Pilowsky et al., 2006; Weissman et al., 2006). The good news is that successful treatment of the mother's depression in many cases caused the children's symptoms to also remit (Weissman et al., 2006), but this is not always the case (Forman et al., 2007).

Long-term follow-up studies are now available on the outcomes of children raised by depressed parents. Offspring from 91 families with depressed parents were assessed 10 years later and showed high rates of depression, phobias, alcohol dependence, and social impairment (Weissman, Warner, Wickramaratne, Moreau, & Olfson, 1997). In the 20 years follow-up study, both the children and the grandchildren were assessed.

If major depression had been present in the previous two generations, 59.2% of the grandchildren (mean age 12 years) already had a psychiatric disorder with anxiety being particularly prominent in the younger children (Weissman et al., 2005). Such studies do not answer the question as to whether the predisposition to depression in the second and third generation is genetic, environmental, or both (see below), but there is clearly an increase in the long-term risk of mood disorder in the children of depressed parents. The risk appears to be greater the longer the mother's depression persists and is greater still if both parents suffer from depression (Milne & Milne, 2002). Table 3.1 summarizes the above age-specific effects reported in the children of depressed mothers.

Table 3.1

POTENTIAL IMPACT OF MATERNAL DEPRESSION ON CHILDREN OF DIFFERENT AGES

INFANTS

Reactive Attachment Disorder: disinhibited vs. inhibited affiliation

Failure to Thrive: child falls below 5% in height and weight for age

Anaclitic Depression: loss of attachment figure causes emotional withdrawal

Behavioral Markers: poor eye contact, reduced smiling and vocalization; lack of reciprocal "turn-taking" and playfulness; colicky, difficult to soothe, poor sleep and appetite; delays in cognitive and social development

Other Issues: Abuse and neglect. Parental failure to implement recommended medical and safety measures such as immunizations and use of car seats.

TODDLERS & PRESCHOOLERS

Anxiety: new onset of insecure attachment; heightened fears of separation, strangers, dogs, etc.; somatic complaints; intensification of nightmares, encopresis, or eneuresis

Depression: Melancholic: sad, tearful, self-isolating, negative affect, low energy, lack of persistence; irritable: tantrums, aggressive behaviors, oppositionality

Other Markers: low self-esteem; change on growth curve; sleep and eating issues; cognitive and social deficits; hyperactivity, impulsiveness, conduct problems

(*continued*)

Table 3.1

POTENTIAL IMPACT OF MATERNAL DEPRESSION ON CHILDREN OF DIFFERENT AGES (CONTINUED)

SCHOOL-AGED CHILDREN
Anxiety: somatic complaints common, school refusal, social anxiety, fears
Depression: irritable or sad, tired, sleep and eating issues, poor concentration, low self-esteem
Behavioral Markers: declining grades and "not working up to potential"; fighting in school and out; oppositional and defiant behavior with adults; conduct issues, social isolation, suicidal thoughts
ADOLESCENTS
Depressive Symptoms: irritability often the predominant presentation. As in adults: sadness and depressed mood, poor concentration, fatigue, loss of interest in activities and friends, and feeling of guilt or worthlessness, thoughts of death and suicide, future seems bleak, sleep and appetite issues
Other Markers: Anxiety, school problems, drugs, promiscuity, irresponsible or illegal activities, anorexia, bulimia, obesity, self-mutilation, somatic complaints, Internet addiction, isolation, intensified parent-child conflict, increasingly parentified role in the home.

CAVEAT: INTERPRETATION OF STATISTICAL CORRELATIONS

The data reviewed above show a strong correlation between maternal depression and poor psychiatric outcomes in the children. It is important, however, to make several observations about such data at this point before guilt is assumed or blame assigned.

1. There is an axiom from behavioral statistics that states that, "*correlation does not imply causation.*" Psychiatric symptoms are indeed more common in the offspring of mothers with PPD than in children of nondepressed mothers, but that is not the same as saying the mother's depression *causes* the child's symptoms. Behavioral systems, including the human family system, are too

complex to make linear assumptions of this sort. The mother's depression may indeed be the cause of the child's distress—or it may not. Alternative explanations for this correlation could be that the out-of-control child may be causing the mother's distress or that both mother and child are responding to an outside stressor (e.g., low socioeconomic status) or that "all of the above are true," which in real life is often the most accurate answer.

2. These studies, by their very nature, cannot distinguish *Nature from Nurture*. If, as most people believe, depression has a genetic component, one would expect the offspring of depressed parents to be more prone to emotional problems, even if parental depression hadn't surfaced during the child's developmental years. In all probability, both nature and nurture contribute to the increased rates of psychiatric symptoms in the offspring of depressed mothers.
3. Correlations are based on statistical averages. If every child of a depressed mother became depressed, we wouldn't need statistical analysis for the data, but we do need statistics precisely because individual outcomes can be quite variable. Some children with depressed mothers become depressed; others do just fine. Inborn resilience, birth order, the availability of outside supports, and therapeutic intervention can all mitigate the effects of maternal PPD on an individual child.

What is perhaps of greatest importance about this body of research correlating maternal symptoms with the children's later psychiatric and behavioral problems is that it identifies a group of children at risk, the magnitude of this risk, and the persistence of this risk over time. The next section discusses diagnosis and treatment for such children.

INTERVENTION: HELPING MOTHER AND CHILD

Identifying Mothers with Postpartum Depression

The single most important measure to protect children of postpartum depressed mothers is to identify the mother's depression early and treat it promptly. Chapters 6 and 13–16 discuss treatment options for women with depression during pregnancy and the postpartum.

Women at high risk for postpartum depression include mothers who are depressed during the pregnancy; those who have had previous episodes of PPD; mothers with major psychiatric diagnoses such as a history of depression, bipolar disorder or schizophrenia, and mothers with a history of premenstrual dysphoric disorder (Bloch, Rodenberg, Koren, & Klein, 2005). Some Axis II personality disorders also confer increased risk, specifically, avoidant, dependent, passive aggressive, obsessive-compulsive, histrionic, narcissistic, and borderline personality disorders (Akman, Uguz, & Kaya, 2007). Substance abuse is associated with an increased risk of postpartum depression as well. Teenage mothers have an increased incidence of PDD, which, in some populations, approaches 50% (Barnet, Duggan, Wilson, & Joffe, 1995). Single mothers and women with troubled marriages or a history of trauma or abuse, women with poor social supports, and women of low socioeconomic status are all at greater risk for PPD. But the truth is, postpartum depression can strike *any woman* after childbirth.

Depressed mothers, however, are unlikely to tell their doctors that they are depressed unless directly asked (Heneghan, Mercer, & DeLeone, 2004). Clinicians therefore need to take the initiative and routinely screen for maternal depression during the postpartum, either informally during the clinical interview, or formally using a screening instrument such as the Edinburgh Postnatal Depression Scale, the Beck Depression Inventory, or the Hamilton Depression Scale (Chaudron, Szilagyi, Kitzman, Wadkins, & Conwell, 2004). Since there can be a delayed onset of depression, monitoring needs to be an ongoing process throughout the postpartum.

A depressed mother's complaints may be quite protean: fatigue, poor sleep, low energy, or irritability. Other common symptoms that need to be tactfully explored are observations of maternal tearfulness, flat affect or speech, apathy or restlessness, expressions of guilt and worthlessness, poor self-care or infant care, and marked changes in appetite or weight. Depressed mothers are more likely to speak negatively of their infants, and complaints that the older children are starting to act up or are showing a new onset of anxiety or depression may also be indicators that the postpartum is not going smoothly.

Unlike postpartum depression, which may develop gradually over several months, postpartum psychosis usually presents dramatically early in the postpartum and is a medical emergency. Hallucinations, delusions, or mania all signal the need for immediate treatment of the mother and sometimes hospitalization. During this crisis, infant care must be assumed by another adult, either in the home or with a temporary surrogate outside the home.

Identifying and Treating Infants Affected by Maternal PPD

Pediatricians, who observe mother-infant interactions from the first well-baby visit on, are in a particularly good position to pick up on an infant's emotional problems. A baby who presents to the pediatrician with failure to thrive or delays in social skills, speech, or cognitive development must be evaluated both medically and emotionally. The clinician should assess the security of the mother-infant bond, and screen for neglect or abuse. If there is any question as to whether the home environment is safe, there should be a home visit.

Diminished eye contact, smiling, or reciprocal interactions between mother and child may suggest impaired bonding. A mother-infant dyad where the mother does not attempt to soothe the crying baby, or where the baby does not "mold" into the mother's embrace or where there is an absence of positive, playful interactions between mother and infant will also raise questions about the mother-infant "fit." Similarly, complaints of severe colic in the infant or reports of new behavioral problems in the older children should promote further inquiry as to the mother's well-being, home supports, and parenting practices.

Several assessment tools are available for screening emotional well-being in infants, including the Infant and Toddler Social and Emotional Assessment (ITSEA). Some clinicians also monitor specific parenting behaviors using questionnaires such as the one developed for the National Evaluation of Healthy Steps for Young Children. An added benefit of administering these questionnaires is that they reinforce the pediatric recommendations for safety, good nutrition, and stimulation of infants.

When an infant is symptomatic, treating the maternal depression is an important first step, but it is often *not sufficient* to reverse the effects on the baby (Forman et al., 2007; Minde & Minde, 2002). Providing in-home supports to the mother can reduce the maternal stress, but again, it is not a substitute for mother-infant therapy. Therapeutic treatment of infants and toddlers is done in the context of the family and focuses on repairing the attachment between mother and infant. Some therapists work one-on-one in the home; others do group work with mother-infant pairs. Parents are educated about normal early development in children and are taught about the importance of eye contact, vocalization, soothing behaviors, and reciprocal interaction. Therapists observe interactions and coach mothers in behaviors that enhance bonding. In therapy, depressed mothers are coached to act "as if" they were not depressed by smiling and talking with their babies, even when they have not fully conquered their own dark mood. Since depressed mothers are often less sensitive to their infant's needs, some therapists use a didactic approach, such as showing pictures of infantile expressions and teaching mothers to differentiate between the sad and an angry child. Therapy can also identify other resources within the family. Edhborg, for instance, noted that in families with depressed mothers, the fathers had often developed warm, joyful relationships with their offspring, a reminder that fathers and other caretakers can play a compensatory role when mothering is impaired by depression (Edhborg et al., 2003).

Identifying and Helping the Toddler or Preschooler with a Depressed Mother

Preschool children between 1 and 5 years of age typically respond to maternal depression with disruptive behaviors, anxiety, and/or depression (Minde & Minde, 2002). Disruptive behaviors range from simple tantrums and hyperactivity to oppositionality and conduct issues. Young children may erupt into aggressive rages in which they bite, hit, or throw things. Oppositional children become willful and refuse to do as adults request and may interrupt, contradict, or show flagrantly disrespectful behavior toward parents, teachers, and other adults. Occasionally conduct issues such as intentional fire-setting or cruelty emerge even at this young age.

Anxiety is reported to be more common than depression in preschoolers with depressed mothers (Pilowsky, Wickramaratne, Nomura, & Weissman, 2006). Common anxieties include separation anxiety, fear of strangers, fear of the dark or of going to bed, shyness, and school refusal. Some preschoolers are afraid they or their parents are going to die or be separated. Sleep problems and fussy eating habits are common in anxious children, as are somatic complaints such as stomachaches or headaches.

A generation ago, the clinical wisdom was that young children do not suffer from "real" depression, but it is now accepted that children of all ages can become depressed, though a depressed preschooler does not look exactly like a depressed infant nor like a depressed adult. Luby has shown that adult *DSM–IV* criteria miss fully three-quarters of preschoolers who are clinically determined to be depressed and has recommended the following five changes to more accurately identify depression in this age group (Luby et al., 2002, 2006):

1. Replacing the adult *DSM–IV* phrasing "diminished interest and pleasure" with "shows low enthusiasm,"
2. Using "change on the growth curve," rather than "change in weight,"
3. Eliminating the subjective criterion "feelings of worthlessness and guilt" with the observer's judgment that the child shows "self-esteem issues,"
4. Replacing "poor concentration and indecisiveness," again a self-report criterion, with "lacks persistence" in activities,
5. Replacing "thoughts of death and dying" with "presence of fears and somatization."

In preschoolers, "irritable" depression is characterized by angry, restless, oppositional behavior and is probably more common than "melancholic" depression, in which the child presents as tearful, listless, and self-isolating. Depressed youngsters sometimes show little spontaneous speech or develop eating and sleep problems. And while young children may not fully understand the concept of death, depressed youngsters can certainly entertain suicidal thoughts and may attempt suicide by available means such as putting a plastic bag over their heads or deliberately running into the path of a car.

Assessment and diagnosis in toddlers and preschoolers is based on parental report, clinical observations, and instruments such as the Behavior Assessment Scale for Children (BASC), the Child Behavior Checklist (CBCL), and the Parents Evaluation of Developmental Status (PEDS). The Ainsworth Strange Situation paradigm is used to assess attachment security in young children, and the Vineland Adaptive Behavior Scale provides a measure of the child's function in relation to others of the same age. Mental health professionals generally use the *DSM–IV* published by the American Psychiatric Association for diagnosis, while pediatricians use the *Diagnostic and Statistical Manual for Primary Care (DSM–PC)*, published by the American Academy of Pediatrics (Wolraich, Felice, & Drotar, 1996).

Therapy for depressed and anxious toddlers and preschool children often includes the parent in sessions, though some therapists do play therapy with the child alone (Cicchetti, Toth, & Rogosch, 1999). Activities such as drawing, building blocks, or engaging in imaginary play with doll families allow young children to express emotional issues. The therapist can then join the child and play out these fantasies or be the observer, commenting on the feelings being expressed to help both parent and child understand what's going on emotionally. The other function of the therapist can be to model supportive and corrective behaviors that the parent can imitate. Parenting skills may also be addressed in separate parenting skills classes that some families prefer because it provides them with the support of other parents who are dealing with similar issues. For children with disruptive behaviors, the parenting skills group may be coupled with a children's social skills group, which teaches the youngster such basic tools as anger management, turn-taking, and fair play.

Identifying and Helping the Troubled School-Aged Child

Like the preschool child, grade school children with depressed mothers may exhibit a mix of anxious, depressive, and disruptive behaviors. In the school-aged child, as in younger children, depression presents as either melancholic withdrawal or with irritability and restlessness. Severely depressed children are more likely to report "hearing voices" than depressed adults are. Depressed schoolchildren sometimes develop eating or sleep problems.

Anxiety is probably more common than depression in the school-aged child with a depressed mother. As with preschoolers, these anxieties include separation anxiety, fear of the dark, specific phobias (e.g., bugs or snakes), fear of death or loss of a parent. Obsessive behaviors (e.g., germ phobia and hand washing) or impulse control problems like trichotillomania may also appear at this age or even younger. Some anxieties such as social phobia (extreme shyness), school refusal, and selective mutism, in which the child typically will speak only to family and close friends but not to outsiders, pose serious impediments to socialization and academic achievement.

Somatic complaints are quite common in depressed and anxious school-aged children. Though some children present with unusual symptoms such as being unable to swallow, the most common complaints are headaches and stomachaches and these often occur in the morning before school, or Sunday evening in anticipation of the impending school week. Though some children are consciously trying to con their parents, most are not: somatization is, for most children, an unconscious expression of their worries. Somatic complaints can lead to missed school days and sometimes to unpleasant or costly medical work-ups. For example, in a study of young patients admitted to an inpatient pediatric neurology unit with severe, unexplained headaches, 40% were found to have depression as their major diagnosis (Ling, Oftedal, & Weinberg, 1970).

Behavioral "acting-out" is perhaps the most frequent presentation in the school-aged child with a depressed mother. Tantrums, disciplinary problems, refusal to do homework, academic difficulties, and trouble with peers are all common. An oppositional-defiant child can frustrate the most patient parent and for a depressed mother, oppositional behavior may trigger despair, anger, or withdrawal. Setting limits becomes a test of wills and without support, the mother may experience a sense of futility and failure. Pathological relationships among sibs are also difficult to control in a household that lacks secure parental leadership. In severely disturbed youngsters, stealing, lying, bullying, hurting people and animals, fire setting, and sexual exploitation may all appear in the grade school years and are diagnostically labeled conduct disorder. Conduct disorder is considered a precursor to antisocial behavior in adulthood, and, as such, demands serious attention.

Treatment strategies for addressing anxiety and depression in the school-aged child range from supportive and insight-oriented therapy, to cognitive behavioral therapy, which targets the child's negative thinking patterns, and to social skills groups that teach children how to cope more effectively with peers by turn-taking, respectful listening, and anger management. Family therapy may be selected if the parent-child or sibling issues are a major focus of concern, and, here again, parenting skills groups may be a useful adjunct. In addition, manual-based public health programs are being developed that specifically seek to prevent depression in children of depressed parents (Beardslee, Gladstone, Wright, & Cooper, 2003). There is no "one-size-fits-all" solution to acting-out behavior in children, but, especially in the lower grades, the parents and school are often encouraged to work jointly to set goals that can be reinforced in both settings.

The question of whether to use antidepressant, antianxiety, or antipsychotic medication with school-aged children is argued on many levels. Public figures such as the Scientologist Tom Cruise have made headlines asserting that antidepressants are never appropriate, even in the treatment of adult women with PPD. Others feel that psychiatric medications are being used too zealously in children to control what are essentially normal childhood behaviors. The FDA became involved in this debate in 2003 when it added a black box warning to the SSRIs (the most common antidepressant/antianxiety medications on the market today), claiming that SSRIs cause increased suicidal thinking in children.

This warning had two effects: within a year there was a precipitous drop in SSRI prescriptions to children and teens in the United States and in Europe. Second, by 2004, the rate of completed suicides in children and teens had risen by 14% in the United States, and, by 2005, the Dutch had experienced a 49% increase in child and adolescent deaths by suicide (Gibbons et al., 2007).

For most child psychiatrists, a recommendation for pharmacotherapy will be based on the severity and duration of the child's symptoms. If a child shows serious symptoms such as psychosis, mania, or suicidality, or when therapy alone has not been effective, or when the child's function is severely compromised (e.g., he or she can't attend school), psychiatrists will prescribe medications to school-aged children and teens as an adjunct to therapy. The parents, unfortunately, still have to negotiate the political and cultural aspects of this debate. For example, some parents are made to feel guilty about "drugging" their children if they choose to go with a recommendation for pharmacotherapy, or conversely, they may be threatened with classification of their child at school if they don't agree to medication. It is an oddly politicized issue, which, in turn, reflects our society's ongoing discomfort with psychiatric illness.

Depression, Anxiety, and Conduct Issues in Teenage Children

Teenagers are not immune from the family disruption caused by a mother's postpartum depression. Teens need well-functioning parents for their own emotional support and guidance. They need to attend school, do homework, and meet other commitments such as filling out college applications or finding work. If a mother is too tired, distracted, or irritable due to depression and a new baby to provide support, the teen's development can easily be derailed. Adolescents may be asked to shoulder more family responsibility when the mother is incapacitated and may resent and rebel against the new responsibilities, or conversely, they may accept an inordinate burden that compromises their academic and social achievement.

As in younger children, teens with depressed parents are themselves at increased risk for depression, anxiety, and behavior problems. But unlike young children, depressed, angry teens are also at increased risk of substance abuse—which, in turn, makes both mood and conduct disorders more intractable. Acting-out teens may get into legal problems, from shoplifting to gang membership and drug dealing, or they may engage in promiscuous or unprotected sex with the concomitant risks of pregnancy, rape, early parenthood, and sexually transmitted disease. Suicidal behaviors, eating disorders, episodic rages, and antisocial behaviors are all relatively common presentations in disturbed adolescents, especially if drugs have entered the picture.

Symptomatically, depressed teens present much as adults do, with sadness, fatigue, poor concentration, feelings of guilt and worthlessness, and changes in sleep and eating habits, but teens tend to exhibit more irritability when depressed than adults typically do. Depressed teens lose their optimism and drive, grades fall, and interest in extracurricular activities and peer relationships may wane. For some, depression brings a paralysis and withdrawal from the outside world that may be exacerbated by intensely absorbing solitary activities such as Internet gaming or pornography.

Treatment of teens with depression and anxiety is similar to that for adults. Therapy can be supportive, insight-oriented, or can focus on cognitive distortions (cognitive behavioral therapy). Some teens prefer group therapy, whereas others are more comfortable in individual sessions. Family therapy may be appropriate if parent-child issues are a core problem. Teens are treated with generally the same set of medications as adults. However, since bipolar disorder and schizophrenia generally don't emerge until the late teens, clinicians treating teens routinely exercise caution when initiating medications lest they inadvertently ignite a first episode of psychotic or manic symptoms.

Treatment for substance abuse is often difficult to initiate in adolescents, first, because adolescents deny and hide their drug use, and, second, because there is strong cultural support for the notion that "everyone does it and it is a normal rite of passage." Parents often share this attitude and have difficulty taking the teen's substance abuse seriously. Alcohol, pot, and other drug use clearly increase the risks of psychiatric disorders, academic failure, and legal problems and must be addressed.

SUMMARY

Postpartum depression robs a woman of her happiness, energy, and ability to parent at a time when her children deeply need her. For infants, the results of maternal depression are potentially devastating because a baby's physical, emotional, and cognitive growth all depend on developing a warm, secure attachment in the first months of life. However, as reviewed above, toddlers, preschoolers, older children, and teens are also at significant risk when a mother becomes depressed and may react to their mother's emotional withdrawal by developing depression and anxiety themselves or by acting out in anger at their loss. Left unsupported, these children are at high risk for psychiatric, behavioral, and academic problems.

Early detection and treatment of maternal depression are essential to the welfare of the whole family. Treating the mother, however, is only part of the story. The children also need to be assessed, and, in some cases, will need additional support and treatment themselves. As reviewed above, depression and anxiety present differently in infants, children, and teens, and there is a variety of treatment options appropriate for different age groups.

Families readily bring children to mental health professionals when there is divorce, illness, or a death in the family, rightly worrying that these events may impact negatively on the child's happiness and development. However, as the literature reviewed in this chapter attests, the children of depressed mothers are also at high risk, but their needs are often not addressed because both family and clinicians focus on the mother and newborn. The high rates of psychopathology in the children of depressed mothers and the persistence of these effects over many years argue that greater attention needs to be paid to these collateral victims of maternal depression.

REFERENCES

Akman, I., Kuscu, K., Ozdemir, N., Yurdakul, Z., Solakoglu, M., Orhan, L., Karabekiroglu, A., & Ozek, E. (2006). Mothers' postpartum psychological adjustment and infantile colic. *Archives of Disease in Childhood, 91,* 417–419.

Akman, I., Uguz, F., & Kaya, N. (2007). Postpartum depression is associated with personality disorders. *Compr Psychiatry, 48,* 343–347.

Barnet, B., Duggan, A. K., Wilson, M. D., & Joffe, A. (1995). Association between postpartum substance use and depressive symptoms, stress, and social support in adolescent mothers. *Pediatrics, 96,* 659–666.

Beardslee, W. R., Gladstone, T. R., Wright, E. J., & Cooper, A. B. (2003). A family-based approach to the prevention of depressive symptoms in children at risk: Evidence of parental and child change. *Pediatrics, 112,* 119–131.

Berkowitz, C. D., & Senter, S. A. (1987). Characteristics of mother-infant interactions in non-organic failure to thrive. *Journal of Family Practice, 25,* 377–381.

Bloch, M., Rodenberg, N., Koren, D., & Klein, E. (2005). Risk factors associated with the development of postpartum depression. *Journal of Affective Disorders, 88,* 9–18.

Chaudron, L. H., Szilagyi, P. G., Kitzman, H. J., Wadkins, H. I., & Conwell, Y. (2004). Detection of postpartum depressive symptoms by screening at well-child visits. *Pediatrics, 113,* 551–558.

Cicchetti, D., Rogosch, F. A., & Toth, S. L. (1998). Maternal depressive disorder and contextual risk: Contributions to the development of attachment insecurity and behavior problems in toddler hood. *Developmental Psychopatholology, 10,* 283–300.

Cicchetti, D., Toth, S. L., & Rogosch, F. A. (1999). The efficacy of toddler-parent psychotherapy to increase attachment security in offspring of depressed mothers. *Attachment and Human Development, 1,* 34–66.

DeCasper, A. J., & Fifer, W. P. (1980). Of human bonding: Newborns prefer their mothers' voices. *Science, 6,* 1174–1176.

Easterbrooks, M. A., & Lamb, M. E. (1979). The relationship between quality of infant-mother attachment and infant competence in initial encounters with peers. *Child Development, 50,* 380–387.

Edhborg, M., Lundh, W., Seimyr, L., & Widstrom, A. M. (2003). The parent child relationship in the context of maternal depressive mood. *Archives of Women's Mental Health, 6,* 211–216.

Farroni, T., Menon, E., & Johnson, M. H. (2006). Factors influencing newborn's preference for faces with eye contact. *Journal of Experimental Child Psychology, 95,* 298–308.

Feldman, R., Keren, M., Gross-Rozval, O., & Tyano, S. (2004). Mother-child touch patterns in infant feeding disorders: Relation to maternal/child and environmental factors. *Journal of the American Academy of Child Adolescent Psychiatry, 43,* 1089–1097.

Field, T., Healy, B., Goldstein, S., Perry, S., Bendell, D., Schanberg, S., Zimmerman, E. A., & Kuhn, C. (1988). Infants of depressed mothers show "depressed" behavior even with nondepressed adults. *Child Development, 59,* 1569–1579.

Forman, D. R., Ohara, M. W., Stewart, S., Gorman, L. L., Larsen, K. E., & Coy, K. C. (2007). Effective treatment for postpartum depression is not sufficient to improve the developing mother-child relationship. *Developmental Psychopathology, 19,* 585–602.

Friedman, S. H., Hrouda, D. R., Holden, C. E., Noffsinger, S. G., & Resnick, P. J. (2005). Child murder committed by severely mentally ill mothers: An examination of mothers found not guilty by reason of insanity. *Journal of Forensic Science, 50,* 1466–1471.

Gibbons, R. D., Brown, C. H., Hur, K., Marcus, S. M., Bhaumik, D. K., Erkins, J. A., Herings, R. M., & Mann, J. J. (2007). Early evidence on the effects of regulator's suicidality warnings on SSRI prescriptions and suicide in children and adolescents. *American Journal of Psychiatry, 164,* 1356–1363.

Goren, C. C., Sarty, M., & Wu, P. Y. (1975). Visual following and pattern discrimination of face-like stimuli by newborn infants. *Pediatrics, 56,* 544–549.

Halligan, S. L., Murray, L., Martins, C., & Cooper, P. J. (2007). Maternal depression and psychiatric outcomes in adolescent offspring: A 13-year longitudinal study. *Journal of Affective Disorders, 97,* 145–154.

Heneghan, A. M., Mercer, M., & DeLeone, N. L. (2004). Will mothers discuss parenting stress and depressive symptoms with their child's pediatrician? *Pediatrics, 113,* 460–467.

Herrera, E., Reissland, N., & Shepard, J. (2004). Maternal touch and maternal child-directed speech: Effects of depressed mood in the postnatal period. *Journal of Affective Disorders, 81,* 29–39.

Kaitz, M., Good, A., Rekem, A. M., & Eidelman, A. I. (1987). Mothers' recognition of their newborns by olfactory cues. *Developmental Psychobiology, 20,* 587–591.

Klinnert, M. D., Nelson, H. S., Price, M. R., Adinoff, A. D., Leung, D. Y., & Mrazek, D. A. (2001). Onset and persistence of childhood asthma: Predictors from infancy. *Pediatrics, 108,* E69.

Ling, W., Oftedal, G., & Weinberg, W. (1970). Depressive illness in children presenting as severe headache. *American Journal of Dis Child, 120,* 122–124.

Luby, J. L., Heffelfinger, A. K., Mrakotsky, C., Hessler, M. J., Brown, K. M., & Hildbrand, T. (2002). Preschool major depressive disorder: Preliminary validation for developmentally modified *DSM–IV* criteria. *Journal of the American Academy of Child and Adolescent Psychiatry, 41,* 928–937.

Luby, J. L., Sullivan, J., Belden, A., Stalets, M., Blankenship, S., & Spitznagel, E. (2006). An observational analysis of behavior in depressed preschoolers: Further validation of early-onset depression. *Journal of the American Academy of Child Adolescent Psychiatry, 45,* 203–212.

Luoma, I., Tamminen, T., Kaukonen, P., Laippala, P., Puura, K., Salmelin, R., & Almqvist, F. (2001). Longitudinal study of maternal depressive symptoms and child well-being. *Journal of the American Academy of Child and Adolescent Psychiatry, 40,* 1367–1374.

Lyons-Ruth, K., Easterbrooks, M. A., & Cibelli, C. D. (1997). Infant attachment strategies, infantile mental lag and maternal depressive symptoms: Predictors of internalizing and externalizing problems at age 7. *Developmental Psychology, 331,* 681–692.

McLearn, K. T., Minkovitz, C. S., Strobino, D. M., Marks, E., & Hou, W. (2006a). Maternal depressive symptoms at 2–4 months postpartum and early parenting practices. *Archives of Pediatric and Adolescent Medicine, 160,* 279–284.

McLearn, K. T., Minkovitz, C. S., Strobino, D. M., Marks, E., & Hou, W. (2006b). The timing of maternal depressive symptoms and mothers' parenting practices with their children. *Pediatrics, 118,* 174–182.

Milgrom, J., Westley, D. T., & McCloud, P. I. (1995). Do infants of depressed mothers cry more than other infants? *Journal of Pediatric Child Health, 31,* 218–221.

Miller, A. R., Barr, R. G., & Eaton, W. O. (1993). Crying and motor behavior of 6-week-old infants and postpartum maternal mood. *Pediatrics, 92,* 551–558.

Minde, K., & Minde, R. (2002). Effect of disordered parenting on the development of children. In M. Lewis (Ed), *Child and adolescent psychiatry—A comprehensive textbook* (3rd ed., pp. 37, 477–493). Philadelphia: Lippincott Williams and Wilkens.

Minkowitz, C. S., Strobino, D., Scharfstein, D., Hou, W., Miller, T., Mistry, K. B., & Swartz, K. (2005). Maternal depressive symptoms and children's receipt of health care in the first three years of life. *Pediatrics, 115,* 306–314.

Minnis, H., Marwick, H., Arthur, J., & McLaughlin, A. (2006). Reactive attachment disorder—A theoretical model beyond attachment. *European Child and Adolescent Psychiatry, 15,* 336–342.

Moehler, E., Brunner, R., Wiebel, A., Reck, C., & Resch, F. (2006). Maternal depressive symptoms in the postnatal period are associated with long-term impairment of mother-child bonding. *Archives of Women's Mental Health, 9,* 273–278.

Paulson, J. F., Dauber, S., & Leiferman, J. A. (2006). Individual and combined effects of postpartum depression in mothers and fathers on parenting behavior. *Pediatrics, 118,* 659–668.

Pilowsky, D. J., Wickramaratne, P., Nomura, Y., & Weissman, M. M. (2006). Family discord, prenatal depression, and psychopathology in offspring: 20-year follow-up. *Journal of the American Academy of Child and Adolescent Psychiatry, 45,* 452–460.

Pilowsky, D. J., Wickramaratne, P. J., Rush, A. J., Huges, C. W., Garber, J., Malloy, E., et al. (2006). Children of currently depressed mothers: A STAR*D ancillary study. *Journal of Clinical Psychiatry, 67,* 126–136.

Polan, H. J., & Ward, M. J. (1994). Role of the mother's touch in failure to thrive: A preliminary investigation. *Journal of the American Academy of Child and Adolescent Psychiatry, 33,* 1098–1105.

Porter, R. H., Cernoch, J. M., & Balogh, R. D. (1984). Recognition of neonates by facial-visual characteristics. *Pediatrics, 74,* 501–504.

Porter, R. H., & Winberg, J. (1999). Unique salience of maternal breast odors for newborn infants. *Neuroscience Bio Behavior Rev, 23,* 439–449.

Rahman, A., Iqbal, Z., Bunn, J., Lovel, H., & Harrington, R. (2004). Impact of maternal depression on infant nutritional status and illness: A cohort study. *Archives of General Psychiatry, 61,* 946–952.

Reck, C., Hunt, A., Fuchs, T., Weiss, R., Noon, A., Moehler, E., Downing, G., Troznick, E. Z., & Mundt, C. (2004). Interactive regulation of affect in postpartum depressed mothers and their infants. *Psychopathology, 37,* 272–280.

Reissland, N., Shepard, J., & Herrera, E. (2003). The pitch of maternal voice: A comparison of mothers suffering from depressed mood and non-depressed mothers reading books to their infants. *Journal of Child Psychology and Psychiatry, 44,* 255–261.

Righetti-Veltema, M., Bousquet, A., & Manzano, J. (2003). Impact of postpartum depressive symptoms on the mother and her 18-month-old. *European Child and Adolescent Psychiatry, 12,* 75–83.

Ross, L. E., & McLean, L. M. (2006). Anxiety disorders during pregnancy and the postpartum period: A systematic review. *Journal of Clinical Psychiatry, 67,* 1285–1298.

Sawicki, J. A. (1997). Sibling rivalry and the new baby: Anticipatory guidance and management strategies. *Pediatric Nursing, 23,* 298–302.

Shaw, D. S., & Vondra, J. I. (1995). Infant attachment security and maternal predictors of early behavior problems: A longitudinal study of low-income families. *Journal of Abnormal Child Psychology, 23,* 335–357.

Smyke, A. T., Dumitrescu, A., & Zeanah, C. H. (2002). Attachment disturbances in young children. I: The continuum of caretaking casualty. *Journal of the American Academy of Child Adolescent Psychiatry, 8,* 972–982.

Sohr-Preston, S. L., & Scaramella, L. V. (2006). Implications of timing of maternal depressive symptoms for early cognitive and language development. *Clinical Child and Family Psychology Review, 9,* 65–83.

Spinelli, M. G. (2001). A systematic investigation of 16 cases of neonaticide. *American Journal of Psychiatry, 160,* 555–562.

Spitz, R. A., & Wolf, K. M. (1946). Anaclitic depression. An inquiry into the genesis of psychiatric conditions in early childhood, II. *Psychoanalytic Study of the Child, 2,* 312–342.

Steward, D. K. (2001). Behavioral characteristics of infants with non-organic failure to thrive during a play interaction. *American Journal of Maternal and Child Nursing, 26,* 79–85.

Teti, D. M., Sakin, J. W., Kucera, E., Corns, K. M., & Eiden, R. D. (1996). And baby makes four: Predictors of attachment security among preschool-age firstborns during the transition to siblinghood. *Child Development, 67,* 579–596.

Touris, M., Kromelow, S., & Harding, C. (1995). Mother-first born attachment and the birth of a sibling. *American Journal of Orthopsychiatry, 65,* 293–297.

U.S. Department of Health and Human Services. (1997). *Child abuse and fatalities in 1995.* Washington, DC: Author.

Weissman, M. M., Pilowsky, D. J., Wickramaratne, P. J., Talati, A., Wisniewski, S. R., Fava, M., et al. (2006). STAR*D-Child team. Remissions in maternal depression and child psychopathology: A STAR*D-Child report. *Journal of the American Medical Association, 295,* 1389–1398.

Weissman, M. M., Warner, V., Wickramaratne, P. J., Moreau, D., & Olfson, M. (1997). Offspring of depressed parents: 10 years later. *Archives of General Psychiatry, 4,* 932–940.

Weissman, M. M., Wickramaratne, P. J., Nomura, Y., Warner, V., Verdeli, H., Pilowsky, D. J., Grillon, C., & Bruder, G. (2005). Families at high and low risk for depression: A 3-generation study. *Archives of General Psychiatry, 62,* 29–36.

Wenzel, A., Haugen, E. N., Jackson, L. C., & Brendle, J. R. (2005). Anxiety symptoms and disorders at eight weeks postpartum. *Journal of Anxiety Disorders, 19,* 295–311.

Wolraich, M. L., Felice, M. E., & Drotar, D. (Eds.). (1996). The classification of child and adolescent mental diagnoses in primary care. *American Academy Pediatrics,* 1–368.

4 Perinatal Mood Disorders: An Introduction

SHAILA MISRI AND KAREN JOE

Down Came the Rain, a book by Brook Shields that takes the reader through the poignant journey of her postpartum depression, brought this disorder out into the open without stigma, shame, and embarrassment. Her personal narration of the frightening thoughts of harming her baby daughter at the American Psychiatric Association meeting in 2007 before a packed audience of health care providers gave this illness the validity, legitimacy, and the attention it has needed since it was first described by Marcé in 1817 in the *Treatise of Insanity.* While postnatal depression has acquired a celebrity status, antenatal depression will need a movement of equal magnitude to bring the illness into the limelight.

Women are hesitant to accept the diagnosis of psychiatric illness in the perinatal period due to the fright, trepidation, denial, and humiliation that goes along with mental illness. This leads to delays in the recognition and treatment of the illness, thereby endangering the mother and the developing baby. The ongoing suffering and the short- and long-term implications of this chronic, relapsing illness in the absence of treatment is detrimental to the pregnant mother and her family. Minimizing the associated morbidity and mortality is vital in ensuring stability and providing a secure environment. The barriers faced by women and caregivers are numerous; to help overcome this obstacle, clinicians must engage in a consensual practice of involving the woman and a significant other in the management of this multifaceted illness and make every attempt to facilitate timely intervention. As yet much work needs to be done to build upon the existing knowledge in caring for mentally ill perinatal woman. What is encouraging, however, is the growing interest and commitment on the part of the caregivers engaged in research and the better quality care of these beleaguered women.

PREVALENCE

The World Health Organization has determined that depression affects approximately 50 million people worldwide (C. Murray & Lopez, 1996). In particular, the prevalence of depression in women is about 20% compared to 10% in men (Kessler, McGonagle, Swartz, Blazer, & Nelson, 1993) with the initial episode often occurring in the childbearing years (Burt & Stein, 2002). Women are particularly prone to experiencing depressive symptomatology during the vulnerable periods of pregnancy, postpartum, pregnancy loss, and infertility (Josefsson et al., 2002).

It is only in the past two decades that clinicians have come to understand that contrary to the traditional belief that pregnancy offers "protection" against mood disorders, depression in pregnancy is indeed a worrisome condition that requires prompt intervention. Because the signs of pregnancy overlap with symptoms of depression, diagnosis is easily missed or dismissed. However, the number of women who actually meet the criteria for major depression is much smaller than those who report depressive symptoms (Bennett, Einarson, Taddio, Koren, & Einarson, 2004; Evans et al., 2001; Kumar & Robson, 1984; Llewellyn, Stowe, & Nemeroff, 1997; Marcus, Flynn, Blow, & Barry, 2003; O'Hara, 1986; Watson, Elliott, Rugg, & Brough, 1984). A meta-analysis by Bennett et al. reported that 7.4% women were found to suffer from depression during the first trimester, 12.85% in the second trimester, and 12% in the third trimester (Bennett et al., 2004). Yet the *DSM–IV–TR* does not acknowledge its existence.

More recently, the continuum and the connection between antenatal and postpartum depression has become evident. Cox, Atkinson, and Gotlib, in three separate studies, demonstrated that depressed mood in pregnancy might presage postpartum depression (Atkinson & Rickel, 1984; Cox, Connor, & Kendell, 1982; Gotlib, Whiffen, Mount, Milne, & Cordy, 1989). In one study, 50% of patients diagnosed in the postpartum period had onset of their symptoms in pregnancy (Gotlib et al., 1989).

Postpartum depression is often minimized and dismissed as "postpartum blues." Postpartum blues is a transient condition with symptoms such as mild mood swings, irritability, anxiety, and insomnia being limited to two weeks postpartum (O'Hara, Schlechte, Lewis, & Wright, 1991). These symptoms, which typically peak within two days postdelivery, affect approximately 50% of women and will resolve with minimal or no treatment (Steiner, 1990). Persistence beyond two weeks is not typical of postpartum blues, nor is suicidal ideation. Symptoms of the blues require close monitoring in women with a prior history of major depression as these may be early indicators of relapse (Lusskin, Pundiak, & Habib, 2007).

Postpartum depression can also be mistakenly used to describe postpartum psychosis. Postpartum psychosis, which affects approximately 0.1%–0.2% of women, generally occurs in the first 1–4 weeks following delivery and involves a rapid decompensation characterized by hallucinations, agitation, delusions, and dramatic mood swings (Cohen, 1998; Lusskin et al., 2007). This acute illness is frequently part of a bipolar disorder and has a significant risk of suicide and infanticide and requires hospitalization (Viguera, Cohen, Baldessarini, & Nonacs, 2002; Yonkers et al., 2004) (see Figure 4.1).

RISK FACTORS

The perinatal period presents a time of increased vulnerability when it pertains to depressive illness. However, there are a variety of biological and psychosocial factors that are believed to influence perinatal depression.

A familial history of psychiatric illness increases the risk for a given patient with first-degree relatives of patients with depression being 1.5–3 times more likely to develop depression when compared to the general population (Beck, 1996; Forty et al., 2006; Kumar & Robson, 1984; Llewellyn et al., 1997; McGuffin, Marusic, & Farmer, 2001; O'Hara, 1986). Women with a prior history of postpartum depression stand a 30%–50% risk of relapse in future pregnancies (Josefsson et al., 2002). The two important biological risk factors for postpartum depression are antenatal depression and postpartum blues (Dennis & Ross, 2006; Evans et al., 2001; Henshaw, 2003; Josefsson, Berg, Nordin, & Sydsjo, 2001; Kitamura et al., 2006; Yonkers et al., 2001). A personal or familial history of depression, depressive symptomatology during pregnancy,

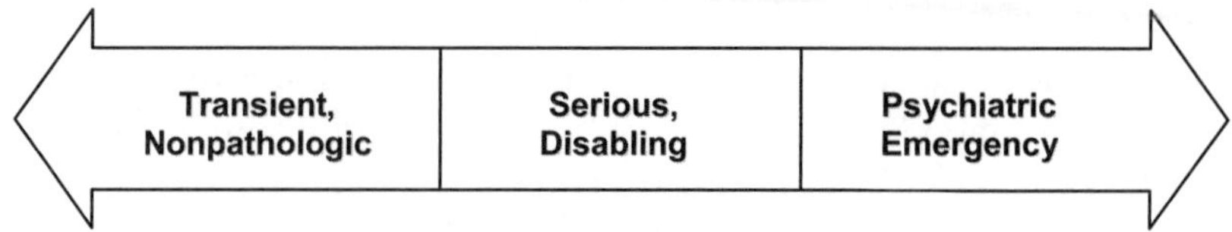

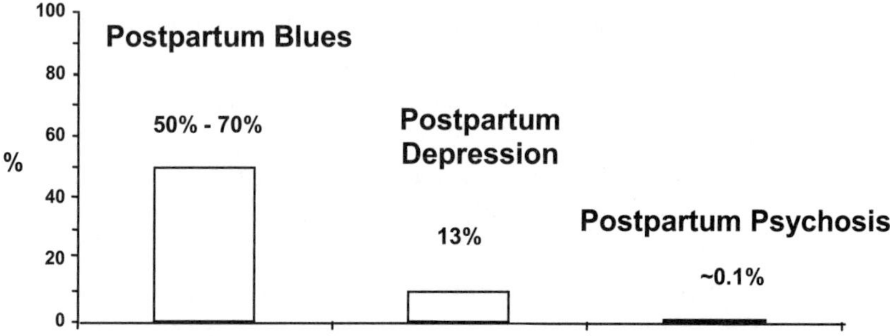

Figure 4.1 Spectrum of postpartum mood changes.

From "Pharmacologic Treatment of Depression in Women: PMS, Pregnancy, and the Postpartum Period," by L. S. Cohen, 1998, *Depression and Anxiety, 8*(Suppl. 1), pp. 18–26. Copyright 1998 Wiley-Liss, Inc. Adapted with permission of the author. Also "Rates and risk of postpartum depression: A meta-analysis," by M. W. O'Hara and A. M. Swain, 1996, *International Review of Psychiatry, 8*(1), pp. 37–54. Copyright 1996. Adapted with permission of the authors.

and premenstrual mood changes are all risk factors for postpartum blues (Bloch, Rotenberg, Koren, & Klein, 2006; O'Hara et al., 1991). Interestingly, while a personal history of depression has been correlated with postpartum depression, a family history has been less consistently associated with this disorder (Brugha et al., 1998; Dennis & Ross, 2006; Forty et al., 2006). A family history does, however, provide valuable clinical information to treating physicians in assessing the presenting episode as well as the possibility of future recurrences. For example, clinical experience shows that patients with a history of psychiatric illness on both sides of the family are at a greater risk of experiencing severe and chronic depression compared to those without.

There are a number of psychosocial risk factors that contribute to perinatal depression, including the lack of a partner, social, or family support. Physical, mental, as well as sexual abuse issues, play a significant role in contributing to the onset of perinatal depression (Stewart, 1994). In one study, a history of sexual abuse was found to be a risk factor for prolonged depression in women who were diagnosed and hospitalized after childbirth (Buist & Janson, 2001). Another crucial factor is the cultural background of the woman. Studies show that stigma is attached to seeking professional help from mental health providers; treatment is not readily sought by immigrant women (Small, Lumley, & Yelland, 2003; Zayas, Cunningham, McKee, & Jankowski, 2002). Clinical experience shows that ethnicity does impact the health-seeking behaviors of mentally ill perinatal women. Unplanned pregnancy is also a vital factor that needs to be considered. This is particularly significant in women who go ahead with the pregnancy despite the lack of partner or social support (Altshuler, Hendrick, & Cohen, 1998; Robertson, Grace, Wallington, & Stewart, 2004). Stressful life events, chronic stressors, and socioeconomic status also contribute to the risk of perinatal depression (Beck, 1996; Kumar & Robson, 1984; O'Hara, 1986; Robertson et al., 2004; Seguin, Potvin, St-Denis, & Loiselle, 1999; Warner, Appleby, Whitton, & Faragher, 1996). A previous pregnancy loss, miscarriage, stillbirth, or abortion is another risk factor for a major depression in the postpartum (Hughes, Turton, & Evans, 1999; Major et al., 2000; Neugebauer, 2003; Neugebauer et al., 1997). Pregnant adolescents are at a higher risk of developing depression. Coincidentally, already depressed adolescents experience a high risk of becoming pregnant (Omar, Martin, & McElderry, 2001).

In recent years, it is noted that discontinuation of antidepressant medications leads to relapse of depressive symptoms upon conception. When patients choose to discontinue their medication during pregnancy, they significantly increase their risk of relapse. Cohen and colleagues in a prospective study of 201 women with major depressive disorder, who were euthymic for at least 3 months prior to conception, found that women who discontinued their antidepressant medication either before pregnancy or during their first trimester experienced a significantly increased risk of relapse compared to those who remained on medications (Cohen et al., 2006). Additionally, of the 65 women who discontinued their medication 68% relapsed compared to 26% of the 82 patients who remained on medication throughout their pregnancies (see Figure 4.2). This study highlights the importance of close monitoring of depressed women throughout pregnancy.

Studies and clinical observations thus far appear to show that biopsychosocial factors are of equal magnitude when it pertains to onset, continuation, and worsening of perinatal depression. Any woman deemed to be at risk early on in pregnancy should be offered appropriate education and support in addition to being followed at frequent intervals to check the course of the depressive illness in pregnancy and postpartum.

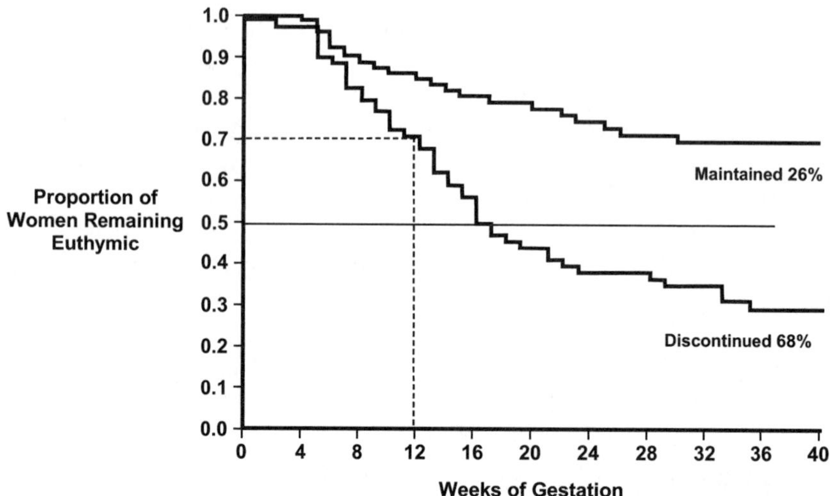

Figure 4.2 Relapse rates with antidepressant discontinuation and maintenance.

From "Relapse of Major Depression During Pregnancy in Women Who Maintain or Discontinue Antidepressant Treatment," by L. S. Cohen, L. L. Altshuler, B. L. Harlow, R. Nonacs, D. J. Newport, A. C. Viguera et al., 2006, *Journal of the American Medical Association, 295*(5), pp. 499–507. Copyright 2006 by American Medical Association. Adapted with permission of the authors.

DIAGNOSIS

It is the timing rather than the symptoms themselves that distinguish the occurrences of perinatal depressive disorders. Although the *DSM–IV–TR* does not recognize the existence of antenatal depression, there is a postpartum-onset specifier (see Figure 4.3). This specifier, however, is limited to the onset of depression within 4 weeks of delivery (American Psychiatric Association, 2000) while clinically, an onset of depression within the first year of delivery is considered postpartum. The reason for this arbitrary definition is that, frequently, symptoms are triggered by onset of menstruation or the process of weaning. The timeline for these events for every woman is highly individual, but frequently tends to fall within 12 months of childbirth.

The notion that impending motherhood is guaranteed to be a wonderful experience often prevents women from reporting accurate symptomatology to their caregivers. Compounding this initial bias is the fact that many perinatal physicians with a high volume of patients can spend a limited amount of time with their patients. Therefore, diagnosis of

Psychological Symptoms	Physical Symptoms
• Depressed mood most of the day, nearly every day • Feeling of guilt, hopelessness, & worthlessness • Reduction of interest and/or pleasure in activities, including sex • Suicidal thoughts • Preoccupation with infant well-being • Severe rumination or delusional thoughts about the infant	• Sleep disturbance: insomnia or hypersomnia • Appetite/weight changes • Decreased energy, unexplained fatigue • Attention/concentration difficulties • Psychomotor disturbances

A. For the diagnosis of major depression, five or more of the above symptoms must be present during the same two-week period, and represent a change from previous functioning. At least one of the symptoms must be either depressed mood or loss of interest or pleasure.

B. The symptoms do not meet criteria for a mixed episode.

C. The symptoms cause significant distress or impairment in social and/or occupational functioning.

D. The symptoms are not due to substance use or a medical condition.

E. The symptoms are not caused by the loss of a loved one, and persist for two months.

F. Postpartum specifier with onset of episode within four weeks postpartum.

Figure 4.3 Symptoms of Clinical Depression.

From the *Diagnostic and Statistical Manual of Mental Disorders,* 4th ed., *Text Revision,* by the American Psychiatric Association, 2000, Washington, DC: American Psychiatric Association. Copyright 2000 by the American Psychiatric Association. Adapted with permission of the publisher.

depression in pregnancy can be easily overlooked. A Swedish study of randomly selected pregnant women determined not only that 14% showed symptoms of psychiatric disorders, but also that the majority of these cases had gone undiagnosed and untreated at that point (Andersson et al., 2003). Additionally, signs of pregnancy mimic symptoms of depression, thus the symptom overlap can further compromise the diagnosis. Sleep and appetite disturbances, weight changes, anergia, increased irritability, and labile mood in the first trimester are all potential symptoms of depression that are confused with normal signs of pregnancy. Distinguishing features of depression include sad, hopeless, or helpless mood, guilt, ruminating negative thoughts, inability to bond, and suicidal ideation. Because very few women will voluntarily disclose their emotional health to their caregivers, asking a simple question such as "How is your mood in the past 2 weeks?" may lead to valuable insight into the patient's mental state. One study found that while only 26% of known antenatal depression cases were identified during prenatal health care visits, shockingly, only 2% of these patients were being referred for treatment (Smith et al., 2004). Depression has substantial comorbidity rates with various anxiety disorders, including panic disorder (PD), generalized anxiety disorder (GAD), obsessive-compulsive disorder (OCD), and posttraumatic stress disorder (PTSD).

While the exact prevalence of perinatal anxiety remains unclear, Anderson and colleagues found that women with no prior psychiatric history reported having anxiety disorders at a rate of 6.6% while attending a routine ultrasound procedure; this is significantly higher than the 2% to 4% found in the nonpregnant population (Andersson et al., 2003; Ross & McLean, 2006).

Panic disorder (PD) in pregnancy occurs at a prevalence rate of 1.3%–2.0%, while the rate of new onset in pregnancy is unknown (Ross & McLean, 2006). Contrary to George and colleagues, who reported on the improvement of panic attacks in pregnancy related to the anxieolytic properties of progesterone metabolites, patients with a prior history of this disorder are seen to be more at risk for worsening of symptoms (George, Ladenheim, & Nutt, 1987). Postpartum onset of PD is common, with existing panic symptoms often worsening during this period (Ross & McLean, 2006). Weaning has also been associated with onset or exacerbation of panic symptoms (Ross & McLean, 2006). Generalized anxiety disorder has a prevalence rate of 8.5% in pregnancy and 4.4%–8.2% in postpartum women (Ross & McLean, 2006). Diagnosis can commonly be overlooked, as it is difficult to differentiate between GAD and common pregnancy-related anxiety. Women with GAD generally tend to be worriers but find the worry associated with GAD to be crippling. One common theme of worry is "what if the baby is damaged?" GAD often occurs comorbidly with OCD. Perinatal OCD has prevalence rates of 0.2%–1.2% in pregnancy and 2.7%–3.9% in the postpartum period (Ross & McLean, 2006). Onset rates of OCD have been reported at 39% in pregnancy and 30% in postpartum (Neziroglu, Anemone, & Yaryuratobias, 1992). Abramowitz and colleagues examined the content of intrusive thoughts in perinatal women and found several common themes, including thoughts of suffocation and accidents, unwanted urges of harm toward the baby, unacceptable sexual thoughts and contaminations (Abramowitz, Schwartz, Moore, & Luenzmann, 2003). Compulsive rituals consist of checking and rechecking the baby, repeated hand washing, etc. Those with a prior history of OCD will experience exacerbation of symptoms in the perinatal period (Buttolph & Holland, 1990; Ingram, 1961). PTSD symptoms in pregnancy have a prevalence rate of 2.3%–7.7% (Ross & McLean, 2006). Previous traumatic life events such as sexual assault, loss of a loved one, or life threats are some of the risk factors that have been associated with PTSD. Avoidance of traumatic reminders may hinder seeking health care services, in particular, physical or gynecological exams in patients with a history of sexual abuse. Chronic PTSD is seen to develop in 1.5% of women as a result of childbirth (Ross & McLean, 2006).

SCREENING

Pregnancy is an optimal time to institute screening given the frequency of contact with the caregiver. Screening for depression should occur early and continue throughout pregnancy (Buist et al., 2006; Gordon, Cardone, Kim, Gordon, & Silver, 2006; Ryan & Misri, 2005; Yonkers et al., 2001). Early detection of depression during pregnancy is important as untreated illness will inevitably continue into postpartum, which has negative consequences for both the mother and infant (Ryan & Misri, 2005).

The Agency for Healthcare Research and Quality (AHRQ) conducted a literature review of depression screening tools used in the perinatal period. The AHRQ found 10 English-language studies involving four different screening tools. Of these 10 studies, 6 were conducted in the United Kingdom, 2 in the United States, 1 in Canada, and 1 in Australia. These studies were limited, however, due to the racial and ethnic mix of the study populations being primarily White and poorly representative of the general population of the United States. The studies also varied in the screening tools used, cut-off scores, and the timing of administration. Studies used one or more of four assessment tools: the Center for Epidemiological Studies Depression Scale (CES-D), the Postpartum Depression Screening Scale (PDSS), the Beck Depression Inventory (BDI), and the Edinburgh Postnatal Depression Scale (EPDS). Both the PDSS and CES-D were used in only 1 study each. The Postpartum Depression Screening Scale was developed more recently but has not yet been studied in pregnancy (Beck & Gable, 2001). The BDI was used in three studies; however, due to its reliance on somatic symptoms, some experts worry that it may produce higher scores and more false-positives in pregnant women compared to other respondents. Eight studies utilized the EPDS, the best-studied screening tool for assessing both antenatal and postpartum depression.

The Edinburgh Postnatal Depression Scale is a self-report questionnaire that has been translated into more than a dozen languages (L. Murray & Carothers, 1990) (see Exhibit 4.1). The EPDS rates depressive symptoms from the previous 7-day period, with higher scores being indicative of more intense symptoms. This scale is a 10-item self report questionnaire with each question scored from 0–3, resulting in total scores ranging from 0–30. Generally, scores of 12 or 13 identify the most severely depressed women (Brouwers, van Baar, & Pop, 2001). While the ideal timing for initiating the screening process has yet to be determined, the EPDS is recommended for use between 28 and 32 weeks of gestation (Austin, 2004; Dennis, 2004) as one meta-analysis found that depressive symptoms (as opposed to major depression) are more prevalent in the second and third trimesters (Bennett et al., 2004). One study found that this self-report questionnaire produced statistically equivalent estimates of prevalence compared with a structured clinical interview (Bennett et al., 2004). The EPDS is easy to read, administer, implement, and can be easily completed in a waiting room setting. A 3-year study in Australia found that 93% of participants found the questionnaire easy to complete with 85% reporting no discomfort with the questions. Researchers noted that reported discomfort with the EPDS was significantly related to scores of ≥13 (Buist et al., 2006).

Screening is increasingly effective if risk factors for the development of depression are identified during the screening process. A population-based study of 594 postpartum women in Canada found that women with EPDS scores of ≥ 10 at 1 week postpartum, indicating depressive symptoms, were more likely to screen positive again at 8 weeks postpartum if they had a history of childhood sexual abuse, were recent immigrants, had a partner with a drug or alcohol abuse problem, or had higher levels of interpersonal conflict, along with other variables (Dennis & Ross, 2006). The United States Preventative Services Task Force (USPSTF) recommends screening adults for depression in clinical practices with systems in place for accurate diagnosis, effective treatment, and follow-up.

EXHIBIT 4.1 OVERVIEW OF THE EDINBURGH POSTNATAL DEPRESSION SCALE (EPDS)

Instructions

1. Women are asked to check the response that is most applicable to them over the **previous 7 days**.
2. All questions must be completed.
3. Encourage women to complete the questionnaire independently, unless language or literacy difficulties are present.

Sample Questions

1. I have looked forward with enjoyment to things:
   - As much as I ever did
   - Rather less than I used to
   - Definitely less than I used to
   - Hardly at all
2. I have been so unhappy that I have had difficulty sleeping:
   - Yes, most of the time
   - Yes, sometimes
   - Not very often
   - No, not at all
3. I have been able to laugh and see the funny side of things:
   - As much as I always could
   - Not quite as much now
   - Definitely not so much now
   - Not at all
4. I have been anxious or worried for no good reason:
   - No, not at all
   - Hardly ever
   - Yes, sometimes
   - Yes, very often

Scoring

Answers are scored from 0–3 in either ascending or descending order, depending on the question.

From "Detection of Postnatal Depression: Development of the 10-Item Edinburgh Postnatal Depression Scale," by J. L. Cox, J. M. Holden, and R. Sagovsky, 1987, *British Journal of Psychiatry, 150,* pp. 782–786. Copyright 1987 by The Royal College of Psychiatrists. Adapted with permission of the authors.

CONSEQUENCES

Untreated perinatal depression has negative consequences for the mother, the developing fetus, and the child. Often, women with antenatal depression do not seek adequate prenatal care potentially leading to compromised obstetrical/medical status. In clinical practice it is not unusual to see a woman with serious depression whose diabetes or hypertension goes unattended due to the all-consuming illness of depression that may prevent her from seeking prenatal visits with her caregiver. The various symptoms of depression that can influence the healthy outcome in pregnancy include insomnia, appetite disturbance, and inappropriate weight gain. Not feeling connected to the growing fetus is the one symptom that is a source of concern to the mother as well as to her caregiver. Antenatal depression has also been associated with spontaneous abortion, gestational bleeding, and preterm delivery (Bonari et al., 2004; Gandhi et al., 2006; Jablensky, Morgan, Zubrick, Bower, & Yellachich, 2005; Kurki, Hiilesmaa, Raitasalo, Mattila, & Ylikorkala, 2000). A prospective population-based study of 623 women found that untreated antenatal depression and anxiety were independently associated with an increased risk of pre-eclampsia (Kurki et al., 2000). Another major complication of antenatal mental illness includes the perpetuation of the condition into the postpartum period with its attendant problems such as impaired bonding with the baby, self-medication, or substance abuse (Marcus et al., 2003; Orr, Miller, James, & Babones, 2000; Stewart, 2006). Suicide always remains a fear; a retrospective study in California found a higher rate of suicide attempts among pregnant women when compared to age-matched nonpregnant women (Gandhi et al., 2006). The risk of suicide in the postpartum period has been well established (Appleby, 1991; Oates, 2003) and identified as one of the leading causes of maternal death (Gandhi et al., 2006; Stewart, 2006). The Confidential Enquiry into Maternal Deaths from 1997–1999 found that suicide accounted for 28% of deaths in the first year postpartum, making it the leading cause of maternal death during this period (Oates, 2003). Young age, multiparity, a history of substance abuse, and a low socioeconomic status are additional contributory factors that increase the risk of suicide attempts. Thus the present knowledge presents a convincing argument for how the untreated maternal depression can affect an unborn child.

Antenatal anxiety frequently coexists with depression and has been linked to premature birth and low birthweight (<2500 grams) (Bonari et al., 2004; Chung, Lau, Yip, Chiu, & Lee, 2001; Halbreich, 2005; Jablensky et al., 2005; Wadhwa, Sandman, Porto, Dunkel-Schetter, & Garite, 1993). Fetal effects of anxiety in pregnancy have been studied extensively providing important information to health care givers; the exact mechanisms of maternal stress on the fetal development remains unclear (Field et al., 2003; O'Connor, Heron, Golding, Beveridge, & Glover, 2002; O'Connor, Heron, Golding, & Glover, 2003; Van den Bergh & Marcoen, 2004; Van den Bergh, Mennes et al., 2005; Van den Bergh, Mulder, Mennes, & Glover, 2005), although a variety of factors appear to be operating at different stages of development. Anxiety in the second and third trimesters of pregnancy has been correlated with changes in fetal movement patterns, sleep/wake cycles, fetal heart rate variability—a marker for fetal distress and increased uterine artery resistance (Bonari et al., 2004; Field et al., 2003; Misri et al., 2006; Teixeira, Fisk, & Glover, 1999; Van den Bergh, Mulder et al., 2005).

Untreated maternal depression can lead to infants with lower APGAR (Activity, Pulse, Grimace, Appearance and Respiration) scores, small gestational age, smaller head circumferences, as well as increased infant cortisol levels relating to lower birthweight (Bonari et al., 2004; Chung et al., 2001; Wadhwa et al., 1993). Interesting biological markers in the newborns of anxious mothers have exhibited lower dopamine and serotonin levels, greater right frontal electroencephalogram activation, and suboptimal performance on the Brazelton Neonatal Behavior Assessment Scale (Field et al., 2003). Infants exposed to antenatal anxiety have been found to be highly reactive, exhibit poorer interactions with their mothers, and perform less optimally on the Bayley Scales of Infant Development (Van den Bergh, Mulder et al., 2005). Mothers reported these infants to exhibit sleeping, activity, and feeding problems at 2 years of age. Evans and colleagues in their Avon Longitudinal Study of Parents and Children found long-term neurobehavioral consequences in children who were exposed to antenatal anxiety (Evans et al., 2001). In this study girls were affected by exposure at both 18 and 32 weeks gestation, while boys only were affected at 32 weeks gestation (O'Connor et al., 2002; O'Connor et al., 2003). These gender differences were noted at both 4 and 6 years of age. Thus these studies demonstrate the far-reaching effects of prenatal exposure to mood and anxiety disorders on toddlers and preschoolers.

In a study examining internalizing behaviors, such as emotional reactivity, depression, anxiety, irritability, and withdrawal, after *in utero* psychotropic medication exposure, researchers found no significant differences between the exposed and nonexposed groups of 4-year-olds (Misri et al., 2006). The results from this study suggest that current maternal mood is a strong predictor of a child's internalizing behaviors. A further investigation examining the externalizing behaviors (attention, aggression, attention deficit/hyperactivity, and oppositional or defiant behaviors) of the same cohort of 4-year-olds found that these behaviors also correlated to maternal depression and anxiety (Oberlander et al., 2007). These results, again, confirm that mothers' current anxiety and depression has an impact on their children's externalizing behaviors (Misri et al., 2006; Oberlander et al., 2007).

Research into the consequences of maternal mental illness on fetal and child development is subject to a variety of limitations. Antenatal studies have yet to control for variables such as partner mental illness, substance abuse, and concomitant medication use. These factors are generally self-reported by the patient and provide an important platform for further investigations to frame the illness in the appropriate context.

REFERENCES

Abramowitz, J. S., Schwartz, S. A., Moore, K. M., & Luenzmann, K. R. (2003). Obsessive-compulsive symptoms in pregnancy and the puerperium: A review of the literature. *Journal of Anxiety Disorders, 17*(4), 461–478.

Altshuler, L. L., Hendrick, V., & Cohen, L. S. (1998). Course of mood and anxiety disorders during pregnancy and the postpartum period. *Journal of Clinical Psychiatry, 59*(Suppl. 2), 29–33.

American Psychiatric Association. (2000). *Diagnostic and statistical manual of mental disorders* (4th ed.). *Text Revision.* Washington, DC: Author.

Andersson, L., Sundstrom-Poromaa, I., Bixo, M., Wulff, M., Bondestam, K., & Astrom, M. (2003). Point prevalence of psychiatric disorders during the second trimester of pregnancy: A population-based study. *American Journal of Obstetric Gynecology, 189*(1), 148–154.

Appleby, L. (1991). Suicide during pregnancy and in the first postnatal year. *British Medical Journal, 302*(67–69), 137–140.

Atkinson, A. K., & Rickel, A. U. (1984). Postpartum depression in primiparous parents. *Journal of Abnormal Psychology, 93*(1), 115–119.

Austin, M. P. (2004). Antenatal screening and early intervention for "perinatal" distress, depression and anxiety: Where to from here? *Archive of Women's Mental Health, 7*(1), 1–6.

Beck, C. T. (1996). A meta-analysis of predictors of postpartum depression. *Nurs Res, 45*(5), 297–303.

Beck, C. T., & Gable, R. K. (2001). Comparative analysis of the performance of the Postpartum Depression Screening Scale with two other depression instruments. *Nursing Research, 50*(4), 242–250.

Bennett, H. A., Einarson, A., Taddio, A., Koren, G., & Einarson, T. R. (2004). Prevalence of depression during pregnancy: Systematic review. *Obstetric and Gynecology, 103*(4), 698–709.

Bloch, M., Rotenberg, N., Koren, D., & Klein, E. (2006). Risk factors for early postpartum depressive symptoms. *General Hospital Psychiatry, 28*(1), 3–8.

Bonari, L., Pinto, N., Ahn, E., Einarson, A., Steiner, M., & Koren, G. (2004). Perinatal risks of untreated depression during pregnancy. *Canadian Journal of Psychiatry, 49*(11), 726–735.

Brouwers, E. P., van Baar, A. L., & Pop, V. J. (2001). Does the Edinburgh Postnatal Depression Scale measure anxiety? *Journal of Psychosomatic Research, 51*(5), 659–663.

Brugha, T. S., Sharp, H. M., Cooper, S. A., Weisender, C., Britto, D., Shinkwin, R., et al. (1998). The Leicester 500 Project. Social support and the development of postnatal depressive symptoms: A prospective cohort survey. *Psychol Med, 28*(1), 63–79.

Buist, A., Condon, J., Brooks, J., Speelman, C., Milgrom, J., Hayes, B., et al. (2006). Acceptability of routine screening for perinatal depression. *Journal of Affected Disorder, 93*(1–3), 233–237.

Buist, A., & Janson, H. (2001). Childhood sexual abuse, parenting and postpartum depression—a 3-year follow-up study. *Child Abuse and Neglect, 25*(7), 909–921.

Burt, V. K., & Stein, K. (2002). Epidemiology of depression throughout the female life cycle. *Journal of Clinical Psychiatry, 63*(Suppl. 7), 9–15.

Buttolph, M., & Holland, A. (1990). Obsessive-compulsive disorders in pregnancy and childbirth. In M. Jenike, L. Baer, & W. Minichielle (Eds.), *Obsessive-compulsive disorders: Theory and management* (pp. 89–97). Chicago: Year Book Medical.

Chung, T. K., Lau, T. K., Yip, A. S., Chiu, H. F., & Lee, D. T. (2001). Antepartum depressive symptomatology is associated with adverse obstetric and neonatal outcomes. *Psychosomatic Medicine, 63*(5), 830–834.

Cohen, L. S. (1998). Pharmacologic treatment of depression in women: PMS, pregnancy, and the postpartum period. *Depression and Anxiety, 8*(Suppl. 1), 18–26.

Cohen, L. S., Altshuler, L. L., Harlow, B. L., Nonacs, R., Newport, D. J., Viguera, A. C., et al. (2006). Relapse of major depression during pregnancy in women who maintain or discontinue antidepressant treatment. *JAMA, 295*(5), 499–507.

Cox, J. L., Connor, Y., & Kendell, R. E. (1982). Prospective study of the psychiatric disorders of childbirth. *British Journal of Psychiatry, 140,* 111–117.

Dennis, C. L. (2004). Can we identify mothers at risk for postpartum depression in the immediate postpartum period using the Edinburgh Postnatal Depression Scale? *Journal of Affected Disorder, 78*(2), 163–169.

Dennis, C. L., & Ross, L. E. (2006). The clinical utility of maternal self-reported personal and familial psychiatric history in identifying women at risk for postpartum depression. *Acta Obstet Gynecol Scand, 85*(10), 1179–1185.

Evans, J., Heron, J., Francomb, H., Oke, S., Golding, O., & Parents, A. L. S. (2001). Cohort study of depressed mood during pregnancy and after childbirth. *British Medical Journal, 323*(7307), 257–260.

Field, T., Diego, M., Hernandez-Reif, M., Schanberg, S., Kuhn, C., Yando, R., et al. (2003). Pregnancy anxiety and comorbid depression and anger: Effects on the fetus and neonate. *Depression and Anxiety, 17*(3), 140–151.

Forty, L., Jones, L., Macgregor, S., Caesar, S., Cooper, C., Hough, A., et al. (2006). Familiality of postpartum depression in unipolar disorder: Results of a family study. *American Journal of Psychiatry, 163*(9), 1549–1553.

Gandhi, S. G., Gilbert, W. M., McElvy, S. S., El Kady, D., Danielson, B., Xing, G., et al. (2006). Maternal and neonatal outcomes after attempted suicide. *Obstetrics and Gynecology, 107*(5), 984–990.

George, D. T., Ladenheim, J. A., & Nutt, D. J. (1987). Effect of pregnancy on panic attacks. *American Journal of Psychiatry, 144*(8), 1078–1079.

Gordon, T. E., Cardone, I. A., Kim, J. J., Gordon, S. M., & Silver, R. K. (2006). Universal perinatal depression screening in an Academic Medical Center. *Obstet Gynecol, 107*(2 Pt 1), 342–347.

Gotlib, I. H., Whiffen, V. E., Mount, J. H., Milne, K., & Cordy, N. I. (1989). Prevalence rates and demographic characteristics associated with depression in pregnancy and the postpartum. *Journal of Consulting and Clinical Psychology, 57*(2), 269–274.

Halbreich, U. (2005). The association between pregnancy processes, preterm delivery, low birth weight, and postpartum depressions—the need for interdisciplinary integration. *American Journal of Obstetrics and Gynecology, 193*(4), 1312–1322.

Henshaw, C. (2003). Mood disturbance in the early puerperium: A review. *Archive of Women's Mental Health, 6*(Suppl. 2), S33–S42.

Hughes, P. M., Turton, P., & Evans, C. D. (1999). Stillbirth as risk factor for depression and anxiety in the subsequent pregnancy: Cohort study. *British Medical Journal, 318*(7200), 1721–1724.

Ingram, I. M. (1961). Obsessional illness in mental hospital patients. *Journal of Mental Science, 107,* 382–402.

Jablensky, A. V., Morgan, V., Zubrick, S. R., Bower, C., & Yellachich, L. A. (2005). Pregnancy, delivery, and neonatal complications in a population cohort of women with schizophrenia and major affective disorders. *American Journal of Psychiatry, 162*(1), 79–91.

Josefsson, A., Angelsioo, L., Berg, G., Ekstrom, C. M., Gunnervik, C., Nordin, C., et al. (2002). Obstetric, somatic, and demographic risk factors for postpartum depressive symptoms. *Obstet Gynecol, 99*(2), 223–228.

Josefsson, A., Berg, G., Nordin, C., & Sydsjo, G. (2001). Prevalence of depressive symptoms in late pregnancy and postpartum. *Acta Obstet Gynecol Scand, 80*(3), 251–255.

Kessler, R., McGonagle, K., Swartz, M., Blazer, D., & Nelson, C. (1993). Sex and depression in the National Comorbidity Survey 1: Lifetime prevalence, chronicity and recurrence. *Journal of Affective Disorders, 29,* 85–96.

Kitamura, T., Yoshida, K., Okano, T., Kinoshita, K., Hayashi, M., Toyoda, N., et al. (2006). Multicentre prospective study of perinatal depression in Japan: Incidence and correlates of antenatal and postnatal depression. *Archives of Women's Mental Health,* 9(3), 121–130.

Kumar, R., & Robson, K. M. (1984). A prospective study of emotional disorders in childbearing women. *British Journal of Psychiatry, 144,* 35–47.

Kurki, T., Hiilesmaa, V., Raitasalo, R., Mattila, H., & Ylikorkala, O. (2000). Depression and anxiety in early pregnancy and risk for preeclampsia. *Obstet Gynecol, 95*(4), 487–490.

Llewellyn, A. M., Stowe, Z. N., & Nemeroff, C. B. (1997). Depression during pregnancy and the puerperium. *Journal of Clinical Psychiatry, 58*(Suppl. 15), 26–32.

Lusskin, S. I., Pundiak, T. M., & Habib, S. M. (2007). Perinatal depression: Hiding in plain sight. *Canadian Journal of Psychiatry,* 52(8), 479–488.

Major, B., Cozzarelli, C., Cooper, M. L., Zubek, J., Richards, C., Wilhite, M., et al. (2000). Psychological responses of women after first-trimester abortion. *General Hospital Psychiatry, 57*(8), 777–784.

Marcus, S. M., Flynn, H. A., Blow, F. C., & Barry, K. L. (2003). Depressive symptoms among pregnant women screened in obstetrics settings. *Journal of Women's Health & Gender-Based Medicine, 12*(4), 373–380.

McGuffin, P., Marusic, A., & Farmer, A. (2001). What can psychiatric genetics offer suicidology? *Crisis, 22*(2), 61–65.

Misri, S., Reebye, P., Kendrick, K., Carter, D., Ryan, D., Grunau, R. E., et al. (2006). Internalizing behaviors in 4-year-old children exposed in utero to psychotropic medications. *American Journal of Psychiatry, 163*(6), 1026–1032.

Murray, C., & Lopez, E. (1996). *A comprehensive assessment of mortality and disability from diseases, injuries, and risk factors in 1990 and projected to 2020.* (Vol. 1). Cambridge, MA: Harvard University Press.

Murray, L., & Carothers, A. D. (1990). The validation of the Edinburgh Postnatal Depression Scale on a community sample. *British Journal of Psychiatry, 157,* 288–290.

Neugebauer, R. (2003). Depressive symptoms at two months after miscarriage: Interpreting study findings from an epidemiological versus clinical perspective. *Depression and Anxiety, 17*(3), 152–161.

Neugebauer, R., Kline, J., Shrout, P., Skodol, A., O'Connor, P., Geller, P. A., et al. (1997). Major depressive disorder in the 6 months after miscarriage. *JAMA, 277*(5), 383–388.

Neziroglu, F., Anemone, R., & Yaryuratobias, J. A. (1992). Onset of Obsessive-Compulsive Disorder in Pregnancy. *American Journal of Psychiatry, 149*(7), 947–950.

Oates, M. (2003). Suicide: The leading cause of maternal death. *British Journal of Psychiatry, 183,* 279–281.

Oberlander, T. F., Reebye, P., Misri, S., Papsdorf, M., Kim, J., & Grunau, R. E. (2007). Externalizing and attentional behaviors in children of depressed mothers treated with a selective serotonin reuptake inhibitor antidepressant during pregnancy. *Archives of Pediatric and Adolescent Medicine, 161*(1), 22–29.

O'Connor, T. G., Heron, J., Golding, J., Beveridge, M., & Glover, V. (2002). Maternal antenatal anxiety and children's behavioural/emotional problems at 4 years. Report from the Avon Longitudinal Study of Parents and Children. *British Journal of Psychiatry, 180,* 502–508.

O'Connor, T. G., Heron, J., Golding, J., & Glover, V. (2003). Maternal antenatal anxiety and behavioural/emotional problems in children: A test of a programming hypothesis. *Journal of Child Psychology and Psychiatry, 44*(7), 1025–1036.

O'Hara, M. W. (1986). Social support, life events, and depression during pregnancy and the puerperium. *Archives of General Psychiatry, 43*(6), 569–573.

O'Hara, M. W., Schlechte, J. A., Lewis, D. A., & Wright, E. J. (1991). Prospective study of postpartum blues: Biologic and psychosocial factors. *Archives of General Psychiatry, 48*(9), 801–806.

Omar, H. A., Martin, C., & McElderry, D. (2001). Screening for depression in adolescents: Association with teen pregnancy. *Journal of Pediatric and Adolescent Gynechology, 14*(3), 129–133.

Orr, S. T., Miller, C. A., James, S. A., & Babones, S. (2000). Unintended pregnancy and preterm birth. *Paediatric and Perinatal Epidemiology, 14*(4), 309–313.

Robertson, E., Grace, S., Wallington, T., & Stewart, D. E. (2004). Antenatal risk factors for postpartum depression: A synthesis of recent literature. *General Hospital Psychiatry, 26*(4), 289–295.

Ross, L. E., & McLean, L. M. (2006). Anxiety disorders during pregnancy and the postpartum period: A systematic review. *Journal of Clinical Psychiatry, 67*(8), 1285–1298.

Ryan, D., & Misri, N. (2005). Depression during pregnancy. *Canadian Family Physician, 51,* 1087–1093.

Seguin, L., Potvin, L., St-Denis, M., & Loiselle, J. (1999). Socio-environmental factors and postnatal depressive symptomatology: A longitudinal study. *Women Health, 29*(1), 57–72.

Small, R., Lumley, J., & Yelland, J. (2003). Cross-cultural experiences of maternal depression: Associations and contributing factors for Vietnamese, Turkish and Filipino immigrant women in Victoria, Australia. *Ethnic Health, 8*(3), 189–206.

Smith, M. V., Rosenheck, R. A., Cavaleri, M. A., Howell, H. B., Poschman, K., & Yonkers, K. A. (2004). Screening for and detection of depression, panic disorder, and PTSD in public-sector obstetric clinics. *Psychiatric Service, 55*(4), 407–414.

Steiner, M. (1990). Postpartum psychiatric disorders. *Canadian Journal of Psychiatry, 35*(1), 89–95.

Stewart, D. E. (1994). Incidence of postpartum abuse in women with a history of abuse during pregnancy. *Canadian Medical Association Journal, 151*(11), 1601–1604.

Stewart, D. E. (2006). A broader context for maternal mortality. *Cmaj, 174*(3), 302–303.

Teixeira, J. M., Fisk, N. M., & Glover, V. (1999). Association between maternal anxiety in pregnancy and increased uterine artery resistance index: Cohort based study. *British Medical Journal, 318*(7177), 153–157.

Van den Bergh, B. R., & Marcoen, A. (2004). High antenatal maternal anxiety is related to ADHD symptoms, externalizing problems, and anxiety in 8- and 9-year-olds. *Child Development, 75*(4), 1085–1097.

Van den Bergh, B. R., Mennes, M., Oosterlaan, J., Stevens, V., Stiers, P., Marcoen, A., et al. (2005). High antenatal maternal anxiety is related to impulsivity during performance on cognitive tasks in 14- and 15-year-olds. *Neuroscience and Biobehavioral Reviews, 29*(2), 259–269.

Van den Bergh, B. R., Mulder, E. J., Mennes, M., & Glover, V. (2005). Antenatal maternal anxiety and stress and the neurobehavioural development of the fetus and child: Links and possible mechanisms. A review. *Neuroscience and Biobehavioral Review, 29*(2), 237–258.

Viguera, A. C., Cohen, L. S., Baldessarini, R. J., & Nonacs, R. (2002). Managing bipolar disorder during pregnancy: Weighing the risks and benefits. *Canadian Journal of Psychiatry, 47*(5), 426–436.

Wadhwa, P. D., Sandman, C. A., Porto, M., Dunkel-Schetter, C., & Garite, T. J. (1993). The association between prenatal stress and infant birth weight and gestational age at birth: A prospective investigation. *American Journal of Obstetrics and Gynecology, 169*(4), 858–865.

Warner, R., Appleby, L., Whitton, A., & Faragher, B. (1996). Demographic and obstetric risk factors for postnatal psychiatric morbidity. *British Journal of Psychiatry, 168*(5), 607–611.

Watson, J. P., Elliott, S. A., Rugg, A. J., & Brough, D. I. (1984). Psychiatric disorder in pregnancy and the first postnatal year. *British Journal of Psychiatry, 144,* 453–462.

Yonkers, K. A., Ramin, S. M., Rush, A. J., Navarrete, C. A., Carmody, T., March, D., et al. (2001). Onset and persistence of postpartum depression in an inner-city maternal health clinic system. *American Journal of Psychiatry, 158*(11), 1856–1863.

Yonkers, K. A., Wisner, K. L., Stowe, Z., Leibenluft, E., Cohen, L., Miller, L., et al. (2004). Management of bipolar disorder during pregnancy and the postpartum period. *American Journal of Psychiatry, 161*(4), 608–620.

Zayas, L. H., Cunningham, M., McKee, M. D., & Jankowski, K. R. (2002). Depression and negative life events among pregnant African-American and Hispanic women. *Women's Health Issues, 12*(1), 16–22.

PART II

Perspectives on Risk Factors, Screening, and Diagnosis

5 Diagnosis and Screening of Perinatal Mood Disorders

LINDA G. KLEMPNER

When Andrea Yates drowned her five children in the bathtub on June 20, 2001, postpartum depression (PPD) etched itself permanently on the national consciousness. Perhaps nothing highlights the need for diagnosis and assessment more vividly than the tragedy of filicide.

Postpartum psychosis is the most heinous form of postpartum mental illness, but by no means the only type. Postpartum depression spans a spectrum of forms from the well-known and common "baby blues" to depression and/or anxiety to psychosis. The husband of my patient, Joyce, said it best, "PPD is *not* a woman's disease—it is a systemic problem. It is a family disease." When PPD hits—whether it manifests as a blue day or as a dark cloud that descends and overtakes a woman's personality—it can lead to potentially catastrophic proportions, especially when left undiagnosed. Similar to premenstrual mood dysphoric disorders and menopause, postpartum depression should be clearly viewed as a biopsychosocial phenomenon. The interplay among the biological and hormonal, the psychological and mental health, and societal aspects combine to affect the degree and severity from individual to individual. As clinicians, it behooves us to pay attention to a woman's story. To understand any single individual's experience, it is useful to grasp the range of factors that potentially affect that experience. Most individuals are unaware or unconscious of many of the physiological, sociocultural, and personal historical forces that contribute to her or his intrapsychic and interpersonal experience (Shapiro, 1988, pp. 69–70).

The importance of early detection and ongoing follow-up is becoming clearer as the call for federally mandated or state-sponsored programs grow. Rapid detection of warning signs during the antepartum or postpartum states benefit both mother and her neonate and subsequent developing child. Early detection reduces the impact of maternal mental illness on the child. Depressed, unresponsive mothers often trigger depressive response in their children. When bonding and attachment are insecure or problematic, future learning and emotional difficulties will emerge in the next generation of children. Edward Tronick's "still-face" classic experiment with mother and child boldly highlights the dilemma facing the baby with an unengaged mother (1998).

The long-term cost of chronic depression and its sequelae on the family system are compelling reasons for all health care professionals to sharpen their diagnostic and screening skills. According to some experts, baby blues is said to impact as many as 75% of all women at some point in the first postnatal year. A sad, labile day, or series of days, when tending to a colicky, crying child leads most women to feel that they are at the end of their rope. Experiencing a bout of the blues, my patient, Arlene said, "Having this baby was a mistake. If I can't think straight anymore, how can I raise a child?" I quipped that Dr. Zachary Stowe (personal communication) often comments that, "part of the new mom's brain was delivered with their placenta." She chuckled and stated, "Wow, that's good to know." A few days later, after much needed rest, her sunny personality reemerged.

Not so with postpartum depression. For those 10% of women with PPD, the hopelessness and helplessness are more profound and enduring. Another patient, Rachel, said, "My husband made a mistake. I am no good to him or to his child. I will never be the mother I thought I would be." Depressed for several months prior to seeking consultation with me, I encouraged Rachel to discuss her fears with her husband. He, in turn, suggested she cut back on her prebaby habits of cleaning the house and doing laundry every day and let him give the baby a supplementary bottle at the 11 P.M. feeding so she could get to bed earlier. Much to her relief, she soon began to feel calmer and think rationally again.

In contrast, my patient, Sara, fell into the one to two in a thousand women with live births who experience postpartum psychosis. At her third session, Sara said, "I have decided to pack a bag and drive away. I may as well be dead. In fact, I might drive into a telephone pole and that will be that." Assessing a psychiatric emergency, I telephoned the patient's husband who immediately drove her over to our local hospital's emergency room where she was admitted for observation. Sara was subsequently prescribed Zoloft and instructed on the "pump and dump" method so she could continue to breastfeed her baby (Burt et al., 2001; Stowe et al., 2003). Despite some initial resistance, she took the medication, joined a support group, and allowed her mother to stay and help with the children until her mood was stabilized.

Without a doubt, quick diagnosis, education, and screening all contribute to identifying and forming an action plan to keep women and their children healthy during this period of hormonal and emotional turmoil. If a woman sometimes hides behind a veil of shame believing she *should* be thrilled with her baby and be happy despite feeling otherwise, our mission as professionals is to detect and treat this disorder as thoroughly and efficiently as possible.

HISTORY

In 1858, French physician Louis Victor Marcé published the first major paper on puerperal mental illness. Puerperal, defined as 6 weeks following childbirth, became synonymous with postpartum-related mental illness. It was not until the endocrine system was studied in the 20th century that more information became available to validate the psychological impact of menstrually related hormonal changes (Benedek, 1952).

At the turn of the 20th century, emergent fields of psychoanalysis and psychiatry dominated views on treating women with mental illness and puerperal diseases. Freud noticed that pregnant women seemed to possess a feeling of calm and well-being (1931/1959b), but suggested that illness of all types could push the instinctive drives beyond the ego's capacity due to "the alteration in women caused by the disturbances of menstruation" (1926/1959a, p. 242). Early psychoanalysts devised a complex metapsychology of female psychosexual development to describe the harm of bad mothering, but did very little to describe what could be done to correct an immediate problem. The unfortunate consequence of this treatment was its emphasis on the past rather than addressing "real time" infant-maternal dyad requiring immediate action.

The late decades of the 20th century realized a shift in attitudes due to changes in psychiatric and neuroscience advances in mental illness.

Benedek observed that biochemical forces seemed to play a role in the maintenance of emotional health and a decline in anxiety in pregnant women (1970). By the 1980s, experimental research and anecdotal evidence suggested that both antenatal and postnatal mental disorders, in either the form of anxiety or depression, have a serious effect on an infant's development and modes of attachment. By 6 months, the infant exposed to a mother's negative affect learns to extrapolate using that behavior with others (Field et al., 1988). Organizing information or "representations of interactions that have been generalized" (RIGS) (Stern, 1985) into normal or pathological expressions begins in early infancy. Neuroscientific researcher Geraldine Dawson (1992a, 1992b) concluded that, "the same event that activates a positive-affect behavior and EEG pattern in normal infants (mother playing peek-a-boo) elicits negative behavior and EEG pattern of activation in infants of depressed mothers. The reverse is also true. Thus by ten months, the emotional responsivity of infants of depressed mothers is already organized differently from that of normal infants" (Beebe & Lachmann, 2002, p. 81).

The danger for babies has become more evident since the 1980s as has the importance of treating maternal depression as early as possible. Meltzer and Kumar (1985), noting confusion about how to classify puerperal mental illness, underscored the urgency to "improve the system for categorizing and registering mental illnesses related to childbirth. Until this is achieved, research into aetiology, outcome, and the provision of services will continue to be impeded" (p. 647).

Here in the United States, it was not until 1994, when the fourth edition of the psychiatric bible known as the *Diagnostic and Statistical Manual of Mental Disorders* or *DSM–IV* was published, that postnatal illnesses were introduced into the lexicon of depression diagnostics as a specifier for mood disorders, including major depression, manic, or mixed episode of major depressive disorder, bipolar I or bipolar II, or brief psychotic disorder (American Psychiatric Association, 1994). The specifying criteria suggests onset of an episode within 4 weeks postnatal, which in the estimation of many health care professional, is not broad enough and demands reassessment in the manual's next revised edition.

Since this period of time, major academic and medical centers focused on the research for prevention and treatment of perinatal disorders. Awareness of these conditions has increased in the form of literature, which is widely available for professionals and the public, and outreach on the permutations of maternal health care, including pregnancy and postpartum (Hendrick & Altschuler, 2002; Misri & Kendrick, 2007; Wisner, Parry, & Piontek, 2002); lactation (Hale, 2006; Kendall-Tackett, 2005); postpartum recovery (Cohen et al., 2006; Corwin, Bozoky, Pugh, & Johnston, 2003; Kennedy, Gardiner, Gay, & Lee, 2007); and depressive outcomes for children with depressive mothers (Minkovitz et al., 2005; Weissman et al., 2006).

PREVALENCE AND RISK FACTORS

Hormonal shifts, which sustain the pregnancy, alter radically in the first 24 hours after delivery. As Chaya, one of my patients said, "Where are those happy hormones?" referring to the estrogen coursing through her body prior to the birth of her son. As Sichel and Driscoll (1999) wrote, "In fact, your estrogen level reaches that of a normal menstrual cycle within twenty-four hours! . . . If this hormone contributes to mood stability, imagine how profoundly its rapid removal can impair mood health in vulnerable women" (p. 203). While it is not the purview of this chapter to outline the complex biochemical and endocrine changes that accompany the antepartum and postpartum stages, suffice it to say that these processes have a cataclysmic, if not always, catastrophic impact on a woman's mental and physical health; and thus on her capacity to carry, deliver, lactate, and bond with an infant. Sichel and Driscoll's *Women's Moods: What Every Woman Must Know About Hormones, the Brain, and Emotional Health* (1999) offers a clear and concise picture of how brain chemistry affects women's moods and reproductive health.

Hormones play a vital role in mood shifts during pregnancy and following delivery, but they are not the only factors needing consideration when assessing patients. Ethnicity and cultural context for birthing and perinatal care should be carefully considered. Lack of a vital community support system and lower socioeconomic status exacerbate perinatal difficulties (Shaw et al., 2006). Risks include medical problems in mother or infant; chronic pain; inflammation; lack of sleep; history of sleep, eating, or substance disorders; breast infections or other lactation issues; abrupt weaning and other baby feeding difficulties. Additional factors to consider include nutrition, genetic influences, maternal age, sensitivity to and type of prescription drugs and/or nutraceuticals being taken, and environmental toxin exposure. Major life stressors include marital or family conflict, feeling isolated, role transition or loss of personal free-

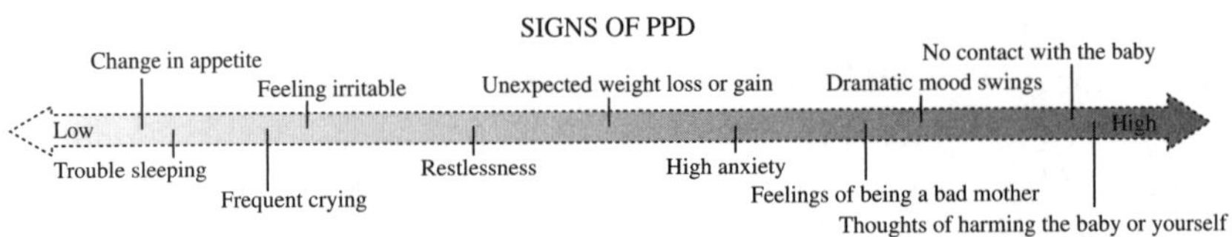

Figure 5.1 Signs of PPD.

dom, number and ages of other children, child care conflict, the absence of a partner or family support system, moving, and leaving a valued place of employment.

In addition, clinicians need to recognize that perinatal mood disorders affect women who have suffered infertility, fetal demise, elective termination, or the loss of a newborn. In my clinical experience, the impact of infertility does not end with successful childbearing. Formerly infertile and adoptive mothers are vulnerable to PPD and feel least entitled to complain. Furthermore, the number of reproductive techniques increasing the number of twins or higher-order multiples and compromised neonates beginning their lives in the neonatal intensive care unit has exploded, subjecting these mothers to intense, and, often, ongoing stress. The Multiple Birth Postpartum Survey undertaken by the Mothers of Supertwins (www.MOSTonline.org) found that these women had a later onset of depression and that women in the 18- to 24-year-old category were extremely vulnerable to serious depression (see Figure 5.1).

Baby Blues

Anywhere from one-half to three-quarters of all new mothers are bound to have a bad day. These women often report feeling labile, anxious, mild mood changes, and short-fused or sensitive reactions to so-called constructive criticism. Additional symptoms include experiencing fatigue, inability to sleep, and lack of appetite.

Reassurance, a little extra sleep, or support with the baby or other children and household chores can reduce these transient feelings. Professionals who educate women on the normalcy of certain feelings can relieve anxiety. However, some symptoms may be severe. When they last more than 2 weeks, it places the woman at risk for a more serious form of postpartum mental distress.

Depression

Approximately 15%–20% of all mothers will develop a postnatal depression. Onset may be rapid, but generally women tend to report noticing a gradual descent into depression lasting 2 weeks or beyond, thus qualifying as a major depressive episode as defined by the *DSM–IV.* In their study, O'Hara and Swain (1996) found that approximately 25% of women who had the blues went on to have a major depressive episode in a subsequent pregnancy. Other strong predictors of a postpartum illness are an episode during pregnancy, a perinatal mood disorder in a first-degree relative, a diagnosis of premenstrual dysphoric disorder (PMDD), or a bout of significant mood change while on oral contraceptives or fertility medications.

Symptoms of Postpartum Depression

Although commonly expected to emerge during the first month postnatal, the following PPD symptoms may occur during pregnancy, shortly after a birth, or within the first year postdelivery. Symptoms for a postpartum depression include the following: (1) feeling sad, irritable, or angry; (2) insomnia; (3) disinterest in activities of daily living; (4) disinterest in the baby or existing children; (5) feeling guilty, hopeless, helpless, and/or worthless; (6) labile moods with or without bouts of uncontrollable and unexplainable crying; (7) anhedonia or lack of pleasure in baby and/or family; (8) constant fatigue and exhaustion; (9) changes in appetite; (10) lack of concentration, difficulty focusing or thinking clearly; (11) excessive and irrational worry; (12) feelings of being a bad or inadequate mother; and (13) changes in sexual desire or significantly lower libido extending beyond the initial 6-week check-up.

Psychosis

The most serious form of postpartum mental illness, psychosis, often emerges prior to a baby's birth. Extreme insomnia or inability to sleep even when given the opportunity, rapid mood swings, confusion, and disorientation are all key signs of psychosis. Postpartum mood disorders with psychotic features occur in 1%–2% of all postdelivery women. But 30%–50% of women have suffered a postpartum depression or psychotic episode in a prior pregnancy relapse. These women have a high rate of postpartum hospitalization. An elevated risk of suicide and infanticide exists, especially when delusions or hallucinations focus on the infant perceived to be evil or pernicious. As the *DSM–IV* states, women may feel as if "the newborn is possessed by the devil, has special powers, or is destined for some terrible fate" (APA, 1994, p. 386).

Postpartum Anxiety Disorders

Even in the most desired of planned pregnancies, worry ranging from minor to obsessive may increase as a mother focuses on her new responsibilities and alterations in roles. The most common complaints of perinatal anxiety disorders include the following: (1) nervousness, anxiety, hypervigilant concerns or attention for the baby; (2) extreme lability; (3) appetite and sleep disturbances; (4) distractibility and inability to concentrate; and (5) a sense of memory loss.

Panic disorder affects approximately 10% of postpartum women. Panic attacks (Metz, Sichel, & Goff, 1998) may accompany anxiety disorder. A more extreme version of anxiety, panic disorder's symptoms include shortness of breath, chest constriction, pains, or heaviness; the sense that this could possibly be a heart attack, chills or fever, trembling, tingling, or numbness of the extremities; inability to think or focus; and terror that this could happen again while driving, holding the baby, or engaged in some other perceived risky activity. Panic disorder is especially disconcerting to most individuals because it appears to come out of the blue, and sufferers fear its return, thus exacerbating anticipatory anxiety.

Posttraumatic stress disorder (PTSD), another form of anxiety disorder, is typically associated with catastrophic experiences, such as assault, rape, and natural disasters. PTSD onset is also linked with sexual, physical, and/or emotional abuse. Women who experience pregnancy, labor and delivery, or postdelivery trauma may manifest posttraumatic stress. Trauma ranges from infant death or medical emergency of mother or infant to a degrading labor and delivery experience. Intrusive thoughts, flashbacks, and nightmares are common symptoms. Beck's (2004) work on PTSD and its interface with PPD is particularly useful in recognizing the effects of iatrogenic trauma. Clinicians should be alert to anniversary grief reactions since the child's birthday is also the corresponding date of the birth trauma. The Web site www.ptsdafterchildbirth.org provides useful information, since this difficulty can significantly impact attachment with the living child and difficulties with subsequent pregnancies.

Postpartum Obsessive Disorders

Obsessive-compulsive disorder (OCD) affects approximately 2%–5% of new mothers and may include a combination of both anxious and depressive symptoms. Since there are women who already have obsessive and/or compulsive tendencies or are diagnosed with an OCD, the numbers experiencing the disorder could possibly be underreported. Frequently, women who experienced a previous bout of postpartum obsessive disorder will suffer with each subsequent pregnancy (Abramowitz, Schiatz, Moore, & Luenzman, 2003). Terrified by the thought of hurting or contaminating a fetus or baby, these women run the risk of maternal-infant attachment difficulties. Symptoms often include intrusive, repetitive thoughts or ritualized actions such as compulsive cleaning, counting, or checking; loss of appetite; or fears of eating. Avoidance of the child or involving a child in ritualistic behaviors often signals a higher level of risk. Recurrent thoughts of harming either oneself or the baby are further complicated by often extreme and/or persistent feelings of shame, guilt, and anxiety.

Such a case involves Melissa who phoned me in a panic. Forced to wean her daughter at 12 weeks due to severe mastitis, Melissa focused on kitchen germs, especially on baby bottles. Spending hours compulsively washing bottles resulted in raw, bleeding hands and mental exhaustion. Nonetheless, she felt she had no choice in order to keep her daughter from harm. She described a family history of OCD and anxiety disorders, and screening clearly suggested an undiagnosed obsessive-compulsive disorder. By acting in tandem with her gynecologist, who prescribed an SSRI, and teaching her cognitive-behavioral thought restructuring, I helped Melissa to finally lead what she considered to be a normal life without fear of causing harm to herself, her child, or another person.

Other Factors to Rule-Out

Women with a history of bipolar disorders have a high rate of complicated postpartum mental difficulties (Viguera et al., 2000). They should be monitored closely, preferably by a psychiatrist in cooperation with the woman's obstetrician. What is most important with bipolar disorder is early intervention to avoid psychiatric emergency. If misdiagnosed, bipolar may be treated with antidepressants instead of mood stabilizers, further exacerbating rapid cycling and depression. Bipolar disease can be treated with medication both before and after the delivery. Some controversy exists in this area, requiring further research on the use of bipolar medications and lactation (Yonkers et al., 2004).

Thyroid disease sometimes masquerades as postpartum depression. Fatigue and irritability, which may be related to thyroid disease, can easily be misdiagnosed as PPD. Health care clinicians need to be alert to the fact that 5%–9% of women (Sichel & Driscoll, 1999) have abnormal thyroid levels postpartum. Having recently adopted an infant after years of fruitless infertility treatments, my patient, Hannah, was immobilized by symptoms of fatigue and exhaustion and inability to concentrate or think clearly. Fearing she had "brought on" a depression due to the many stressors in her life, she was enormously relieved to learn that she had a thyroid disorder, easily remedied with medication.

Anemia, a physical illness, may also contribute to postpartum depressive symptoms. Both pregnancy and blood loss following delivery can contribute to an iron deficiency. Common symptoms include fatigue, weakness, cognitive impairment, chest pains, rapid heart rate, and shortness of breath. These symptoms can trigger feelings of anxiety or depression misdiagnosed as a postpartum mood disorder. Simple blood work confirms anemia for quick treatment of a serious health risk.

ASSESSMENTS

The Face-to-Face Interview

Nothing replaces the value of the face-to-face personal interview. Allowing the mother an opportunity to narrate her story in a semistructured or open-ended conversation proves invaluable to diagnosis and treatment. Having a comfortable relationship with a nurse in a physician's office, hospital social worker, or group support facilitator enables a woman to ideally unlock the fear, shame, or guilt she may feel of becoming a bad or even crazy mother. Giving her the time to unravel her story and reveal her thoughts or feelings is not always easy given the time constraints of most busy physicians, hospital staff, or private practice clinicians. However, offering a woman safety and space to share concerns enables detection and avenues for treatment that are vital to short-circuit a harmful and/or protracted depressive episode.

Reading body language and affect (the woman who says she's fine while speaking in flat tones with shoulders slumped or a leg in restless motion) are clinically indispensable assessment tools. Additionally, having the clinical skills to detect nuances of verbal or nonverbal signs may capture important, but potentially, unnoticed symptoms. Knowledge of risks and vigilant recognition of the troubling signs of perinatal mood disorders enables a clinician to provide a quick response to educate and offer solutions. The recognition and support clinicians provide can be enormously reassuring no matter the degree of distress, ranging from the blues to a psychiatric emergency.

Some of the questions worth asking in a semistructured interview, which may not be captured on a written screening instrument, include: (1) personal history of depression and anxiety prior to, during, or following a previous pregnancy; (2) family history of depression, bipolar, and anxiety disorders; (3) major stressors (good or bad) in one's life, which may have significant impact in the present; (4) recent life changes of a physical or emotional nature; (5) marital satisfaction and quality of relationship; (6) parenting style conflict; (7) family and friend support system; and (8) history of sleep patterns.

Many women need reinforced practical encouragement from an expert to justify changing former behaviors, such as insisting on adhering to the routine of checking e-mail, doing household chores, or making dinner despite feeling overwhelmed or debilitated. Asking for help in changing routine is difficult. I remind every new mother that the first 3 months are the hardest, showering with a neonate at home rates as a victory, and that women who do not sleep often feel crazy and may truly run the risk of psychosis. If a new mother is not good at napping, I recommend abundant rest and skipping chores.

Clinically, I find it useful to ask for a baseline self-description of how each woman formerly perceived herself as compared to "who she's become" at this point in time. Ascertaining whether she views her core self as resilient or rigid, optimistic or pessimistic, introverted or extraverted, passive or active are all key indicators as to how she may problem-solve and resolve this current difficulty.

Validated and Reliable Instruments

Clinicians, particularly those in doctor's offices, clinics, and hospital settings, are likely to find standardized psychometric tools a simple and effective diagnostic procedure. Quick to administer and score and requiring little exertion on the individual's part, these instruments offer basic feedback for evaluation and diagnosis. They offer a good baseline for physician's office, clinic, and maternity hospital unit personnel to judge the population. Ideally, all patients should be assessed for perinatal mood disorders. An abundance of valid and reliable tools is available either at cost or free of charge.

Zung Depressive Inventory, Beck Depression Inventory-II, and Hamilton Rating Scale for Depression

These three screening tools are reliable and valid self-report scales. While pinpointing major depression using *DSM–IV* criteria, none of these instruments diagnose perinatal-specific changes. The Zung Depressive Inventory, a tool commonly relied upon in the early 1980s, is rarely used. It has been surpassed by the Beck Depression Inventory-Revised (BDI-II), which continues to be used in many settings for diagnosing major depression. Solidly reliable and valid, the 21-item scale BDI-II assesses the intensity of depressive mood over the past 2-week period in clinically depressed and normal patients. The test materials may be purchased through Harcourt Assessments, Inc. at www.harcourt assessment.com in English and Spanish.

Widely used with other assessments, the Hamilton Rating Scale for Depression (HAM-D) focuses on the presence and severity of a depressive illness already diagnosed. Unlike the Zung and BDI-II, the HAM-D is conducted in a semistructured interview format by a health care professional. Completion of the 21-item questionnaire requires approximately 30 minutes. The HAM-D may be downloaded courtesy of GlaxoWellcome (now GlaxoSmithKline) at healthnet.umass.edu/mhealth/HAMD.pdf.

Postpartum Depression Predictors Inventory-Revised

Developed in 1986 and subsequently revised, Cheryl Beck (2002) developed the Postpartum Depression Predictors Inventory-Revised (PDPI-R) to help identify women at risk. As a result, it is a more sensitively drawn instrument than the above-mentioned assessment tools diagnosing major depression. Marital status and socioeconomic status are required. These are viewed as significant since women who are single and have low socioeconomic status are more vulnerable. During the antenatal period, 10 predictors are assessed: (1) prenatal depression, (2) prenatal anxiety, (3) planned/unplanned pregnancy, (4) history of previous depression, (5) lack of social support, (6) marital dissatisfaction, and (7) life stress. During the postnatal period three additional predictors,

(8) child care stress, (9) infant temperament, and (10) maternity blues, are assessed.

The PDPI-R is not a self-report but utilizes a semistructured interview procedure between a health care professional and a woman. Beck suggests that the PDPI-R be completed once per trimester and periodically for the first year following delivery. The PDPI-R identifies women who can be referred for help immediately. In the public domain, the inventory includes "Guide Questions for Its Use" and several blank lines for "Comments," which allow the professional to notate thoughts on a woman's evaluation or allow for a treatment plan.

Antenatal Psychosocial Health Assessment

Developed in Ontario, Canada, by a group of physicians, midwives, and antepartum nurses (Reid, Carroll, Wilson, & Stewart, 1998), the Antenatal Psychosocial Health Assessment (ALPHA) comes in two forms. Two pages in length, the ALPHA Self-Report Questionnaire for Women instructs a woman to evaluate the changes in her life, which she might wish to discuss with a health care provider. The categories include family life, her own life, and concerns in her life. The four factors evaluated in the assessment are (1) family factors, (2) maternal factors, (3) substance abuse, and (4) family violence. The ALPHA form has a handy follow-up plan checklist useful to professionals and a space for comments. It is designed to highlight areas of "low, some, or high" concern, which, when identified, allow for follow-up and referral. Available in English and French, the ALPHA forms, an ALPHA video, and "Professional Guide" and "Provider's Summary for Self-Report" are available for purchase through the Department of Family & Community Medicine, University of Toronto at family.healthcare@utoronto.ca.

Postpartum Depression Checklist

Developed by Cheryl Beck (1995), the Postpartum Depression Checklist (PDC) (1999, Appendix A) offers a checklist of symptoms derived from 11 themes, including (1) lack of concentration, (2) loss of interest, (3) loneliness, (4) insecurity, (5) obsessive thinking, (6) lack of positive emotions, (7) loss of self, (8) anxiety attacks, (9) loss of control, (10) guilt, and (11) contemplating death. The checklist comes with a "Suggested Questions to Elicit Responses from the Postpartum Depression Checklist" (Beck, 1999, Appendix B). The process in which the health care professional administers the semistructured questions with a mother allows for a deeper and broader interview than a self-administered checklist. The PDC is useful in assisting professionals to determine what type of intervention is advantageous. It helps to pinpoint specific troubling areas of a woman's life, including obsession, anxiety, and depression. The woman responding affirmatively to questions regarding "contemplating death" can be referred for help immediately.

Postpartum Depression Screening Scale

Developed by Cheryl Beck and Robert Gable, the Postpartum Depression Screening Scale (PDSS) is a self-administered tool requiring 5 to 10 minutes to complete. This measure uses simple, easily comprehensible language. (See Exhibit 5.1.) Utilizing a five-point Likert-type scale,

---

EXHIBIT 5.1 POSTPARTUM DEPRESSION SCREENING SCALE

Below are sample items describing how a mother may be feeling after the birth of her baby. The mother is to indicate how much she agrees or disagrees with each statement during the past two weeks, using the following scale:

1	2	3	4	5
Strongly Disagree	**Disagree**	**Neither Agree nor Disagree**	**Agree**	**Strongly Agree**

I get anxious over even the littlest things that concerned my baby

1 2 3 4 5

I was scared that I would never be happy again

1 2 3 4 5

I felt like I had to hide what I was thinking or feeling toward the baby

1 2 3 4 5

I started thinking that I would be better off dead

1 2 3 4 5

---

the PDSS examines seven symptom areas: sleeping/eating disturbances, anxiety/insecurity, emotional lability, mental confusion, loss of self, guilt/shame, and suicidal thoughts. The test scoring system falls into three ranges: normal adjustment, significant symptoms of PPD, and positive screening for major postpartum depression. Its authors suggest that it be administered 2 weeks postdelivery and intermittently after that. The PDSS offers clinicians an approach for formulating a treatment plan.

In addition to English and Spanish versions of the PDSS, there is a Continuing Education Questionnaire and Evaluation, which offers two continuing education credits for mastering the tool. These can be purchased by contacting Western Psychological Services at 1-800-648-8857 or www.wpspublish.com.

Edinburgh Postnatal Depression Scale

Developed by Cox, Holden, and Sagovsky in 1987, the Edinburgh Postnatal Depression Scale (EPDS), noted for its reliability and validity, consists of 10 short items. Requiring less than 5 minutes' completion time, it is easy to complete and the scoring system is easily mastered by the health professional. The EPDS' authors permit free use of the scale, provided that the names of the authors, the title, and journal name are given credit in all reproductions. The Edinburgh Postnatal Depression Scale can be found easily via an Internet search. In addition to English and Spanish, translations of the EPDS, including Arabic, Mandarin Chinese, Czech, Dutch, French, German, Greek, Punjab, Slovenian, Swedish, Urdu, and Vietnamese, are also available (Cox & Holden, 2006).

Consisting of 10 statements, the EPDS asks the mother to underline which of the four responses most closely matches how she has been feeling for the past week. (See Exhibit 5.2.) An answer of "Yes, quite often" to question 10, which states, "The thought of harming myself has occurred to me," is a signal for immediate intervention by the professional. A score of 12 or more indicates depression but not its severity. Further evaluation by means of face-to-face screening with a professional trained in assessing perinatal mood disorders should be employed. The EPDS usually takes less than 5 minutes to complete and is easy to score. The instrument is not designed to diagnose mothers with anxiety neurosis, phobias, or character disorder, but rather it is viewed as having strong utility for the detection of perinatal depression. It can be repeated at various intervals to track changes in the mother's mood and may be introduced antenatally to track suspected depression.

EXHIBIT 5.2 THE EDINBURGH POSTNATAL DEPRESSION SCALE

How are you feeling?

As you have recently had a baby, we would like to know how you are feeling now. Please underline the answer which comes closest to how you have felt in the past 7 days, not just how you feel today. Here is an example, already completed.

I have felt happy:
Yes, most of the time
Yes, some of the time
No, not very often
No, not at all

This would mean: 'I have felt happy some of the time during the past week'. Please complete the other questions in the same way.

CONCLUSION

Logistically, time and staff are in short supply in many hospital and clinical settings. This is regrettable because nothing can replace the importance of the face-to-face interview using relevant psychometric antenatal and postnatal mental status screening tools. Ideally, these tools, released with informed consent, would move across disciplines and medical settings along with the postnatal mother's treatment, increasing the probability of rapid diagnosis and quick intervention. Undiagnosed postpartum mood disorder presents in women long after a neonate develops into a full-fledged human being. The problem with the standard, postdelivery 6-week check-up in the gynecologist's office is that PPD may not have fully emerged. In addition, a woman in denial or feeling shame or guilt may not take advantage of the check-up to share her thoughts or feelings.

Although beset with the responsibility for their newly born charges, pediatricians should be aware of the mother's health as well. The pediatrician or his or her nurse, who detects the pernicious effects of the depressed, overanxious, or obsessive mother, may impact long-term welfare of the children. Albeit an additional task on the part of the pediatrician's staff, prevention, intervention, and referral for a mother's treatment may be of significant benefit to mother and child.

Equally important is coordination of communication and referral among the physicians and their staff, mental health professionals, doulas, or lactation specialists who may have access to the mother's mental health status. Flagging concerns and enlisting the aid of a partner, close family relative, or good friend to monitor signs and symptoms is instrumental to facilitate a well-coordinated and effective treatment plan.

This process of identifying a woman at risk allows for rapid intervention whether it be medication evaluation, psychotherapy, or group support. Likewise, mental health professionals with easy access to medical caregivers offer more accurate and streamlined coordination of treatment. Open lines of communications between ancillary disciplines can mitigate or prevent a full-blown depressive episode. The rewards of a team approach justify the effort and should be encouraged.

The Internet enhances diagnosis and treatment through its ability to provide instantaneous information. Concerned laypeople and professionals must be selective about choosing sites that provide correct and up-to-date information so they avoid inaccuracies and potentially harmful errors in judgment. Many states have valuable sites listing local resources, as does the Canadian Web site pregnets (www.pregnets.org). Respected university medical centers conducting research and offering education include Emory University School of Medicine (www.emorywomensprogram.org) and Massachusetts General Hospital Center for Women's Mental Health (www.womensmentalhealth.org). Health care professionals may find valuable resources such as educational opportunities and information on prescription products to treat perinatal depression at http://www.psych.uic.edu/research/perinatalmentalhealth/ or through the UIC Perinatal Mental Health Consultation Line at 1-800-573-6121. The national organization, Postpartum Support International (www.postpartum.net), offers a wide array of services for professionals and concerned mothers, including a nonemergency-oriented line, otherwise known as a warm line, staffed by English- and Spanish-speaking volunteers.

Considering the consequences for the entire family, it is imperative to understand risk factors and improve diagnosis and assessment of those at risk for postpartum mood disorders. Rapid response enabling prevention and treatment benefits families in the short run and society in the long run. As so many new mothers say when they feel better: "I have me back again"—that is the goal of diagnosis and screening.

REFERENCES

Abramowitz, J., Schiatz, S., Moore, K., & Luenzman, K. (2003). Obsessive-compulsive symptoms in pregnancy and the puerperium: A review of the literature. *Journal of Anxiety Disorders, 17,* 461–478.

American Psychiatric Association. (1994). *Diagnostic and statistical manual of mental disorders* (4th ed.). Washington, DC: Author.

Beck, C. (1995). Screening methods for postpartum depression. *Journal of Obstetrics, Gynecologic, and Neonatal Nursing, 24*(4), 308–313.

Beck, C. (1999). *Postpartum depression: Case studies, research, and nursing care.* Washington, DC: Association of Women's Health Obstetric and Neonatal Nurses.

Beck, C. (2002). Revision of the postpartum depression predictors inventory. *Journal of Obstetrics, Gynecologic, and Neonatal Nursing, 31,* 394–402.

Beck, C. (2004). Birth trauma: In the eye of the beholder. *Nursing Research, 53,* 28–35.

Beebe, B., & Lachmann, F. (2002). *Infant research and adult treatment: Co-constructing interactions.* Hillsdale, NJ: The Analytic Press.

Benedek, T. (1952). *Studies in psychosomatic medicine.* New York: Ronald Press.

Benedek, T. (1970). The psychobiology of pregnancy. In E. Anthony & T. Benedek (Eds.), *Parenthood: Its psychology and psychopathy* (pp. 137–151). Boston: Little, Brown.

Burt, V. K., Suri, R., Altshuler, L., Stowe, Z., Hendrick, V., & Muntean, E. (2001). The use of psychotropic medications during breast-feeding. *The American Journal of Psychiatry, 158*(7), 1001–1009.

Cohen, L., Altshuler, L., Harlow, B., et al. (2006). Relapse of major depression in women who maintain or discontinue antidepressant medication. *Journal of the American Medical Association, 295,* 499–507.

Corwin, E., Bozoky, I., Pugh, L., & Johnston, N. (2003). Interleukin-lbeta elevation during the postpartum period. *Annals of Behavioral Medicine, 25,* 41–47.

Cox, J., & Holden, J. (2006). *Perinatal mental health: A guide to the Edinburgh Postnatal Depression Scale.* London: Gaskill.

Cox, J., Holden, J., & Sagovsky, R. (1987). Detection of postnatal depression: Development of the 10-item Edinburgh Postnatal Depression Scale. *British Journal of Psychiatry, 150,* 782–786.

Dawson, G. (1992a). Infants of mothers with depressive symptoms: Neurophysiological and behavioral findings related to attachment status. *Infant Behavior and Development, Abstracts Issue, 15,* 117.

Dawson, G. (1992b). Frontal lobe activity and affective behavior of infants of mothers with depressive symptoms. *Child Development, 63,* 725–737.

Field, T., et al. (1988). Infants of depressed mothers show "depressed" behavior even with non-depressed adults. *Child Development, 59,* 1569–1579.

Freud, S. (1959a). The question of lay analysis. In J. Strachey (Trans.), *The standard edition of the complete psychological works of Sigmund Freud* (20, pp. 179–258). London: Hogarth Press. (Original work published 1926).

Freud, S. (1959b). Female sexuality. In J. Strachey (Trans.), *The standard edition of the complete psychological works of Sigmund Freud* (21, pp. 221–243). London: Hogarth Press. (Original work published 1931).

Hale, T. (2006). *Medications and mothers' milk* (12th ed.). Amarillo, TX: Hale Publishing.

Hendrick, V., & Altschuler, L. (2002). Management of major depression during pregnancy. *American Journal of Psychiatry, 159,* 1667–1673.

Kendall-Tackett, K. (2005). *Depression in new mothers: Causes, consequences and treatment options.* Binghamton, England: Haworth Press.

Kennedy, H., Gardiner, A., Gay, C., & Lee, K. (2007). Negotiating sleep: A qualitative study of new mothers. *Journal of Perinatal Nursing, 21,* 114–122.

Meltzer, E., & Kumar, R. (1985). Puerperal mental illness, clinical features and classification: A study of 142 mother-and-baby admissions. *British Journal of Psychiatry, 147,* 647–654.

Metz, A., Sichel, D., & Goff, D. (1998). Postpartum panic disorder. *Journal of Clinical Psychiatry, 49,* 278–279.

Minkovitz, C., Strobino, D., Scharfstein, D., Hou, W., Miller, T., Mistry, K., & Swartz, K. (2005). Maternal depressive symptoms and children's receipt of health care in the first 3 years of life. *Pediatrics, 2,* 306–314.

Misri, S., & Kendrick, K. (2007). Treatment of perinatal mood and anxiety disorders: A review. *The Canadian Journal of Psychiatry, 52,* 489–498.

O'Hara, M., & Swain, A. (1996). Rates and risk of postpartum depression—a meta-analysis. *International Review of Psychiatry, 8,* 37–54.

Reid, A., Carroll, J., Wilson, L., & Stewart, D. (1998). Using the ALPHA form in practice to assess antenatal psychosocial health. *Canadian Health Association Journal, 6,* 677–684.

Shapiro, S. (1988). Menarche and menstruation: Psychoanalytic implications. In J. Zuckerberg (Ed.), *Critical psychophysical passages in the life of a woman: A psychodynamic perspective* (pp. 69–91). New York: Plenum.

Shaw, E., Levitt, C., Wong, S., Kaczorowski, J., & McMaster University Postpartum Research Group. (2006). Systematic review of the literature on postpartum care: Effectiveness of postpartum support to improve maternal parenting, mental health, and quality of life, and physical health. *Birth, 33,* 210–220.

Sichel, D., & Driscoll, J. (1999). *Women's moods: What every woman must know about hormones, the brain, and emotional health.* New York: William Morrow.

Stern, D. (1985). *The interpersonal world of the infant.* New York: Basic Books.

Stowe, Z., Hostetter, A., Owens, M., Ritchie, J., Sternberg, K., Cohen, L., & Nemeroff, C. (2003). The pharmacokinetics of sertraline excretion into human breast milk: Determinants of infant serum concentrations. *Journal of Clinical Psychiatry, 64,* 73–80.

Tronick, E. (1998). Dyadically expanded states of consciousness and the process of therapeutic change. *Infant Mental Health Journal, 19,* 290–299.

Viguera, A., Nonacs, R., Cohen, L., Tondo, L., Murray, A., & Baldessarini, R. (2000). Risk of recurrence of bipolar disorder in pregnant and nonpregnant women after discontinuing lithium maintenance. *American Journal of Psychiatry, 157,* 179–184.

Weissman, M., Pilowsky, D., Wickramaratne, P., et al. for the STAR*D-Child Team. (2006). Remissions in maternal depression and child psychopathology: A STAR*D-Child report. *Journal of the American Medical Association, 295,* 774–781.

Wisner, K., Parry, B., & Piontek, C. (2002). Postpartum depression. *New England Journal of Medicine, 347,* 194–199.

Yonkers, K., et al. (2004). Management of bipolar disorder during pregnancy and the postpartum period. *American Journal of Psychiatry, 161,* 608–620.

6 Omega-3s, Exercise, and St. John's Wort: Three Complementary and Alternative Treatments for Postpartum Depression

KATHLEEN KENDALL-TACKETT

Depression in new mothers is common in many cultures, affecting anywhere from 10% to 20% of postpartum women (Kendall-Tackett, 2005). Because of postpartum depression's devastating effects on mother and baby, it's vital that it be identified and treated promptly. As other chapters in this volume describe, frontline treatments for postpartum depression include both antidepressants and psychotherapy. Increasingly, however, women are turning to alternative modalities to treat their depression. These modalities can be used alone, and sometimes in combination with standard treatments. In this chapter, three of the most common alternative treatments for depression are described: long-chain Omega-3 fatty acids (EPA and DHA), exercise, and St. John's wort. The impact of each of these on breastfeeding is also considered, as are women's reasons for seeking out alternative treatments in the first place.

WHY PATIENTS USE ALTERNATIVE AND COMPLEMENTARY TREATMENTS

From the patient's perspective, alternative treatments offer a number of advantages. If you understand why women might prefer to use these modalities, you can talk more comfortably with them. And they are more likely to be forthcoming about using them. Below are some reasons women have shared about why they use alternative treatment approaches.

- *Control:* One reason patients prefer alternative medicine is that they can control their own health care. Instead of having to wait for a doctor's appointment, they can address their depression right away.
- *Privacy:* Patients may be ashamed to admit that they are depressed and are frightened by the possibility that their employers or others will find out that they are taking antidepressants. Unfortunately, on occasion, medication information *does* get released to employers via insurance forms or just plain gossip—even with confidentiality regulations in place. And antidepressant use can influence hiring and promotion decisions in some types of jobs. Even if that's not the case, patients may still not want others to know.
- *Costs:* Newer and name-brand antidepressants can be expensive, especially if not covered by insurance. In contrast, alternative treatments are generally reasonably priced and can be purchased at discount and warehouse stores. The savings each month can be substantial compared with name-brand nongeneric prescription drugs.
- *Side Effects and Safety:* The side-effect and safety profiles of alternative treatments are generally better than those associated with medications (Klier et al., 2006; Schultz, 2006). For example, the tricyclic antidepressants have a host of anticholinergic side effects including dry mouth, constipation, and blurred vision. The selective serotonin reuptake inhibitors (SSRIs) have sexual side effects, such as inorgasmia. Many patients find these side effects intolerable and may stop taking their medications. In one recent study, only 28% of patients prescribed antidepressants were still taking them 3 months later (Olfson, Marcus, Tedeschi, & Wan, 2006). Side effects were a common reason for patients stopping their medications. The incidence of adverse effects of Omega-3s and exercise are almost nonexistent unless used at very high levels. And, according to one recent review, risk of adverse effects associated with St. John's wort is 10 times lower than with standard antidepressants (Schultz, 2006).

The discussion above highlights why women might choose alternative treatment approaches for postpartum depression. In the next section, current research is presented on a new approach to the etiology of depression. This new research explains why a wide variety of treatments are all effective. (For a full review of this literature, see Kendall-Tackett, 2007, 2008).

INFLAMMATION AND DEPRESSION

Over the past decade, researchers have found that systemic inflammation plays a key role in the etiology of depression. Inflammation is due to activity of the immune system and is part of our physiological stress response. Inflammation is generally assessed in these studies by measuring serum levels of proinflammatory cytokines, the messenger molecules of the immune system. The proinflammatory cytokines identified most often in depression are interleukin-1β (IL-1β), interleukin-6 (IL-6), and tumor necrosis factor-α (TNF-α).

There are a number of plausible explanations for why inflammation might increase the risk for depression (Maes & Smith, 1998). First, when inflammation levels are high, people experience classic symptoms of depression, such as fatigue, lethargy, and social withdrawal. Researchers discovered this connection when using cytokines as a treatment for cancer or hepatitis. Depression increases in patients receiving cytokine therapy, and it increases in a dose-responsive way: the greater the dose of cytokines, the higher their depression (Konsman, Parnet, & Dantzer, 2002). Second, inflammation activates the hypothalamic-pituitary-adrenal (HPA) axis, dysregulating levels of cortisol. Cortisol is designed to keep inflammation in check. However, when someone is either severely stressed or depressed, cortisol levels are either too high or too low. In either case, cortisol does not restrain the inflammatory response (Dhabhar & McEwen, 2001). Finally, inflammation decreases the neurotransmitter serotonin by lowering levels of its precursor, tryptophan (Maes & Smith, 1998).

Our bodies "translate" physical and psychological stress into inflammation, and inflammation underlies all the other risk factors for depression. This means that inflammation is not simply *a* risk factor; it is *the* risk factor that ties the others together (Kendall-Tackett, 2007).

Pregnant and postpartum women are particularly vulnerable to this effect because their inflammation levels normally rise during the last trimester of pregnancy—a time when they are also at high risk for depression (Kendall-Tackett, 2005, 2007). Inflammation serves several important functions in pregnant women, including ripening the cervix and protecting them from infection postpartum (Coussons-Read, Okun, Schmitt, & Giese, 2005). Moreover, stressors common to new mothers, such as sleep disturbance, pain, and psychological trauma, also increase inflammation (Kendall-Tackett, 2007).

Another line of evidence relevant to our discussion is that most effective treatments for depression are also anti-inflammatory. For example, standard antidepressants, especially SSRIs, lower inflammation, and this may partially explain their efficacy. For example, a recent study compared C-reactive protein levels in patients with major depression before and after treatment with SSRIs. C-reactive protein is an acute-phase protein and another marker of inflammation. In these patients, C-reactive protein dropped significantly after treatment, independent of whether depression resolved (O'Brien, Scott, & Dinan, 2006).

Although evidence is preliminary, two forms of psychotherapy—cognitive therapy and interpersonal psychotherapy—are also arguably anti-inflammatory. For example, two recent studies have demonstrated that negative beliefs, such as hostility, can increase the levels of pro-inflammatory cytokines—especially IL-6 (Kiecolt-Glaser et al., 2005; Suarez, Lewis, Krishnan, & Young, 2004). The primary goal of cognitive therapy is to reduce negative cognitions (Rupke, Blecke, & Renfrow, 2006). Since negative cognitions increase inflammation, reducing their occurrence will have physical effects as well—primarily reducing inflammation. Similarly, interpersonal therapy is an effective treatment for postpartum depression and focuses on helping women with the role changes involved in becoming a mother. It also helps women increase the amount of social support they have (Grigoriadis & Ravitz, 2007). Social support, by attenuating the stress response, lowers inflammation (see Kendall-Tackett, 2008).

These findings provide a backdrop to understanding the three alternative treatments I describe—Omega-3s, exercise, and St. John's wort. All are effective, at least in part, because they decrease inflammation. The first modality is Omega-3 fatty acids.

OMEGA-3 FATTY ACIDS

A number of recent studies have demonstrated that Omega-3 fatty acids are effective for preventing and treating mood disorders. Researchers have documented these effects in population studies, randomized controlled trials, and in prevention studies. With regard to depression, it is the long-chain Omega-3 fatty acids that are of interest: eicosapentenoic acid (EPA) and docosahexanoic acid (DHA). These fatty acids must be consumed as part of our diets because humans are quite inefficient at converting them from other foods. Unfortunately, the diets of many living in Western industrialized countries are deficient in EPA and DHA.

The health impact of Western diets has been observed in a series of epidemiologic studies. For more than 100 years, an increasing number of people have developed major depression, heart disease, diabetes, and other conditions related to inflammation (Kiecolt-Glaser et al., 2007). This rise in depression and other conditions corresponds to a rather striking change in our consumption of fats. We now consume more Omega-6 fatty acids and fewer Omega-3s than we did a century ago. Omega-6s are found in vegetable oils, such as corn and safflower oils, and are a staple of many processed foods. Omega-3 fatty acids are polyunsaturated fats found in plant and marine sources (Kiecolt-Glaser et al., 2007). In previous centuries, our ratio of Omega-6s to Omega-3s has been approximately 2 to 3:1. In contrast, the ratio the average North American consumes ranges from 15 to 17:1 (Kiecolt-Glaser et al., 2007). This dramatic change is affecting our physical and mental health. Researchers first documented these effects via population studies, examining rates of fish consumption (Kiecolt-Glaser et al., 2007; Maes & Smith, 1998).

The Mental Health Effects of EPA and DHA in Population Studies

Several recent studies have found that people who eat more fatty, cold-water fish have higher levels of EPA and DHA, and lower rates of several affective disorders, including major depression (Tanskanen et al., 2001), bipolar disorder (Noaghiul & Hibbeln, 2003), and suicide risk (Sublette, Hibbeln, Galfalvy, Oquendo, & Mann, 2006). Summarizing these studies, Kiecolt-Glaser et al. (2007) noted that depression is 10 times more common in countries where people don't eat fish, or eat a small amount. Fish consumption has a similar effect on postpartum depression. In a large population study, with more than 14,000 women from 22 countries, Hibbeln (2002) noted that postpartum depression was up to 50 times more common in countries with low fish consumption. Mothers who ate high amounts of seafood during pregnancy, and who had high levels of DHA in their milk postpartum, had lower levels of postpartum depression.

Treatment With EPA

Researchers have also studied the efficacy of EPA and DHA in treating depression (Parker et al., 2006; Peet & Stokes, 2005). In these clinical trials, researchers gave either a placebo, EPA alone, or EPA/DHA supplements to people who were currently depressed. Investigators found that EPA is the most effective Omega-3 for treating depression. When EPA was added to patients' medications, they were significantly less depressed than those who received a placebo (Peet & Horrobin, 2002; Peet & Stokes, 2005). In a recent review, EPA had efficacy in treating depression in four of the six studies reviewed (Peet & Stokes, 2005).

In a study of childhood depression, children who received EPA and DHA had significantly improved depression compared with children who received a placebo (Nemets, H., Nemets, B., Apter, Bracha, & Belmaker, 2006). EPA also helped stabilize symptoms of bipolar disorder in a 12-week double-blind trial (Frangou, Lewis, & McCrone, 2006). Peet and Stokes (2005) found that 1 gram of EPA per day was the effective dose for treatment. Doses higher than 2 grams seemed to have the reverse effect. DHA alone is not an effective treatment for depression (Akabas & Deckelbaum, 2006). However, DHA is useful for prevention (see below). These and other findings led an expert panel of the American Psychiatric Association to conclude that EPA was a promising treatment for mood disorders (Freeman et al., 2006a).

DHA in the Perinatal Period

In Western cultures, pregnant women's diets are often deficient in DHA. This is unfortunate given babies' high need for it in utero. Writing about mothers in Australia, Rees and colleagues (2005) noted that during the last trimester of pregnancy, babies accumulate an average of 67 mg/day of DHA. The average intake for Australian mothers is 15 mg/day. In contrast, DHA consumption among Japanese, Koreans, and Norwegians is about 1,000 mg/day. Because babies need DHA for brain and vision development, women's bodies will preferentially divert DHA to the baby, and the baby will take the DHA it needs from maternal stores. With each subsequent pregnancy, mothers are further depleted (Freeman et al., 2006b). Mothers' deficiency increases their risk for depression.

In the Adelaide Mothers' and Babies' Iron Trial, a 1% increase in plasma DHA was related to a 59% decrease in depressive symptoms postpartum (Rees et al., 2005). As noted earlier, Hibbeln's (2002) population study found that mothers who ate high amounts of seafood during pregnancy, and who had high levels of DHA in their milk postpartum, had lower levels of postpartum depression. The same preventative effect was not found for EPA. Current recommended minimum intake is 200 to 400 mg/day.

DHA may have another effect that could help prevent depression postpartum. In a study of infant sleep, mothers with high levels of DHA during pregnancy had babies who exhibited more mature sleep patterns in the first few days of life. With a sample of 17 neonates, the investigators examined the ratio of quiet to active sleep using a monitor placed beneath the crib mattress. A higher percentage of quiet sleep is characteristic of older babies, and researchers consider this a marker of more mature sleep. Babies whose mothers had high levels of DHA during pregnancy exhibited more mature sleep patterns as neonates. The investigators concluded that babies of high-DHA mothers had more mature central nervous systems than babies of mothers who were low in DHA. Although a small sample, the findings are intriguing. Babies with more mature sleep patterns allow their mothers to get more uninterrupted sleep—and this could have an indirect effect on maternal mental health (Cheruku, Montgomery-Downs, Farkas, Thoman, & Lammi-Keefe, 2002).

Why They Work: The Anti-Inflammatory Effects of EPA and DHA

The above-cited studies indicate that EPA and DHA have a role in the prevention and treatment of postpartum depression. The intriguing question is why. It wasn't until recently that researchers confirmed what they suspected: that EPA and DHA are anti-inflammatory.

In a large population study, high levels of EPA and DHA were related to lower levels of proinflammatory cytokines (IL-1α, IL-1β, IL-6, and TNF-α) and higher levels of anti-inflammatory cytokines, such as IL-10. For people with low levels of EPA and DHA, the opposite was true: high levels of proinflammatory cytokines and low levels of anti-inflammatory cytokines (Ferrucchi et al., 2006). The sample in this study was representative of the population—not a specific subgroup. The fatty acids were directly measured in the plasma rather than estimated from patient dietary reports. And it was the first study that specifically examined the relationship between fatty acids and cytokines.

In a study of older adults, the combination of depression and a high ratio of Omega-6s to Omega-3s dramatically increased levels of proinflammatory cytokines (IL-6 and TNF-α). Patients who were depressed *and* had low levels of Omega-3s had the highest levels of proinflammatory cytokines. The authors noted that a diet that is low in EPA/DHA increases the risk of both depression and other diseases related to chronic inflammation (Kiecolt-Glaser et al., 2007).

Relevant to our discussion of postpartum depression is the impact of Omega-3s on stress. EPA and DHA may increase resilience to stress by regulating and attenuating the stress response. When college students had a high ratio of Omega-6s to Omega-3s (indicating a deficiency in Omega-3s), they were more likely to secrete proinflammatory cytokines when stressed in the laboratory. When Omega-3 levels were higher, the levels of proinflammatory cytokines were reduced in response to stress.

Safety Concerns During Pregnancy and Lactation

One concern about any type of supplementation is whether it is safe for pregnant and breastfeeding women. Several recent studies of either pregnant or breastfeeding women have noted no teratogenic effects with a wide range of dosages (Marangell, Martinez, Zboyan, Chong, & Puryear, 2004; Shoji et al., 2006; Smuts et al., 2003). A few of these findings are summarized below. (For a complete review, see Kendall-Tackett, 2008.)

Most studies of EPA/DHA's impact on pregnancy are population studies examining fish or fish-oil consumption. One study sampled 182 women from the Faroe Islands: a community between Shetland and Iceland (Grandjean, Bjerve, Weihe, & Steuerwald, 2001). The average fish consumption in this sample was 72 grams of fish, 12 grams of whale muscle, and 7 grams of blubber per day. The researchers found that DHA was the best predictor of gestational length, with a 1% increase in relative concentration related to a 1.5-day increase in gestation. However, an increase of 1% in relative EPA concentration was related to a 246-gram decrease in birthweight. This effect was independent of the effects of environmental contaminants and did not appear related to infant outcomes.

A randomized trial of 341 women compared cod liver oil supplementation (803 mg EPA, 1,183 mg DHA) to corn oil from 18 weeks gestation to 3 months postpartum (Hellend, Smith, Saarem, Saugstad, & Drevon, 2003). All the babies in this study were breastfed for at least

3 months. There were no teratogenic effects noted. At 4 years of age, children whose mothers had taken cod liver oil during pregnancy and lactation had a higher Mental Processing Composite score. This score correlated with head circumference at birth, but not birthweight or gestational age. Only pregnancy intake of DHA was significantly related to mental abilities at age 4. There are some cautions to mention with cod liver oil. Since it contains three fat-soluble vitamins (A, D, & E), it is possible to take too much. Unless supervised by a health care provider, mothers are safer if they take a fish-oil supplement that contains EPA and DHA only rather than cod liver oil.

Another clinical trial (Malcolm, McCulloch, Montgomery, Shepherd, & Weaver, 2003) randomly assigned 100 mothers to either fish oil (200 mg DHA) or a placebo from 15 weeks gestation to delivery. Fatty acids were measured in plasma and red blood cells at 15, 28, and 40 weeks, and in umbilical cord blood. Infant visual evoked potentials were measured at birth and at 50 and 66 weeks. Interestingly, there was no impact of maternal supplementation on level of DHA on umbilical cord blood or visual evoked potentials. However, infant DHA status (regardless of group) did make a difference. High-DHA infants showed increased maturation of the central visual pathways. The authors noted that their findings suggested that infants accrue sufficient amounts, in spite of and/or at the expense of their mothers, to meet the needs of their developing neural and visual systems. There were no teratogenic effects of supplementation noted.

Hawkes and colleagues (2002) conducted a double-blind trial with women who were 3 days postpartum. Women received either a placebo; 700 mg EPA/300 mg DHA; or 140 mg EPA/600 mg DHA for 12 weeks. Supplementation with EPA/DHA did not alter cytokine levels in breast milk. The authors concluded that these levels of supplementation did not cause perturbations in cytokine concentrations and were thus safe for breastfeeding women, without harm to the baby.

At very high dosages of EPA/DHA supplementation, there has been some concern about changes in breast milk fatty acid composition. In one study where 83 mothers were supplemented from 20 weeks gestation to delivery, there were significant changes to the fatty acid composition of breast milk. But these changes may, indeed, prove beneficial—not harmful. Fish oil supplementation significantly increased EPA and DHA concentrations in breast milk (Dunstan, Roper et al., 2004), and in the erythrocytes of mothers and babies in the fish-oil group (Dunstan, Mori et al., 2004). There were no differences between the treatment and control groups in immune parameters in breast milk. But higher levels of EPA/DHA were related to increased levels of IgA (an antibody) and sCD14 (immune cell). The researchers identified these higher levels as potentially protective. The dosage used in this study was very high (2.2 g DHA, 1.5 g EPA): *11 times* the recommended minimum of DHA. Even with this large dose, EPA/ DHA might also help promote beneficial probiotic Lactobacilli, which can help protect against the development of allergic disease.

Sources of EPA and DHA

Fish is the most common dietary source of EPA and DHA. However, this can be a problem for pregnant and breastfeeding women as they often need to limit the amount of fish they eat because of contaminants in seafood. Fortunately, there are alternative sources of EPA and DHA that are tested for contaminants and are contaminant-free. These include supplements, prenatal vitamins, and fortified foods. Some of these sources of DHA are vegetarian and Kosher. There is currently no vegetarian source of EPA; fish or fish oil are the only sources. Table 6.1 lists current recommended dosages, and sources of information on EPA/ DHA that are safe for pregnant and breastfeeding women.

Table 6.1

DOSAGES OF EPA/DHA

200–400 mg DHA for prevention of depression

1,000 mg EPA for treatment of depression
(with medication and/or DHA)

FDA GRAS (generally recognized as safe) Levels:
1,500 mg DHA
3,000 mg DHA/EPA

For a listing of brands of fish oil verified by the U.S. Pharmacoepia as contaminant-free:
www.USP.org

For a listing of other products with added DHA:
www.BreastfeedingMadeSimple.com

What About Flaxseed?

For people who do not want to take fish oil or fish-oil products, many have turned to flaxseed as an alternative. The principal Omega-3 in flaxseed is alpha-linolenic acid (ALA). ALA is an essential fatty acid and is the parent Omega-3. Although our bodies can convert ALA to EPA and DHA, they do so inefficiently. Only 10% to 15% of ALA is converted to EPA and DHA (Parker et al., 2006). Supplementation with ALA does not increase EPA and DHA levels and has no impact on depression (Bratman & Girman, 2003; Kendall-Tackett, 2005, 2007). Flaxseed does, however, have cardiovascular benefits. And it is not harmful. It simply does not prevent or treat depression.

Summary

Increasing evidence suggests that DHA can help prevent depression in new mothers and that EPA can be a useful treatment—alone, or in combination with medications and/or DHA. EPA and DHA also appear to be helpful in the treatment of bipolar disorder, but should not be used alone: only as an adjunct to treatment with standard medications. A recent review in the *British Journal of Psychiatry* summarized these findings as follows:

> There is good evidence that psychiatric illness is associated with the depletion of EFAs [essential fatty acids] and, crucially, that supplementation can result in clinical amelioration. . . . The clinical trial data may herald a simple, safe and effective adjunct to our standard treatments. (Hallahan & Garland, 2005, p. 276)

EPA and DHA are one promising intervention for mothers—especially those who are at risk for postpartum depression. And there is little apparent risk to their use. The next modality I describe—exercise—has similar benefits with no apparent negative side effects.

EXERCISE

Exercise is another effective treatment for postpartum depression (Daley, Macarthur, & Winter, 2007). Traditionally, exercise has been recommended for people with mild to moderate depression. But exercise is an effective, nonpharmacologic intervention for people with major depression as well. It can also be safely combined with other modalities.

Exercise for Depressed People

Several recent studies have demonstrated the effectiveness of exercise in improving mood. In a large study from Finland ($N = 3{,}403$), exercise lowered depression and helped with feelings of anger, distrust, and stress. Two to three times a week was enough to achieve this mood-altering effect (Hassmen, Koivula, & Uutela, 2000). Men and women who exercised perceived their health and fitness as better than nonexercisers. Exercise also increased their social connections with others.

In a study of 70 women with fibromyalgia, Da Costa and colleagues (2000) examined the relationship between depressed mood and weekly exercise. Women were evaluated at baseline and 3 years later. The authors found that women who engaged in more weekly leisure activity had lower depressed mood at the 3-year follow-up.

Subjects in the previously cited studies had mild to moderate depression. But Babyak et al.'s (2000) study demonstrated that exercise can be helpful for major depression too. In this randomized clinical trial, depressed older adults were randomly assigned to one of three groups: exercise alone; sertraline alone; or a combination of exercise and sertraline. After 4 months, all the patients improved, and there were no differences between the groups. People in the exercise-only group did as well as people in the two medication groups. In addition, people in the exercise-only group were significantly less likely to relapse. Six months after completion of treatment, 28% of the exercise-only group became depressed again vs. 51% of the medications-only and medications-exercise groups. The authors concluded that exercise is an effective intervention, even in patients with major depression. And it helps prevent relapse.

In a sample of 32 older adults (ages 60 to 84 years), subjects were randomized to one of two conditions; 10 weeks of supervised weight-lifting exercise followed by 10 weeks of unsupervised exercise. The control group attended lectures for 10 weeks. The patients all had major or minor depression. There was no contact with any study participant until the end of the research period at 26 months. Individuals in the exercise group had significantly lower scores on the Beck Depression Inventory at 20 weeks, and at follow-up at 26 months, than the nonexercisers. Moreover, at the 26-month follow-up, 33% of the exercisers were still regularly weight lifting vs. 0% of the controls (Singh, Clements, & Fiatarone Singh, 2001).

In another sample, older adults were randomly assigned to either exercise classes or health education for 10 weeks (Mather et al., 2002). All participants were depressed, but their depression was not being adequately controlled by medication. Exercise was proposed as an adjunct to treatment. Blind assessments were made before the study started, at 10 and 34 weeks. Fifty-five percent of the exercise group became less depressed compared with 33% of the group who received education.

The mood-altering effects of exercise appear fairly quickly. In a study of 26 women, Lane and colleagues (2002) measured anger, confusion, depression, fatigue, tension, and vigor before and after two exercise sessions. There was significant mood enhancement after each exercise session. Depressed mood was especially sensitive to exercise and decreased significantly after each session.

Why It Works

Exercise works as a treatment for several reasons. First, it changes brain chemistry. Specifically, exercise elevates serotonin and dopamine levels and releases endorphins that relieve pain and create a sense of well-being. Both aerobics and strength training achieve this effect. Second, it increases self-efficacy. Increasing self-efficacy via exercise decreased depressive symptoms in a sample of older adults (McAuley, Blissmer, Katula, Duncan, & Mihalko, 2000). Third, in moderate amounts, it too was recently found to lower inflammation. For example, in one study of older adults, an exercise program accelerated wound healing (Emery, Kiecolt-Glaser, Glaser, Malarky, & Frid, 2005). This is an indirect indication that exercise lowered systemic inflammation. When systemic inflammation is high, wound healing is impaired because proinflammatory cytokines are in the bloodstream and not at the wound site where they belong (Kiecolt-Glaser et al., 2005). However, the intervention lowered perceived stress and improved wound healing, suggesting lower systemic levels of proinflammatory cytokines.

Another study with older adults had similar findings. After a 10-week exercise intervention, the subjects had lower stress and improved mood and quality of life. They also had a significant decrease in serum IL-6 (Starkweather, 2007). It is important to note that too much exercise can actually increase both IL-6 and TNF-α (Goebel, Mills, Irwin,

& Ziegler, 2000). But a moderate amount appears to have an anti-inflammatory effect.

Exercise and Breastfeeding

One concern mothers may raise is the impact of exercise on breastfeeding. Does exercise cause lactic acid to build up in their milk so that babies won't breastfeed or refuse their mothers' milk? A study of 12 lactating women sought to answer this question (Quinn & Carey, 1999). In this study, milk and blood samples were taken after a nonexercise session (control), after maximal exercise, and after a session that was 20% below the maximal range. They found that in women with an adequate maternal caloric intake, moderate exercise did not increase lactic acid in breast milk nor cause babies to reject it. When women were exercising in a range that they considered "hard" (using the perceived-exertion scale), lactic acid increased. The authors recommended exercise in a moderate range because it does not lead to lactic acid accumulation in the breast milk nor does it alter babies' willingness to breastfeed.

What Mothers Can Do

Exercise can be helpful treatment for depression and can be used in combination with other treatment modalities. To achieve an antidepressant effect, mothers should exercise at least two to three times a week for at least 20 minutes. For severe depression, women should exercise three to five times a week, for 30 to 45 minutes. In summary, exercise is a highly effective treatment for depression—alone or in combination with other treatments. And it can be a viable alternative treatment if mothers refuse medications.

ST. JOHN'S WORT

St. John's wort (*Hypericum perforatum*) is the most widely used herbal antidepressant in the world (Dugoua, Mills, Perri, & Koren, 2006). Use of St. John's wort dates back to the Middle Ages, when it was used to treat insanity resulting from "attacks of the devil." It was named *St. John's* in reference to St. John's Day on the medieval church calendar because it blooms near that day (June 24). *Wort* is the old English word for a medicinal plant. It is native to Great Britain, Wales, and northern

Europe. Settlers brought it to North America in the 1700s (Balch, 2002), and it is now a common wildflower in the northeastern and north central United States.

Efficacy of St. John's Wort

There is a large body of evidence that indicates that St. John's wort is an effective treatment for depression (Sarris, 2007). Most of the earlier research has been done in Germany, where St. John's wort is the preferred treatment for depression, and where standard antidepressants are tried only after St. John's wort has failed (Linde et al., 1996; Ufer et al., 2007; Wurglies & Schubert-Zsilavecz, 2006). Evidence for St. John's wort's effectiveness can be found in both review articles and in results of randomized clinical trials.

Review Articles

In a meta-analysis of 23 randomized trials, Linde and colleagues (1996) found that *hypericum* extracts were significantly superior to placebos, and were as effective as standard antidepressants in treating depression. They indicated that the rate of study drop-outs and side effects was lower for St. John's wort than antidepressants. Placebo groups (across 13 studies) had an average response rate of 22.3%, compared with 55% of the *hypericum* groups.

A review of 22 studies had similar findings (Whiskey, Werneke, & Taylor, 2001). The authors found that St. John's wort was more effective than a placebo, and as effective as antidepressants. They also concluded that side effects were more common with standard antidepressants than with St. John's wort.

Two recent reviews reached similar conclusions. One review noted that St. John's wort was more effective than a placebo, and comparable to antidepressants, in its effectiveness in 27 trials (Lawvere & Mahoney, 2005). The other review indicated that there was "very strong evidence" of St. John's wort effectiveness for mild to moderate depression (Duguoa et al., 2006).

Data From Clinical Trials

A number of clinical trials have compared the efficacy of St. John's wort to either a placebo or an antidepressant. One trial compared St. John's wort (*Hypericum* Extract STEI 300) to a placebo and the tricyclic antidepressant imipramine. The subjects were 263 primary-care patients with moderate depression. The authors found that St. John's wort was effective for moderately depressed patients after 4, 6, and 8 weeks of treatment (Philipp, Kohnen, & Hiller, 1999). They also found that St. John's wort was as effective as imipramine, and that patients tolerated St. John's wort better, thereby increasing patient compliance.

In another trial (Lecrubier, Clerc, Didi, & Kieser, 2002), 375 patients were randomized to receive either St. John's wort (*Hypericum perforatum* Extract WS 5570) or a placebo for 6 weeks to treat mild to moderate depression. At the end of 6 weeks, patients receiving St. John's wort had significantly lower scores on the Hamilton Depression Rating Scale, and significantly more patients were in remission or had a response to treatment than patients receiving the placebo. Interestingly, both groups had similar rates of adverse effects. Fifty-three percent of the patients in the St. John's wort group responded to treatment compared with 42% of the placebo group. The authors concluded that St. John's wort was safe and effective for the treatment of mild to moderate depression.

Anghelescu and colleagues (2006) compared the efficacy and safety of *Hypericum* Extract WS 5570 to paroxetine for patients with moderate to severe depression. The acute phase of treatment lasted for 6 weeks, with another 4 months follow-up to prevent relapse. The patients improved on both treatments with no significant difference in efficacy. The authors noted that St. John's wort was an important alternative to standard antidepressants for depressed patients.

A 2002 clinical trial had wide press coverage, but unfortunately, much of it was inaccurate regarding the efficacy of St. John's wort (*Hypericum* Depression Trial Study Group, 2002). In this study, 340 adults with major depression were randomly assigned to receive *H Perforatum,* a placebo, or sertraline for 8 weeks. Subjects responding to the medication could opt to receive still-blinded treatment for another 18 weeks. Depression was assessed at baseline and again at 8 weeks. The researchers found no significant difference in depression levels or rate of response between the placebo and St. John's wort. That much was widely reported. What the media did not report was that the same was true for sertraline. The rate of full response was almost identical for the St. John's wort and sertraline groups (24% vs. 25%). The low response rates for both medications suggest some limitations to the study. Eight weeks may not have been sufficient for patients with severe depression to recover. Or the dosages may have been too low. The authors noted that their findings were not unusual in that approximately 35% of studies of standard antidepressants show no greater efficacy than the placebo.

Another study of patients that same year with major depression had opposite findings. This study (Van Gurp, Meterissian, Haiek, McCusker, & Bellavance, 2002) included 87 patients with major depression recruited from Canadian family practice physicians. Patients were randomly assigned to receive either St. John's wort or sertraline. At the end of the 12-week trial, both groups improved, and there was no difference between the two groups. But there were significantly more side effects in the sertraline group at 2 and 4 weeks. The authors concluded that St. John's wort, because of its effectiveness and benign side effects, was a good *first choice* for a primary-care population.

Mechanism for Efficacy

Researchers still do not understand the exact mechanism for St. John's wort's antidepressant effect. Linde et al. (1996) noted that *hypericum* extracts have at least 10 groups of components that may cause its pharmacological effects. St. John's wort is standardized by percentage of hypericin, one of the active constituents. Hypericin was once considered the primary antidepressant component. But that is no longer true (Bratman & Girman, 2003). Hyperforin, another component, is in more recent research hypothesized as the antidepressant constituent (Lawvere & Mahoney, 2005; Muller, 2003; Wurglies & Schubert-Zsilavecz, 2006; Zanoli, 2004). Hyperforin appears to inhibit the reuptake of serotonin, GABA, and L-glutamate (Kuhn & Winston, 2000), and may relieve depression by preventing the reuptake of serotonin, the same mechanism as the selective serotonin reuptake inhibitors (SSRIs). Indeed, Muller (2003) noted that only hyperforin (and its structural analogue, adhyperforin) inhibit neurotransmitter reuptake.

St. John's wort, and particularly hyperforin, also appears to be anti-inflammatory (Balch, 2002; Kuhn & Winston, 2000; Wurglies & Schubert-Zsilavecz, 2006). Hyperforin has antinociceptive (antipain) and anti-inflammatory effects in animal studies (Abdel-Salam, 2005). It inhibits the expression of another inflammatory marker—intercellular adhesion molecule (Zhou et al., 2004). In vitro effects show that St. John's wort is antioxidant, anticyclooxygenase-1, and anticarcinogenic (Zanoli, 2004). In humans, its effects are anti-inflammatory, antibacterial, and antitumor (Dell'Aica, Caniato, Biggin, & Garbisa, 2007).

Only recently has St. John's wort been shown to specifically lower levels of the proinflammatory cytokines involved in depression (Hu et al., 2006). The study used an animal model to test whether St. John's wort could counter the toxic side effects of chemotherapy. The investigators specifically investigated whether St. John's wort had an impact on the levels of proinflammatory cytokines, including IL-1β, IL-2, IL-6, IFN-γ, and TNF-α. They found that St. John's wort did protect rats receiving chemotherapy medications by inhibiting proinflammatory cytokines and intestinal epithelium apoptosis. Although not a study of depression, it was the first to demonstrate that St. John's wort inhibits the cytokines that are high in depression.

Dosage

The dosage is 900 mg of St. John's wort per day (300 mg/three times per day), standardized to 0.3% hypericin and/or 2% to 4% hyperforin (Lawvere & Mahoney, 2005). It generally takes 4 to 6 weeks to take effect (Bratman & Girman, 2003; Ernst, 2002; Kuhn & Winston, 2000). It reaches peak level in the plasma in 5 hours, with a half-life of 24 to 48 hours. Herbalists often combine it with other herbs to address the range of symptoms that depressed people have. Some of these herbs include lemon balm, kava, schisandra, rosemary, black cohosh, and lavender (Kuhn & Winston, 2000).

Safety Concerns

Taken by itself, St. John's wort has an excellent safety record, with a very low frequency of adverse reactions (Ernst, 2002; Muller, 2003). Approximately 2.4% of patients who take St. John's wort develop side effects. The most common are mild stomach discomfort, allergic reactions, skin rashes, tiredness, and restlessness. Like other antidepressants, St. John's wort can trigger an episode of mania in vulnerable patients or patients with bipolar disorder (Bratman & Girman, 2003). St. John's wort can also cause photosensitivity. A review of 38 controlled clinical trials and two meta-analyses on St. John's wort found its safety and side-effect profile to be better than standard antidepressants. The incidence of adverse events ranged from 0% to 6%, which is 10 times less than adverse effects associated with antidepressants (Schultz, 2006).

More concerning is that St. John's wort interacts with several classes of medications, and accelerates the metabolism of anticonvulsants, cyclosporins, birth control pills, and others, leading to lower serum levels of the medication than prescribed (Duguoa et al., 2006; Ernst, 2002; Hale, 2006). It can also interact with prescription antidepressants, and cause a potentially fatal episode of serotonin syndrome (Bratman & Girman, 2003). Prescription antidepressants should not be taken while taking St. John's wort (Harkness & Bratman, 2003). Always encourage mothers who are taking St. John's wort to tell their health care providers that they are taking the herb.

Finding Quality Herbs

Practitioners are often concerned about how consumers can find good quality herbs. That remains a challenge, as the U.S. Pharmacoepia has not yet verified brands of St. John's wort. The U.S. Pharmacopeia (USP) is expected to publish a monograph on St. John's wort in 2008. Until then, there are other ways for consumers to know which brand to buy. ConsumerLabs.com, an independent organization that tests supplements, does rate specific brands. To use its Web site, patients must pay a small subscription fee. Table 6.2 lists additional sources of reliable information on herbs.

Consumers can also closely read the information about the product on the package. While not a guarantee, more reputable companies generally provide more information on how the herbs were processed and the amount of active ingredients in each capsule. Types of information to look for are listed in Table 6.3.

Table 6.2

WHERE TO GO FOR INFORMATION ON HERBS AND HERB SAFETY

WEB SITES ON HERBS/SUPPLEMENTS
www.ConsumerLab.com (rates quality of nutritional products through independent testing)
Institute for Natural Products Research: www.naturalproducts.org
Herbs for Health magazine: www.discoverherbs.com
The Complete German Commission E Monographs available online and for purchase from the American Botanical Council: www.herbalgram.org

Table 6.3

WHAT TO LOOK FOR ON A SUPPLEMENT LABEL
STANDARDS FOR HERBAL PREPARATIONS
Statement of % standardization of the extract
Statement describing which compounds are standardized
Statement describing which parts of the plant are used in the formulation
Extract ratio (the ratio of extract concentration to crude plant materials, e.g., 1:4)
Recommended daily dosage
Weight and number of capsules or tablets per package
Substantiated structure/function claims
Product expiration date to confirm freshness
A toll-free number and/or Website address for company information and contact
USP: Notation that the manufacturer followed standards of the U.S. Pharmacopeia.

From *Pocket Reference Guide to Botanical and Dietary Supplements,* by Dennis McKenna, PhD, 2000, p. 77. Marine on St. Croix, MN: Institute for Natural Products Research. Copyright 2000. Reprinted with permission.

St. John's Wort and Breastfeeding

St. John's wort is generally safe to take while breastfeeding (Dugoua et al., 2006; Hale, 2006). In a case study, Klier and colleagues (2002) examined the pharmacokinetics of St. John's wort in four breast milk samples (including both fore and hind milk) from a mother taking the standard dose of St. John's wort (300 mg/three times per day). They tested the samples for both hypericin and hyperforin and found that only hyperforin was excreted into breast milk, at a low level. Both hyperforin and hypericin were below the level of quantification in the infant's plasma. The authors recommended caution in prescribing this herb to breastfeeding mothers until long-term effects are clear.

More recently, Klier and colleagues (2006) tested 36 breast milk samples from five mothers taking 300 mg of St. John's wort, three times a day.

They also tested the plasma of the five mothers and two infants. As with their earlier case study, they found that only hyperforin was excreted into breast milk, at low levels. Hyperforin was at the limit of quantification in the infants' plasma, with the relative infant doses being 0.9% to 2.5% of the mother's dose. This level of infant exposure is comparable to that of antidepressants. No side effects were noted in either mothers or babies.

A recent review found that there is good evidence to support use of St. John's wort while breastfeeding, but it raised some cautions about St. John's wort during pregnancy (Dugoua et al., 2006). The authors found that taking St. John's wort while breastfeeding affects neither milk supply nor infant weight. They noted that it could cause colic, drowsiness, or lethargy, although only a few cases have been reported. The authors concluded that common and traditional use of St. John's wort caused minimal risk for breastfeeding women and their babies (Dugoua et al., 2006).

When mothers ask about St. John's wort, it is important to suggest that they discuss their options with their health care providers to determine the best approach. Normal use of this medication does not appear to be harmful for mothers or babies. Although hyperforin is excreted into breast milk, it appears in very low levels in infant plasma (in some cases, undetectable).

CONCLUSION

EPA, exercise, and St. John's wort are all effective treatments for even major depression. These modalities are low-cost, well tolerated, and mothers can initiate them themselves. They are also generally safe and have minimal impact on breastfeeding. Omega-3s and exercise can be combined with antidepressants; St. John's wort never should be. In addition, Omega-3s, exercise, and St. John's wort can all be offered as alternatives to mothers who refuse to take medications. As with other treatments for depression, mothers should be monitored to determine whether these techniques are reducing their depression. If not, other options should be added, or tried instead.

REFERENCES

Abdel-Salam, O. M. (2005). Anti-inflammatory, antinociceptive, and gastric effects of *Hypericum perforatum* in rats. *Scientific World Journal, 5*, 586–595.

Akabas, S. R., & Deckelbaum, R. J. (2006). Summary of a workshop on n-3 fatty acids: Current status of recommendations and future directions. *American Journal of Clinical Nutrition, 83,* 1536–1538.

Anghelescu, I. G., Kohnen, R., Szegedi, A., Klement, S., & Kieser, M. (2006). Comparison of *Hypericum* extract WS 5570 and paroxetine in ongoing treatment after recovery from an episode of moderate to severe depression: Results from a randomized multicenter study. *Pharmacopsychiatry, 39,* 213–219.

Babyak, M., Blumenthal, J. A., Herman, S., Khatri, P., Doraiswamy, M., Moore, K., Craighead, W. E., Baldewicz, T. T., & Krishnan, R. R. (2000). Exercise treatment for major depression: Maintenance of therapeutic benefit at 10 months. *Psychosomatic Medicine, 62,* 633–638.

Balch, P. (2002). *Prescription for herbal healing.* New York: Avery.

Bratman, S., & Girman, A. M. (2003). *Handbook of herbs* and *supplements and their therapeutic uses.* St Louis: Mosby.

Cheruku, S. R., Montgomery-Downs, H. E., Farkas, S. L., Thoman, E. B., & Lammi-Keefe, C. J. (2002). Higher maternal plasma docosahexaenoic acid during pregnancy is associated with more mature neonatal sleep-state patterning. *American Journal of Clinical Nutrition, 76,* 608–613.

Coussons-Read, M. E., Okun, M. L., Schmitt, M. P., & Giese, S. (2005). Prenatal stress alters cytokine levels in a manner that may endanger human pregnancy. *Psychosomatic Medicine, 67,* 625–631.

Da Costa, D., Larouche, J., Dritsa, M., & Brender, W. (2000). Psychosocial correlates of prepartum and postpartum depressed mood. *Journal of Affective Disorders, 59,* 31–40.

Daley, A. J., Macarthur, C., & Winter, H. (2007). The role of exercise in treating postpartum depression: A review of the literature. *Journal of Midwifery and Women's Health, 52,* 56–62.

Dell'Aica, I., Caniato, R., Biggin, S., & Garbisa, S. (2007). Matrix proteases, green tea, and St. John's wort: Biomedical research catches up with folk medicine. *Clinical Chimica Acta, 381,* 69–77.

Dhabhar, F. D., & McEwen, B. S. (2001). Bidirectional effects of stress and glucocorticoid hormones on immune function: Possible explanations for paradoxical observations. In R. Ader, D. L. Felten, & N. Cohen (Eds.), *Psychoneuroimmunology* (3rd ed.) (Vol. 1, pp. 301–338). New York: Academic Press.

Dugoua, J-J., Mills, E., Perri, D., & Koren, G. (2006). Safety and efficacy of St. John's wort (*Hypericum*) during pregnancy and lactation. *Canadian Journal of Clinical Pharmacology, 13,* e268–e276.

Dunstan, J. A., Mori, T. A., Barden, A., Beilin, L. J., Holt, P. G., Calder, P. C., Taylor, A. L., & Prescott, S. L. (2004). Effects of n-3 polyunsaturated fatty acid supplementation in pregnancy on maternal and fetal erythrocyte fatty acid composition. *European Journal of Clinical Nutrition, 58,* 429–437.

Dunstan, J. A., Roper, J., Mitoulas, L., Hartmann, P. E., Simmer, K., & Prescott, S. L. (2004). The effect of supplementation with fish oil during pregnancy on breast milk immunoglobulin A, soluble CD14, cytokine levels and fatty acid composition. *Clinical & Experimental Allergy, 34,* 1237–1242.

Emery, C. F., Kiecolt-Glaser, J. K., Glaser, R., Malarky, W. B., & Frid, D. J. (2005). Exercise accelerates wound healing among healthy older adults: A preliminary investigation. *The Journals of Gerontology. Series A, Biological Sciences and Medical Sciences, 60,* 1432–1436.

Ernst, E. (2002). The risk-benefit profile of commonly used herbal therapies: Ginkgo, St. John's wort, ginseng, echinacea, saw palmetto, and kava. *Annals of Internal Medicine, 136,* 42–53.

Ferrucci, L., Cherubini, A., Bandinelli, S., Bartali, B., Corsi, A., Lauretani, F., Martin, A., Andres-Lacueva, C., Senin, U., & Guralnik, J. M. (2006). Relationship of plasma polyunsaturated fatty acids to circulating inflammatory markers. *Journal of Clinical Endocrinology & Metabolism, 91,* 439–446.

Frangou, S., Lewis, M., & McCrone, P. (2006). Efficacy of ethyl-eicosapentaenoic acid in bipolar depression: Randomized double-blind placebo-controlled study. *British Journal of Psychiatry, 188,* 46–50.

Freeman, M. P., Hibbeln, J. R., Wisner, K. L., Davis, J. M., Mischoulon, D., Peet, M., Keck, P. E., Jr., Marangell, L. B., Richardson, A. J., Lake, J., & Stoll, A. L. (2006a). Omega-3 fatty acids: Evidence basis for treatment and future research in psychiatry. *Journal of Clinical Psychiatry, 67,* 1954–1967.

Freeman, M. P., Hibbeln, J. R., Wisner, K. L., Brumbach, B. H., Watchman, M., Gelenberg, A. J. (2006b). Randomized dose-ranging pilot trial of omega-3 fatty acids for postpartum depression. *Acta Psychiatrica Scandanavica, 113,* 31–35.

Goebel, M. U., Mills, P. J., Irwin, M. R., & Ziegler, M. G. (2000). Interleukin-6 and tumor necrosis factor-alpha production after acute psychological stress, exercise, and infused isoproterenol: Differential effects and pathways. *Psychosomatic Research, 62,* 591–598.

Grandjean, P., Bjerve, K. S., Weihe, P., & Steuerwald, U. (2001). Birthweight in a fishing community: Significance of essential fatty acids and marine food contaminants. *International Journal of Epidemiology, 30,* 1272–1278.

Grigoriadis, S., & Ravitz, P. (2007). An approach to interpersonal psychotherapy for postpartum depression: Focusing on interpersonal changes. *Canadian Family Physician, 53,* 1469–1475.

Hale, T. W. (2006). *Medications and mothers' milk* (12th ed.). Amarillo, TX: Hale Publishing.

Hallahan, B., & Garland, M. R. (2005). Essential fatty acids and mental health. *British Journal of Psychiatry, 186,* 275–277.

Harkness, R., & Bratman, S. (2003). *Handbook of drug-herb and drug-supplement interactions.* St. Louis, MO: Mosby.

Hassmen, P., Koivula, N., & Uutela, A. (2000). Physical exercise and psychological well-being: A population study in Finland. *Preventative Medicine, 30,* 17–25.

Hawkes, J. S., Bryan, D-L., Makrides, M., Neumann, M. A., & Gibson, R. A. (2002). A randomized trial of supplementation with docosahexaenoic acid-rich tuna oil and its effects on the human milk cytokines interleukin 1-β, interleukin 6, and tumor necrosis factor α. *American Journal of Clinical Nutrition, 75,* 754–760.

Helland, I. B., Smith, L., Saarem, K., Saugstad, O. D., & Drevon, C. A. (2003). Maternal supplementation with very-long-chain n-3 fatty acids during pregnancy and lactation augments children's IQ at 4 years of age. *Pediatrics, 111,* e39–e44.

Hibbeln, J. R. (2002). Seafood consumption, the DHA content of mothers' milk and prevalence rates of postpartum depression: A cross-national, ecological analysis. *Journal of Affective Disorder,* 69, 15–29.

Hu, Z. P., Yang, X. X., Chan, S. Y., Xu, A. L., Duan, W., Zhu, Y. Z., et al. (2006). St. John's wort attenuates irinotecan-induced diarrhea via down-regulation of intestinal proinflammatory cytokines and inhibition of intestinal epithelial apoptosis. *Toxicology & Applied Pharmacology, 216,* 225–237.

Hypericum Depression Trial Study Group. (2002). Effect of *Hypericum perforatum* (St. John's wort) in major depressive disorder. *Journal of the American Medical Association, 287,* 1807–1814.

Kendall-Tackett, K. A. (2005). *Depression in new mothers.* Binghamton, NY: Haworth.

Kendall-Tackett, K. A. (2007). A new paradigm for depression in new mothers: The central role of inflammation and how breastfeeding and anti-inflammatory treatments protect maternal mental health. *International Breastfeeding Journal,* 2(6), http://www.internationalbreastfeedingjournal.com/content/2/1/6

Kendall-Tackett, K. A. (2008). *Non-pharmacologic treatments for depression in new mothers: The antidepressant effects of omega-3s, exercise, bright light therapy, social support, psychotherapy, and St. John's wort.* Amarillo, TX: Hale Publishing.

Kiecolt-Glaser, J. K., Belury, M. A., Porter, K., Beversdoft, D., Lemeshow, S., & Glaser, R. (2007). Depressive symptoms, omega-6, omega-3 fatty acids, and inflammation in older adults. *Psychosomatic Medicine, 69,* 217–224.

Kiecolt-Glaser, J. K., Loving, T. J., Stowell, J. R., Malarky, W. B., Lemeshow, S., Dickinson, S. L., & Glaser, R. (2005). Hostile marital interactions, proinflammatory cytokine production, and wound healing. *Archives of General Psychiatry, 62,* 1377–1384.

Klier, C. M., Schafer, M. R., Schmid-Siegel, B., Lenz, G., & Mannel, M. (2002). St. John's wort (*Hypericum perforatum*)—Is it safe during breastfeeding? *Pharmacopsychiatry, 35,* 29–30.

Klier, C. M., Schmid-Siegel, B., Schafer, M. R., Lenz, G., Saria, A., Lee, A., & Zernig, G. (2006). St. John's wort (*Hypericum perforatum*) and breastfeeding: Plasma and breast milk concentrations of hyperforin for 5 mothers and 2 infants. *Journal of Clinical Psychiatry, 67,* 305–309.

Konsman, J. P., Parnet, P., & Dantzer, R. (2002). Cytokine-induced sickness behaviour: Mechanisms and implications. *Trends in Neuroscience, 25,* 154–158.

Kuhn, M. A., & Winston, D. (2000). *Herbal therapy and supplements: A scientific and traditional approach.* Philadelphia: Lippincott.

Lane, A. M., Crone-Grant, D., & Lane, H. (2002). Mood changes following exercise. *Perceptual & Motor Skills, 94,* 732–734.

Lawvere, S., & Mahoney, M. C. (2005). St. John's wort. *American Family Physician, 72,* 2249–2254.

Lecrubier, Y., Clerc, G., Didi, R., & Kieser, M. (2002). Efficacy of St. John's wort extract WS 5570 in major depression: A double-blind, placebo-controlled trial. *American Journal of Psychiatry, 159,* 1361–1366.

Linde, K., Ramirez, G., Mulrow, C. D., Pauls, A., Weidenhammer, W., & Melchart, D. (1996). St. John's wort for depression: An overview and meta-analysis of randomized clinical trials. *British Medical Journal, 313,* 253–258.

Maes, M., & Smith, R. S. (1998). Fatty acids, cytokines, and major depression. *Biological Psychiatry, 43,* 313–314.

Malcolm, C. A., McCulloch, D. L., Montgomery, C., Shepherd, A., & Weaver, L. T. (2003). Maternal docosahexaenoic acid supplementation during pregnancy and visual evoked potential development in term infants: A double-blind, prospective, randomized trial. *Archives of Diseases of Childhood, Fetal, and Neonatal Education, 88,* 383–390.

Marangell, L. B., Martinez, J. M., Zboyan, H. A., Chong, H., & Puryear, L. J. (2004). Omega-3 fatty acids for the prevention of postpartum depression: Negative data from a preliminary, open-label pilot study. *Depression & Anxiety, 19,* 20–23.

Mather, A. S., Rodriguez, C., Guthrie, M. F., McHarg, A. M., Reid, I. C., & McMurdo, M.E.T. (2002). Effects of exercise on depressive symptoms in older adults with poorly responsive depressive disorder: Randomized controlled trial. *British Journal of Psychiatry, 180,* 411–415.

McAuley, E., Blissmer, B., Katula, J., Duncan, T. E., & Mihalko, S. L. (2000). Physical activity, self-esteem, and self-efficacy relationships in older adults: A randomized controlled trial. *Annals of Behavioral Medicine, 22,* 131–139.

Muller, W. E. (2003). Current St. John's wort research from mode of action to clinical efficacy. *Pharmacology Research, 47,* 101–109.

Nemets, H., Nemets, B., Apter, A., Bracha, Z., & Belmaker, R. H. (2006). Omega-3 treatment of childhood depression: A controlled, double-blind pilot study. *American Journal of Psychiatry, 163,* 1098–1100.

Noaghiul, S., & Hibbeln, J. R. (2003). Cross-national comparisons of seafood consumption and rates of bipolar disorders. *American Journal of Psychiatry, 160,* 2222–2227.

O'Brien, S. M., Scott, L. V., & Dinan, T. G. (2006). Antidepressant therapy and C-reactive protein levels. *British Journal of Psychiatry, 188,* 449–452.

Olfson, M., Marcus, S. C., Tedeschi, M., & Wan, G. J. (2006). Continuity of antidepressant treatment for adults with depression in the United States. *American Journal of Psychiatry, 163,* 101–108.

Parker, G., Gibson, N. A., Brotchie, H., Heruc, G., Rees, A-M., & Hadzi-Pavlovic, D. (2006). Omega-3 fatty acids and mood disorders. *American Journal of Psychiatry, 163,* 969–978.

Peet, M., & Horrobin, D. F. (2002). A dose-ranging study of the effects of ethyl-eicosapentaenoate in patients with ongoing depression despite apparently adequate treatment with standard drugs. *Archives of General Psychiatry, 59,* 913–919.

Peet, M., & Stokes, C. (2005). Omega-3 fatty acids in the treatment of psychiatric disorders. *Drugs, 65,* 1051–1059.

Philipp, M., Kohnen, R., & Hiller, K-O. (1999). *Hypericum* extract versus imipramine or placebo in patients with moderate depression: Randomized multicenter study of treatment for eight weeks. *British Medical Journal, 319,* 1534–1539.

Quinn, T. J., & Carey, G. B. (1999). Does exercise intensity or diet influence lactic acid accumulation in breast milk? *Medicine and Science in Sports and Exercise, 31,* 105–110.

Rees, A-M., Austin, M-P., & Parker, G. (2005). Role of omega-3 fatty acids as a treatment for depression in the perinatal period. *Australia & New Zealand Journal of Psychiatry, 39,* 274–280.

Rupke, S. J., Blecke, D., & Renfrow, M. (2006). Cognitive therapy for depression. *American Family Physician, 73,* 83–86.

Sarris, J. (2007). Herbal medicines in the treatment of psychiatric disorders: A systematic review. *Phytotherapy Research, 21,* 703–716.

Schultz, V. (2006). Safety of St. John's wort extract compared to synthetic antidepressants. *Phytomedicine, 13,* 199–204.

Shoji, H., Franke, C., Campoy, C., Rivero, M., Demmelmair, H., & Koletzko, B. (2006). Effect of docosahexaenoic acid and eicosapentaenoic acid supplementation on oxidative stress levels during pregnancy. *Free Radical Research, 40,* 379–384.

Singh, N. A., Clements, K. M., & Fiatarone Singh, M. A. (2001). The efficacy of exercise as a long-term antidepressant in elderly subjects: A randomized, controlled trial. *Journal of Gerontology, 56A,* M497–M504.

Smuts, C. M., Huang, M., Mundy, D., Plasse, T., Major, S., & Carlson, S. E. (2003). A randomized trial of docosahexaenoic acid supplementation during the third trimester of pregnancy. *Obstetrics & Gynecology, 101,* 469–479.

Starkweather, A. R. (2007). The effects of exercise on perceived stress and IL-6 levels among older adults. *Biological Nursing Research, 8,* 1–9.

Suarez, E. C., Lewis, J. C., Krishnan, R. R., & Young, K. H. (2004). Enhanced expression of cytokines and chemokines by blood monocytes to in vitro lipopolysaccharide stimulation are associated with hostility and severity of depressive symptoms in healthy women. *Psychoneuroendocrinology, 29,* 1119–1128.

Sublette, M. E., Hibbeln, J. R., Galfalvy, H., Oquendo, M. A., & Mann, J. J. (2006). Omega-3 polyunsaturated essential fatty acid status as a predictor of future suicide risk. *American Journal of Psychiatry, 163,* 1100–1102.

Tanskanen, A., Hibbeln, J. R., Tuomilehto, J., Uutela, A., Haukkala, A., Viinamaki, H., Lehtonen, J., & Vartiainen, E. (2001). Fish consumption and depressive symptoms in the general population of Finland. *Psychiatric Service, 52,* 529–531.

Ufer, M., Meyer, S. A., Junge, O., Selke, G., Volk, H. P., Hedderich, J., & Gleiter, C. H. (2007), Patterns and prevalence of antidepressant drug use in the German state of Baden-Wuerttemberg: A prescription-based analysis. *Pharmacoepidemiology & Drug Safety, 16*(10), 1153–1160.

Van Gurp, G., Meterissian, G. B., Haiek, L. N., McCusker, J., & Bellavance, F. (2002). St. John's wort or sertraline?: Randomized controlled trial in primary care. *Canadian Family Physician, 48,* 905–912.

Whiskey, E., Werneke, U., & Taylor, D. (2001). A systematic review and meta-analysis of *Hypericum perforatum* in depression: A comprehensive clinical review. *International Clinical Psychopharmacology, 16,* 239–252.

Wurglies, M., & Schubert-Zsilavecz, M. (2006). *Hypericum perforatum:* A "modern" herbal antidepressant: Pharmacokinetics of active ingredients. *Clinical Pharmacokinetics, 45,* 449–468.

Zanoli, P. (2004). Role of hyperforin in the pharmacological activities of St. John's wort. *Clinical Nurse Specialist, 10,* 203–218.

Zhou, C., Tabb, M. M., Sadatrafiei, A., Grun, F., Sun, A., & Blumberg, B. (2004). Hyperforin, the active component of St. John's wort, induces IL-8 expression in human intestinal epithelial cells via a MAPK-dependent, NF-kappaB-independent pathway. *Journal of Clinical Immunology, 24,* 623–636.

7 Stress System Dysregulation in Perinatal Mood Disorders

SANDRA N. JOLLEY AND TRICIA SPACH

Most research into the etiology of perinatal mood disorders (PMD) has been conducted over the last 30 years and has focused primarily on psychosocial risk factors, such as marital discord, history of life stress, stress in the previous year, history of depression, family history of depression, and poor social support (Beck & Indman, 2005). Most clinicians who work with women with perinatal mood disorders, however, feel strongly that there is a biological basis for perinatal mood disorders, a premise based on dramatic changes in a woman's mood during pregnancy and postpartum. Various hypotheses posit neuroendocrine dysfunction in the perinatal period as the likely culprit. Studies seeking to elucidate differences between depressed and nondepressed groups have focused on progesterone and estrogen with conflictual results. Fewer studies have focused on the role of cortisol, a principal hormone of the stress system (Hypothalamic-Pituitary-Adrenal Axis (HPA). The stress system (HPA axis) has been the focus of much research in general depression and anxiety literature with significant findings when differences between depressed and nondepressed groups are compared. Because of the dramatic hormonal increases (particularly estrogen and progesterone) during pregnancy and rapid postpartum drops affecting HPA axis regulation, perinatal women may be at increased risk for HPA dysregulation resulting in mood disorders. The purpose of this chapter is to provide the clinician with an overview of brain physiology of the stress system as a foundation for understanding how the hormonal changes in the perinatal period may make some women more vulnerable to mood disorders.

HYPOTHALAMIC-PITUITARY-ADRENAL AXIS

Before the complex hormonal changes of pregnancy and postpartum are discussed, it is important to understand the normal physiologic functioning of the HPA axis in mentally healthy women. The HPA axis, in conjunction with other neurological systems, promotes adaptation and regulation of stress and effect (Elenkov & Chrousos, 2006). When the stress system is activated, physical and emotional stressors set into motion central and peripheral responses designed to respond appropriately to stress, regulate homeostasis, and increase the woman's chances for survival. The behavioral responses to stress include arousal, alertness, and heightened attention. Energy in the form of oxygen and nutrients are directed to the stressed body site and to the central nervous system (CNS) where they are needed most. The HPA axis interacts with many other systems and constantly receives information from higher centers of the CNS, the periphery, the environment, and peripheral actions. Accordingly, this system, a highly complex physiologic network, regulates the dynamic equilibrium of humans. In healthy women (those without psychiatric illness), this system is well regulated by appropriate stimulation and inhibition systems that work in concert to maintain homeostasis during stressful situations. (See Figure 7.1.)

Corticotrophin releasing hormone (CRH, also called CRF, corticotrophin releasing factor) primarily controls the HPA axis. It also serves as the driver of the stress-induced adrenocorticotropin hormone (ACTH)-cortisol secretion (Strauss & Barbieri, 2004), as well as mediates and integrates endocrine, visceral, behavioral, and immune responses to stress; as such, it plays a pivotal role in regulating the stress system. CRH, a polypeptide derived from the paraventricular nucleus of the hypothalamus (brain), stimulates secretion of ACTH from the anterior pituitary (brain), which results in cortisol release from the adrenal cortex (abdomen). (See Figure 7.2.) In healthy adults, CRH, ACTH, and cortisol are released in a pulsatile fashion within a circadian rhythm (Buckley & Schatzberg, 2005). CRH is under negative feedback regulation by circulating cortisol, which inhibits CRH release and thus decreases ACTH and cortisol levels to keep the system in balance. In times of stress, cortisol

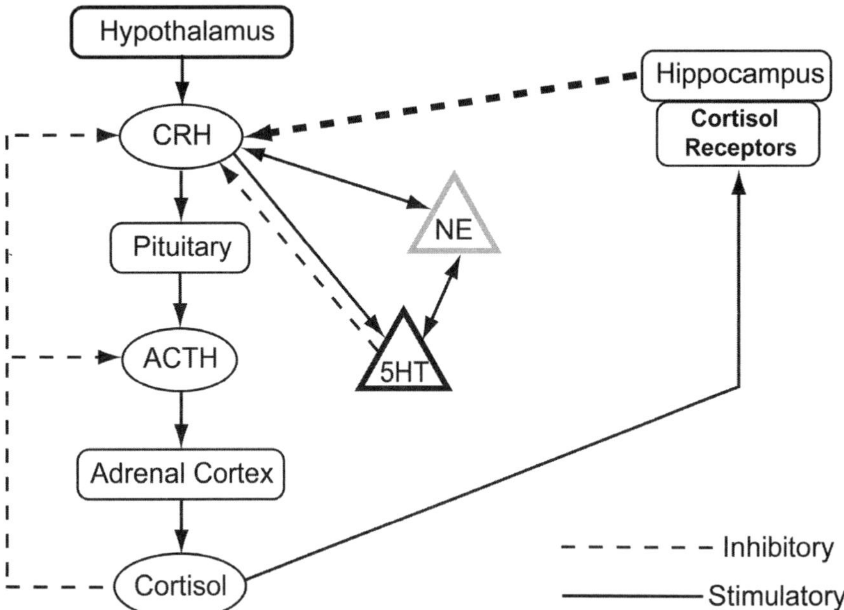

FIGURE 7.1 Normal regulation of HPA.

is released from the adrenal cortex, after stimulation by ACTH, which is released from the anterior pituitary via the bloodstream. Cortisol helps support the increased metabolic needs during "flight or fight" and the need for heightened arousal responses (Carlson, 2006). The adaptive function of the HPA axis is critically dependent on glucocorticoid (cortisol) feedback mechanisms to dampen the stressor-induced activation of the HPA axis and to shut off further glucocorticoid secretion (Jacobson & Sapolosky, 1991). Hence, once a stressor abates, the systems returns to a prestressful-event state of homeostasis.

The HPA axis interacts and influences a large array of neurological, hormonal, and immune systems, including reproductive hormones (GNRH, LH, FSH, estrogen, progesterone), neurotrophins, thyroid hormone, growth hormone, opioids, catecholamines, serotonin, neuropeptides, and cytokines. The HPA axis system also interfaces with many other neurological systems. Collectively, this broad influence of the HPA axis is even more important as it provides a primary link and perhaps interplays between constitutional and psychosocial influences in the development of mood states.

One of the most important systems that affect the regulation of the HPA axis is the limbic system. The limbic system is a set of interconnected

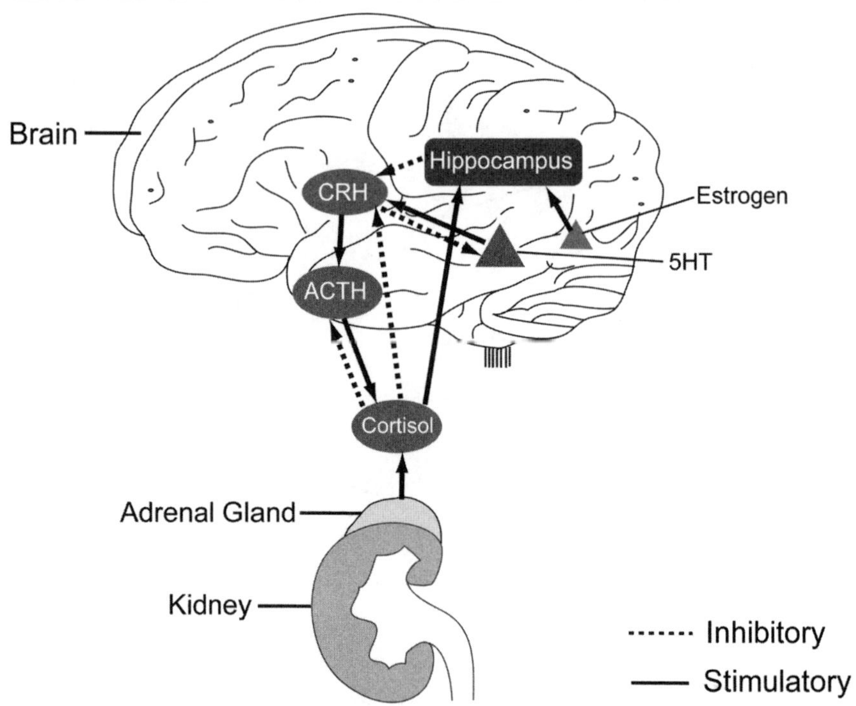

FIGURE 7.2 The brain and mood.

brain structures that includes the limbic cortex, the hippocampus, and the amygdala. The primary function of the limbic system is to process experiences by connecting lower vegetative brain areas and higher cortical centers. Past experiences help them determine whether an event is threatening or otherwise stressful and help to determine the behavioral, neuroendocrine, and autonomic responses. The amygdala is important in the memory of fearful and emotionally laden events, whereas the hippocampus is concerned with determining the context in which such events take place as well as other aspects of episodic and declarative memory (Carlson, 2006; Charney & Nestler, 2004).

Stimulators of the HPA Axis

Norepinephrine (NE)

Norepinephrine is released from the Locus coeruleus (LC) and affects widespread regions in the brain (Carlson, 2006), including CRH. NE and CRH have a positive feedback loop whereby NE stimulates CRH and CRH stimulates NE. Norepinephrine plays a critical role in organizing the behavioral state, particularly in arousal, vigilance, activation of the stress response, and modulation of memory systems, especially to aversive stimuli.

Amygdala

The amygdala is a part of the limbic system and acts as a primary stimulator of the stress response (Charney & Nestler, 2004). Specifically, the amygdala plays a role in identifying feelings and expressions of emotions, formation of emotional memories, and recognition of emotional cues expressed by other people. CRF in the hypothalamus (HPA axis) and NE in the locus coeruleus are both stimulated by the central nucleus of the amygdala. The amygdala responds positively to glucocorticoids and activates the NE component of the stress system (Herman, Ostrander, Mueller, & Figueiredo, 2005). Functionally, stress results in increased CRF concentrations in the amygdala. Several studies have shown that CRF when administered directly into the amygdala induces many fearful and anxious behaviors.

Estrogen

It is well known that estrogens regulate the hypothalamus for reproductive function. However, it was discovered that estrogens also function as neurotransmitters in the brain. Estrogens stimulate the HPA axis through the direct stimulation of CRH and NE systems (Elenkov & Chrousos, 2006). During her reproductive years, a normal cycling woman experiences monthly fluctuation of circulating estrogen that may affect her behavior and mood. Studies have shown that the period of peak estrogen (estradiol) secretion immediately before ovulation is associated with elevations in mood whereas the lowest period of estrogen at estrous is associated with depressed mood and more suicide attempts (Mastorakos & Ilias, 2003). Estrogen also stimulates the serotonergic system resulting in improved mood and cognition, and thus may affect mood changes in childbearing women.

Estrogen also acts as a promoter of neurogenesis (making new neurons), particularly in the hippocampus (Tanapat, Hastings, Reeves, & Gould, 1999), and high estrogen levels during pregnancy are thought to have a protective effect on the dentate gyrus, when cortisol levels are higher. Certain types of acute and chronic stress, including high cortisol levels, inhibit neurogenesis including depression and posttraumatic stress disorder (Herman et al., 2005).

Inhibitors of the HPA Axis

Prefrontal Cortex

The prefrontal cortex is also thought to inhibit the release of CRH and the amygdala. The prefrontal cortex is involved in executive function such as formulating plans and strategies. It also functions as a break or inhibitor of the HPA axis, helping to keep it regulated.

Hippocampus

The primary role of the hippocampus in the HPA system is terminating the stress response through the inhibition of CRH. Research has shown that the hippocampal formation controls the stress axis in a complex manner by modulating basal levels, controlling the magnitude of the initial stress response, and by terminating this response. Functionally, the hippocampus, as a central component of the limbic circuitry, plays a fundamental role in controlling aspects of cognitive and behavioral functions through integration of both the psychological and physiological responses to stress. The hippocampus also inhibits the amygdala, a region that stimulates both CRF in the hypothalamus and NE in the LC (Kaufman & Charney, 2000).

The hippocampus contains an abundance of two corticosteroid receptors: type I and type II receptors (Jacobson & Sapolsky, 1991). These work to inhibit ACTH secretion and play a central role in regulating the adrenocortical activity at the hypothalamic level (Jacobson & Sapolsky, 1991). This high concentration of corticosteroid receptors functions not only to modulate the stress response at a cellular level, but also induces cellular memory formation called long-term potentiation (LTP), a process essential to certain types of learning and memory formation (Kim, Song, & Kosten, 2006). Under normal conditions, the abundance of corticosteroid receptors enables humans to efficiently adapt to stress and to form memories that aid in cognitive adaptations. As the level of stress increases, either in duration or intensity, these same receptors play a role in durable changes within the hippocampus, including modifications to synaptic plasticity, suppression of adult neurogenesis, and changes to the neuronal cell size (Kim et al., 2006). Hence, there exists a window or optimal level of stress whereby receptors serve adaptively; levels beyond that window imbue a cytotoxic environment, resulting in long-term changes at both a cellular and functional level (Kim et al., 2006). These changes are thought to lead to loss of feedback inhibition of the HPA axis, atrophy of the hippocampus, and perhaps to the cognitive deficits seen in depression (Warner-Schmidt & Duman, 2006).

HPA Axis Regulation in Response to Challenge

Psychological or physiological challenges stimulate increased release of CRH from the hypothalamus, initiating a cascade of events that include increased secretion of ACTH from the anterior pituitary and subsequently increased cortisol from the adrenal cortex. The HPA axis is stringently constrained by negative feedback systems, including cortisol receptors and ATCH receptors in the anterior pituitary, hypothalamus, hippocampus, and CRH autoreceptors in the hypothalamus. This abundance of regulation supports HPA homeostasis, including a return to baseline after perturbation (Gold & Chrousos, 2002).

HPA Regulation in General Depression and Anxiety Disorders

Depression research consistently demonstrates changes in the responsiveness and regulation of the HPA axis (Gold & Chrousos, 2002). HPA regulation (the return to normal homeostasis after an episode of activation) relies on properly functioning negative and positive HPA feedback systems (Berntson & Cacioppo, 2000; Ramsay & Lewis, 2003). Failure of these systems and thus of the HPA axis to respond to negative feedback is termed *dysregulation*. Increased CRH, ACTH, and cortisol levels are among the strongest biological findings in major depression, also called *melancholic depression* (Gold & Chrousos, 2002). These changes in HPA axis hormones are associated with symptoms of depression, dysphoria, increased levels of anxiety, anhedonia, and loss of cognitive and affective flexibility, hyperarousal, decreased concentration, decreased sleep, and weight loss (Gold & Chrousos, 2002). Moreover, elevations in CRH result in decreased responsiveness of CRH receptors located in the anterior pituitary. Elevations in cortisol result in attenuated hippocampal glucocorticoid receptor function leading to disinhibition of the hypothalamus (Lee, Ogle, & Sapolsky, 2002). HPA function seen in melancholic depression is an example of HPA dysregulation. Baseline ACTH and cortisol levels generally do not differ between groups of research participants with and without major depression, but significant differences are reported when ACTH and cortisol release are stimulated with either psychologic or physiologic stressors (Holsboer, 2001; Reidel et al., 2002). The most common physiologic methods used in human depression research to stimulate ACTH and cortisol levels are Dexamethasone, ovine CRH, or a combination of both (Ising et al., 2005; Kunzel et al., 2003).

HPA Regulation During Pregnancy

Dramatic changes in the HPA axis occur during pregnancy as a result of the tremendous changes in estrogen and progesterone in pregnancy (Mastorakos & Ilias, 2003). An appreciation of HPA axis regulation during pregnancy and postpartum is critical to our understanding of PPD (Charmandari, Tsigos, & Chrousos, 2005; Gold & Chrousos, 2002). During pregnancy, part of the complexity of the hormonal increases of estrogen, progesterone, CRH, and cortisol is the integrated role and constant interaction of the fetus, placenta, and mother. The placenta is an incomplete producer of these hormones and must rely on precursors reaching it from the fetus and the mother, conceptually termed the feto-placental-maternal unit. Maternal concentrations of estrogen (especially estriol) levels increase during pregnancy at least 800-fold, and are at the highest levels ever in humans. Progesterone levels increase about 15 times during pregnancy.

During pregnancy the placenta secretes increasingly greater amounts of CRH (de Weerth & Buitelaar, 2005), with a 20- to 25-fold increase in placental CRH through 31 weeks of gestation (Sandman et al., 2006). The bioactivity of the increasing placental CRH, which does not have a circadian rhythm, is controlled through most of the pregnancy by CRH-binding protein. However, CRH-binding protein is significantly reduced (by two-thirds) in the third trimester (Strauss & Barbieri, 2004), releasing elevated levels of placental CRH. Cortisol levels normally increase 3-fold, maternal hypothalamic CRH and placental CRH both stimulate the anterior pituitary to increase ACTH, which in turn stimulates the secretion of maternal cortisol from the adrenal cortex. Maternal plasma CRH levels are positively correlated to plasma ACTH and cortisol levels, which are also correlated to CRH, resulting in the hypercortisolism of

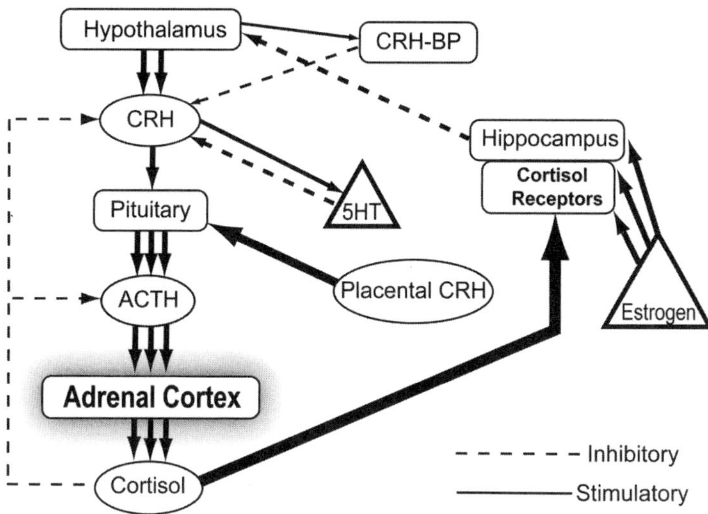

FIGURE 7.3 Regulation of HPA in month 8–9 of pregnancy.

pregnancy (de Weerth & Buielaar, 2005; Strauss & Barbieri, 2004; Wadhwa, Sandman, Chicz-DeMet, & Porto, 1997).

Increased glucocorticoids initiate the negative loop feedback of the HPA axis, inhibiting the maternal release of ACTH and CRH. But the same cortisol released from the adrenal cortex has a positive feedback loop with placental CRH, which continues to stimulate the pituitary ACTH and cortisol secretion (de Weerth & Buitelaar, 2005; Jones, Brooks, & Challis, 1989; Robinson, Emanuel, Frim, & Majzoub, 1988). Cortisol levels peak at 34–36 weeks gestation and correlate with fetal lung maturation due to hypertrophy of the adrenal cortex. Postpartum, the cortisol levels decrease to normal levels in 4–5 days (Strauss & Barbieri, 2004). This information suggests that the elevated CRH levels of pregnancy have the opportunity to affect the regulation of the maternal HPA axis. (See Figure 7.3.)

Birth and Postpartum

With the removal of the placenta at birth, progesterone, estrogen, and CRH levels drop dramatically, reaching prepregnancy levels by the 5th postpartum day. Cortisol levels also fall abruptly after delivery, but the hypertrophied adrenal cortex returns to normal at about 4–5 days postpartum. (See Figure 7.4.)

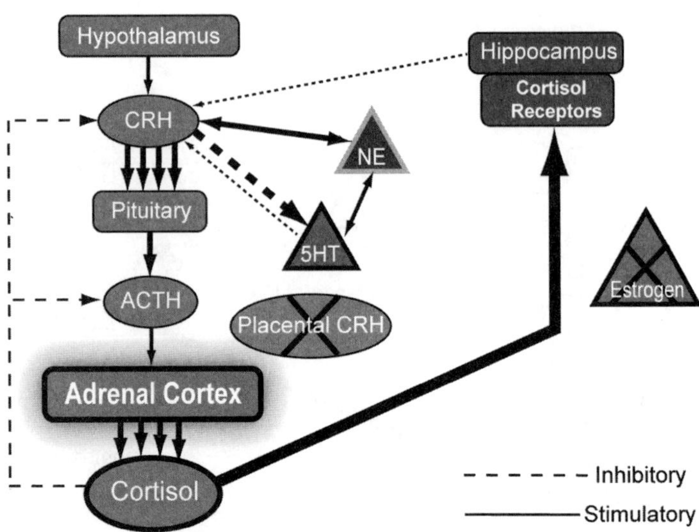

FIGURE 7.4 Regulation of HPA early postpartum.

HPA IN PERINATAL MOOD DISORDERS

Pregnancy

The hormonal changes during pregnancy affect other neurological systems, including serotonin, norepinephrine, and dopamine, which have been implicated in the pathogenesis of depression and anxiety disorders (Garlow & Nemeroff, 2004). It may be that the effects of placental CRH are more troublesome in individuals predisposed to depression from either constitutional factors or prior experience. Most of the research describing the neurobiology of mood disorders in pregnancy has focused on the effects of the stress system (HPA axis) on infant neurodevelopment and behavioral outcomes, which is not the topic of this discussion (de Weerth & Buitelaar, 2005).

Only a few studies have compared cortisol levels during pregnancy between women with mood disorders and those without mood disorders. Total 24-hour urinary cortisol measured between the 16th and 29th week of gestation was significantly correlated with NE, depression (CES-D; Radloff, 1977), state anxiety (STAI; Edicott & Spitzer, 1978), and stress (Daily Hassles Scale), measured at the same time (Diego et al., 2006).

In another recent study, anxiety state and mood state were compared with a series of stimulated cortisol in pregnant women who had no evidence of mood disorders (Nierop, Bratsikas, Zimmermann, & Ehlert, 2006). Comparisons were made across two groups: identified between 2 and 27 days (mean 13 days) postpartum as probable cases and non-probable cases from results of the Edinburgh Postpartum Screening Scale (EPDS; Cox, Holden, & Sagovsky, 1987). The Trier Social Stress Test (TSST; Kirschbaum, Pirke, & Hellhammer, 1993), a psychosocial stimulation, consists of an unprepared speech (5 minutes), and a mental arithmetic task performed in front of an audience. A series of salivary cortisols were taken, one at baseline before the TSST was introduced, one 10 minutes before the test began, one immediately before and after the TSST, and then an additional five samples taken at 10, 20, 30, 45 and 60 minutes. There was no difference at baseline between the two groups, but the salivary cortisol reactivity (mean and standard deviation) in probable cases was significantly higher than the nonprobable cases. This study demonstrates that women who have psychological stress during pregnancy (but an absence of a psychiatric diagnosis) exhibit elevated cortisol levels during pregnancy and may be at risk for developing postpartum depression (Nierop et al., 2006).

Postpartum

Research on the biologic underpinnings of PPD has focused on the HPA axis; however, it has been hindered by simplistic conceptual models that obscure the complexity of physiology in the transition from pregnancy to postpartum (Rubinow, 2005). Studies of the HPA axis in postpartum women are few in number and focus primarily on cortisol. Several studies have measured postpartum cortisol levels and found no relationship with mood (Abou-Saleh, Ghubash, Karim, Krymski, & Bhai, 1998; Corwin, Brownstead, Barton, Heckhard, & Morin, 2005; Groer et al., 2005; Harris et al., 1996; Hohlagschwandtner, Husslein, Klier, & Ulm, 2001; Nappi et al., 2001; O'Hara, Lewis, Schlechte, & Varner, 1991; Taylor, Dore, & Glover, 1996). The sampling of cortisol (blood or saliva) in these studies occurred only on one occasion from day 1 to day 35 postpartum, but the samples were taken only once a day, usually in the morning. In a seminal study by O'Hara, salivary cortisol was measured at 1, 2, 3, 4, 6, 8 days postpartum (O'Hara, 1995) with no differences found in daily cortisol between the depressed and nondepressed groups. But when a P.M. salivary cortisol measure was added to an A.M. cortisol level and measured daily for the first 35 postpartum days, significant differences between the depressed and nondepressed groups were found (Harris et al., 1996). The postpartum depressed women ($n = 7$) had significantly lower evening cortisol levels when compared with the nondepressed postpartum women ($n = 113$). Single or daily samples of cortisol may not be adequate to fully describe HPA axis regulation. Multiple samples of ACTH and cortisol at 10–20 minute intervals are optimal to measure the ACTH to cortisol relationship, required to assess the regulation or dysregulation of the HPA axis and associated mood (Keenan, Roelfsema, & Veldhuis, 2004).

A recent study used maximal treadmill exercise to stimulate ACTH and cortisol levels at 6 and 12 weeks postpartum (Jolley, Elmore, Barnard, & Carr, 2007). In a sample of 22 postpartum women who were not depressed during pregnancy, a significant difference in the relationship of lag ACTH to cortisol was found between the depressed and nondepressed postpartum women. Women who experienced postpartum depression had dysregulated ACTH and cortisol relationships due to higher ACTH levels and lower cortisols. The nondepressed group had the expected, regulated correlation between lag ACTH and cortisol; as ACTH increased, cortisol also increased (Jolley et al., 2007). (See Figure 7.5.)

Dysregulation of the HPA axis may influence immune system changes in women with PPD (Groer & Morgan, 2007). Evidence suggests that

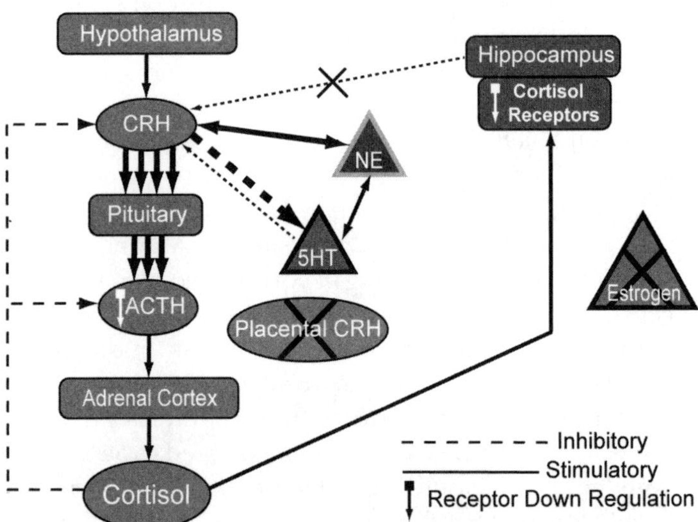

FIGURE 7.5 Regulation of HPA early postpartum depression.

women with lower salivary cortisol levels at 4–6 weeks postpartum who also met the criteria for PPD reported more symptoms of infection, more fatigue, more daytime sleepiness, and higher levels of perceived stress, postpartum stress, and negative life events ($n = 25$). They also tended to be younger with a mean age of 23 ($p < .06$) and only 32% breastfed their newborns compared to 55% of the nondepressed mothers. In addition, these same women had lower serum and whole blood levels of Interferon-gamma (INF-γ) and lower INF-γ/Interleukin-10 ratios, implying changes to the Th1/Th2 ratio (T-cells involved in cellular and humoral immunity, respectively). These findings point to a link between dysregulation of the HPA axis and altered cellular immunity in women with PPD (Groer & Morgan, 2007). The interaction between mood and the immune system should therefore be considered in planning treatment for women with PPD as altered cellular immunity may compromise a woman's ability to fight viral illnesses or fungal infections, which could add to the physiological stress seen in new mothers and women with PPD.

CASE STUDY ILLUSTRATING POSTPARTUM DEPRESSION AND HPA DYSREGULATION

Krista is a 27-year-old family practice resident who participated in a study measuring cortisol levels in postpartum women (for protocol details, see Jolley et al., 2007). Since the birth of her daughter, Krista has experienced the following symptoms: anhedonia, sleep disturbance, feelings of guilt and worthlessness, low energy, difficulty concentrating, feeling overwhelmed, weight loss, and intense feelings of maternal inadequacy. Her scores on the Postpartum Depression Screening Scale at intervals 3, 6, and 12 weeks postpartum and at 6 and 12 months postpartum (Beck & Gable, 2002) indicate significant symptoms of postpartum depression. The following narrates significant aspects of her life history and provides clinical details of the events surrounding the birth of her baby.

Krista grew up in a small town in Arkansas as the fourth child in a family of six children. At age 15, her family moved to New Mexico where she completed high school and attended college. She describes her childhood as rather typical, with a close-knit immediate and extended family. She denies any family history of psychiatric illness. She also denies any physical, emotional, or sexual abuse, although she recalls one incident where her father whipped her with a belt at age 4. As a child, she felt closer to her dad despite his strict disciplinary style and threats to "use the belt" when she misbehaved. She describes her relationship with her mother as distant and lacking in affection. She notes that her maternal grandmother provided more closeness and warmth than her own mother and to this day feels quite close to her grandmother. Currently, she reports a good relationship with both her parents and visits them twice a year. She also talks to her mother by phone twice per week.

An assessment of past trauma and losses reveals several significant life events. At age 9, Krista's three teenage sisters were in a car accident that resulted in the death of a close family friend. All her sisters were injured, and the one closest to her in age sustained a severe head injury and was comatose for 2 weeks. At age 12, Krista's grandfather died. During his illness, Krista spent hours in the intensive care unit waiting room, but wasn't allowed visitation. Krista and her brother were home alone when they received the news of his death. At age 16, Krista miscarried an unplanned first trimester pregnancy. Unaware of her pregnancy, the miscarriage came as a surprise. She cried in response to the loss but also knew it was a blessing. Shortly thereafter, she and her boyfriend separated. In college, Krista's close girlfriend died in a car accident and Krista was not able to attend the funeral because of work obligations in another state. This was devastating and to this day Krista struggles with unresolved feelings about her close friend's death and her failure to attend the funeral.

One year prior to the birth of her baby, Krista's former boss and mentor was killed in an automobile accident. Krista felt quite close to this man as he was instrumental in her decision to attend medical school and she had hoped to join his family practice in Wyoming upon completion of her residency. Because of the demands of her residency, however, she did not attend his funeral. She describes this experience as "blowing me away."

Krista and her husband of 2 years were overjoyed at the news of this planned pregnancy. The timing, though challenging, seemed ideal. Her pregnancy was uneventful and without medical complications. At 40 weeks gestation, she began bleeding and was taken immediately to the hospital where she had an emergency cesarean section because of a placental abruption. Krista was awake for the delivery with her husband and friend in attendance. She gave birth to a healthy infant daughter. On a scale of 1 to 16 that rates a mother's overall birth experience, she recorded a 5.1 on a line with "traumatic" at one end (0) and "ecstasy" at the other end (16).

Krista breastfed her daughter for 1 year and pumped breast milk while at work. She continued with her medical training and sustained PPDS scores reflective of depression. These scores were highest at 3 weeks postpartum (92) and stabilized at 6 weeks postpartum, between 60–65 where they remained for the next 11 months. Scores from 60–79 indicate significant symptoms of postpartum depression, and scores of 80 and above indicate major postpartum depression (Beck & Gable, 2000).

At 6 and 12 weeks postpartum Krista's baseline cortisol levels were 4.8 ug/dl and 5.4 ug/dl, respectively, and were similar to other median levels in the group of women with postpartum depression (4.8 ug/dl and 5.5 ug/dl). The nondepressed group medians were higher at baseline, with the median level of 7.2 ug/ml and 6.6 ug/ml, respectively. After stress induction (exercise at 90% VO_2 max), Krista's *peak* cortisol level at 32 minutes was 7.6 ug/ml, a level that correlates with the *baseline* levels of the nondepressed group. These findings indicate not only a lower baseline cortisol level but also a blunted response to stress challenges, therefore suggesting dysregulation of the HPA axis.

Krista's baseline levels of ACTH at 6 weeks postpartum (13.4 pg/ml) were similar to the nondepressed baseline median (13.4 pg/ml) in the nondepressed group, but her peak ACTH levels were considerably higher (27.8 pg/ml) than the nondepressed group median (21.1 pg/ml). It is expected in a normal, regulated HPA axis that as ACTH rises, cortisol also rises accordingly. In this case, lower cortisols and higher ACTH levels could indicate that increasingly, CRH is being released and thus stimulating more and more ACTH, but the adrenal gland is not producing the expected amount of cortisol; less cortisol results in less negative feedback to inhibit CRH and ACTH and thus, dysregulation ensues.

The clinical application of Krista's cortisol and ACTH levels are best achieved by viewing them in the context of her life narrative. Her history of trauma, multiple losses, and attachment relationships collectively add to her mood state going into pregnancy. Additionally the fear and physical trauma from her emergency surgical birth (secondary to an abruptio placenta) could act as additional stressors, possibly increasing CHR release from the amygdala and further compounding perturbations in her HPA axis during the postpartum. All these events can and should be viewed as stressors, whose potency can activate the HPA axis and lead to physiologically derived symptoms of depression.

Therapist and counselors providing care for women with postpartum mood disorders can integrate this knowledge into their work with women in several key ways. Central to this knowledge is the understanding that all stress, whether physical or psychological, can activate the HPA axis; psychological stress can stimulate the HPA axis as robustly as physical stress. Because research suggests that women with PPD have diminished capacity to physiologically cope with stress regardless of the source, every effort should be made to help the woman structure her daily routines and cognitions such that they are stress-reducing. On a practical level, this may mean that the entire family rallies behind the mother to help her get adequate sleep, exercise, rest, and nutrition, variables known to promote stress reduction. In addition, it may be helpful to correct cognitive distortions, to facilitate expressions of grief and loss, and to teach self-soothing and stress-reducing techniques such as progressive relaxation. Moreover, therapists should assess for a history of loss; unresolved grief; trauma from physical, sexual, or emotional abuse; and trauma from more unusual sources such as early childhood major medical illnesses or procedures, car accidents, severe burns, domestic violence, rape, witness to violence or gruesome accidents, and/or military service. Care should be supportive and consistent with the evidence-based practice and treatment guidelines for those individuals exposed to traumas. In some cases, treatment could include grief counseling for complicated or unresolved grief. In the event that a woman with PPD needs an evaluation for medication, therapists can work in conjunction with a psychiatrist or psychiatric nurse practitioner to coordinate this care and to address the mother's concerns regarding medication use while breastfeeding.

SUMMARY

Caring for women with postpartum depression requires a sophisticated understanding of the myriad factors underpinning the illness. HPA axis dysregulation represents one physiologic aspect of the illness where much more research needs to be conducted to fully understand the relationship between PPD and the HPA axis regulation.

REFERENCES

Abou-Saleh, M., Ghubash, R., Karim, L., Krymski, M., & Bhai, I. (1998). Hormonal aspects of postpartum depression. *Psychoneuroendocrinology, 23*, 465–475.

Beck, C. T., & Gable, R. K. (2000). Postpartum Depression Screening Scale: Development and psychometric testing. *Nursing Research*, *49*(5), 272–282.

Beck, C. T., & Gable, R. K. (2002). *Postpartum Depression Screening Scale (PDSS) manual.* Los Angeles: Western Psychological Services.

Beck, C. T., & Indman, P. (2005). The many faces of postpartum depression. *Journal of Obstretic, Gynecologic, and Neonatal Nursing, 34*(5), 569–576.

Berntson, G., & Cacioppo, J. (2000). From homeostasis to allodynamic regulation. In J. Cacioppo, L. Tassinary, & G. Berntson (Eds.), *Handbook of psychophysiology* (pp. 459–481). Cambridge, England: Cambridge University Press.

Buckley, T. M., & Schatzberg, A. F. (2005). On the interactions of the hypothalamic-pituitary-adrenal (HPA) axis and sleep: Normal HPA axis activity and circadian rhythm, exemplary sleep disorders *Journal of Clinical Endocrinology and Metabolism, 90*(5), 3106–3114.

Carlson, N. R. (2006). *Physiology of behavior.* Boston: Allyn and Bacon.

Charmandari, E., Tsigos, C., & Chrousos, G. P. (2005). Endocrinology of the stress response. *Annual Reviews of Physiology, 67,* 259–284.

Charney, D. S., & Nestler, E. (2004). *Neurobiology of mental illness.* Oxford, England: Oxford University Press.

Corwin, E. J., Brownstead, J., Barton, N., Heckhard, S., & Morin, K. (2005). The impact of fatigue on postpartum depression. *J Obstet Gyneocol Neonatal Nurs, 34*(5), 577–586.

Cox, J. L., Holden, J. M., & Sagovsky, R. (1987). Detection of postnatal depression: Development of the 10-item Edinburgh Postnatal Depression Scale. *British Journal of Psychiatry, 150,* 782–786.

Diego, M. A., Jones, N. A., Field, T., Hernandez-Reif, M., Scjanberg, S., Kuhn, C., & Gonzalez-Garcia, A. (2006). Maternal psychological distress, prenatal cortisol and fetal weight. *Psychosomatic Medicine, 68*(5), 747–753.

de Weerth, C., & Buitelaar, J. (2005). Physiological stress reactivity in human pregnancy—a review. *Neuroscience and Biobehavioral Reviews, 29,* 295–312.

Edicott, J., & Spitzer, R. (1978). A diagnostic review: The Schedule for Affective Disorders and Schizophrenia. *Arch Gen Psychiatry, 35,* 837–844.

Elenkov, I. J., & Chrousos, G. P. (2006). Stress system—organization, physiology and immunoregulation. *Neuroimmunomodulation, 13*(5–6), 257–267.

Garlow, S. J., & Nemeroff, C. B. (2004). The neurochemistry of depressive disorders: Clinical studies. In D. S. Charney & E. J. Nestler (Eds.), *Neurobiology of mental illness* (pp. 440–460). Oxford, England: Oxford University Press.

Gold, P. W., & Chrousos, G. P. (2002). Organization of the stress system and its dysregulation in melancholic and atypical depression, high vs. low CRH/NE states. *Molecular Psychiatry, 7*(3), 254–275.

Groer, M., Davis, M., Casey, K., Short, B., Smith, K. C., & Groer, S. (2005). Neuroendocrine and immune relationships in postpartum fatigue. *MCN Am J Matern Child Nurs, 30*(2), 133–138.

Groer, M. W., & Morgan, K. (2007). Immune, health and endocrine characteristics of depressed postpartum mothers. *Psychoneuroendocrinology, 32*(2), 133–139.

Harris, B., Lovett, L., Smity, J., Read, G., Walker, R., & Newcombe, R. (1996). Cardiff puerperal mood and hormone study. III. Postnatal depression at 5 to 6 weeks postpartum, and its hormonal correlates across the peripartum period. *British Journal of Psychiatry, 168*(6), 739–744.

Herman, J. P., Ostrander, M. M., Mueller, N. K., & Figueiredo, H. (2005). Limbic system mechanisms of stress regulation: Hypothalamo-pituitary-adrenal axis. *Progress in Neuro-Psychopharmacology and Biological Psychiatry, 29*(8), 1201–1213.

Hohlagschwandtner, M., Husslein, P., Klier, C. M., & Ulm, B. (2001). Correlation between serum testosterone levels and peripartal mood states. *Acta Obstet Gynecol Scand, 80,* 326–330.

Holsboer, F. (2001). Stress, hypercortisolism and corticosteroid receptors in depression: Implications for therapy. *Journal of Affective Disorders, 62,* 77–91.

Ising, M., Kunzel, H. E., Binder, E. B., Nickel, T., Modell, S., & Holsboer, F. (2005). The combined dexamethasone/CRH test as a potential surrogate marker in depression. *Progress in Neuro-Psychopharmacology and Biological Psychiatry, 29,* 1085–1093.

Jacobson, L., & Sapolosky, R. (1991). The role of the hippocampus in feedback regulation of the hypothalamic-pituitary-adrenocortical axis. *Endocrine Reviews, 12,* 118–134.

Jolley, S. N., Elmore, S., Barnard, K., & Carr, D. R. (2007). Dysregulation of the hypothalamic-pituitary-adrenal axis in postpartum depression. *Biological Research in Nursing, 8,* 210–222.

Jones, S. A., Brooks, A. N., & Challis, J. R. (1989). Steroids modulate corticotropin releasing hormone production in human fetal membranes and placenta. *Journal of Clinical Endocrinology and Metabolism, 68,* 825–830.

Kaufman, J., & Charney, D. (2000). Comorbidity of mood and anxiety disorders. *Depression and Anxiety 12*(Suppl. 1), 69–76.

Keenan, D. M., Roelfsema, F., & Veldhuis, J. D. (2004). Endogenous ACTH concentration-dependent drive of pulsatile cortisol secretion in the human. *American Journal of Physiology-Endocrinology and Metabolism, 287,* E652–E661.

Kim, J. J., Song, E. Y., & Kosten, T. (2006). Stress effects in the hippocampus: Synaptic plasticity and memory. *Stress, 9*(1), 1–11.

Kirschbaum, C., Pirke, K. M., & Hellhammer, D. H. (1993). The "Trier Social Stress Test"—a tool for investigating psychobiological stress responses in a laboratory setting. *Neuropsychobiology, 28,* 76–81.

Kunzel, H. E., Binder, E. B., Nickel, T., Ising, M., Fuchs, B., Majer, M., Pfennig, A., Ernst, G., Kern, N., Schmid, D. A., Uhr, M., Holsboer, F., & Modell, S. (2003). Pharmacological and nonpharmacological factors influencing hypthalamic-pituitary-adrenocortical axis reactivity in acutely depressed psychiatric in-patients, measured by the Dex-CRH test. *Neuropsychopharmacology, 28,* 2169–2178.

Lee, A. L., Ogle, W. O., & Sapolsky, R. M. (2002). Stress and depression: Possible links to neuron death in the hippocampus. *Bipolar Disorders, 4,* 117–128.

Mastorakos, G., & Ilias, I. (2003). Maternal and fetal hypothalamic-pituitary-adrenal axes during pregnancy and postpartum. *Annals of the New York Academy of Sciences, 997,* 136–149.

Nappi, R. E., Petraglia, F., Luisi, S., Polatti, F., Farina, C., & Genazzani, A. R. (2001). Serum allopregnanolone in women with postpartum "blues." *Obstetrics and Gynecology, 97*(1), 77–80.

Nierop, A., Bratsikas, A., Zimmermann, R., & Ehlert, U. (2006). Are stress-induced cortisol changes during pregnancy associated with postpartum depressive symptoms? *Psychosomatic Medicine, 68,* 931–937.

O'Hara, M. W. (1995). *Postpartum depression: Causes and consequences.* New York: Springer-Verlag.

O'Hara, M. W., Lewis, D. A., Schlechte, J. A., & Varner, M. W. (1991). Controlled prospective study of postpartum mood disorders: Psychological, environmental, and hormonal variables. *Journal of Abnormal Psychology, 100*(1), 63–73.

Radloff, L. S. (1977). The CES-D Scale: A self-report depression scale for research in the general population. *Applied Psychological Measurement, 1*(3), 385–401.

Ramsay, D., & Lewis, M. (2003). Reactivity and regulation in cortisol and behavioral responses to stress. *Child Development, 74*(2), 456–464.

Reidel, W. J., Klassen, T., Griez, E., Honig, A., Menheere, P. P., & van Praag, H. M. (2002). Dissociable hormonal, cognitive and mood responses to neuroendocrine challenge: Evidence for receptor-specific serotonergic dysregulation in depressed mood. *Neuropsychopharmacology, 26*(3), 358–367.

Robinson, B. G., Emanuel, R. L., Frim, D. M., & Majzoub, J. S. (1988). Glucocorticoid stimulates expression of corticotropin-releasing hormone gene in human placenta. *Proceedings of the National Academy of Sciences, 85,* 5244–5248.

Rubinow, D. R. (2005). Reproductive steroids in context. *Archives of Women's Mental Health, 8,* 1–5.

Sandman, C. A., Glynn, L., Schetter, C. D., Wadhwa, P., Garite, T., Chicz-DeMet, A., & Hobel, C. (2006). Elevated maternal cortisol early in pregnancy predicts third trimester levels of placental cortitropin releasing hormone (CRH): Priming the placental clock. *Peptides, 27,* 1457–1463.

Strauss, J., & Barbieri, R. L. (2004). *Yen & Jaffe's reproductive endocrinology: Physiology, pathophysiology, and clinical management.* Philadelphia: W. B. Saunders.

Tanapat, P., Hastings, N. B., Reeves, A. J., & Gould, E. (1999). Estrogen stimulates a transient increase in the number of new neurons in the dentate gyrus of the adult female rat. *Journal of Neuroscience, 19,* 5792–5801.

Taylor, A., Dore, C., & Glover, V. (1996). Urinary phenylethylamine and cortisol levels early in the puerperium. *J Affect Disorders, 37*(2–3), 137–142.

Wadhwa, P. D., Sandman, C. A., Chicz-DeMet, A., & Porto, M. (1997). Placental CRH modulates maternal pituitary adrenal function in human pregnancy. *Ann NY Acad Sci, 814,* 276–281.

Warner-Schmidt, J. L., & Duman, R. S. (2006). Hippocampal neurogenesis: Opposing effects of stress and antidepressant treatment. *Hippocampus, 16,* 239–249.

8 Infertility: Challenges and Complications in Pregnancy and Postpartum

ANDREA MECHANICK BRAVERMAN

Infertility has significant emotional and psychosocial challenges for the women and men who experience it. Infertility is described as a roller coaster ride—each month brings peaks of hope and then valleys of disappointment and loss when menses begins. Throughout the journey, patients carry overriding feelings of anxiety about whether they will ever get to be parents. In addition, feelings of inadequacy, depression, hopelessness, and social isolation often accompany the infertility journey. These issues often do not immediately resolve upon achieving a pregnancy or even with the birth of a much-wanted child. This chapter will address many of the clinical issues and challenges that present to clinicians when working with these women and their partners during pregnancy and the postpartum period.

REVIEW OF THE LITERATURE

There have been few studies following up on women and men who have achieved a pregnancy after infertility. However, there has been much discussion about whether, once pregnancy is achieved, there are any substantive differences in the pregnancy and postpartum experience. Certainly, variables such as the duration of pregnancy attempts, history of pregnancy loss, age, and the demands and intrusiveness of treatment may affect the pregnancy and/or postpartum experience.

Pregnancy after infertility treatment has been referred to as "a premium pregnancy: precious, priceless, and precarious" (Covington & Burns, 2006, p. 440). The literature overall shows that, even if infertility experience does not translate into differences between women who conceived spontaneously and those who conceived through treatment, there are emotional differences between these two expectant parent groups. Certainly, the lay literature articulates these anticipated feelings, as described in the popular book *How to Be a Successful Fertility Patient:*

> Women who can conceive easily probably will think you are being overconcerned, or even paranoid about your pregnancy, but they didn't go through what you went through to get to this point. It may be okay for other pregnant women to keep jogging five miles a day, or work overtime at nights and on weekends, or have a couple of cups of caffeinated coffee a day, but you will want to be more cautious. To give yourself maximum peace of mind, you will probably want to take it easy as much as possible during the first trimester. (Robin, 1993, p. 408)

There have been attempts to compare the experiences of women who conceived after fertility treatment with those who conceived spontaneously. In a study of 74 women who conceived via assisted reproductive technologies (ART) and 40 women who conceived spontaneously, the authors found that the two groups were similar psychologically on dimensions of self-esteem, depression, and anxiety at 12 and 28 weeks of pregnancy (Klock & Greenfield, 2000). Improved self-esteem and decreased anxiety as the pregnancy progressed was found in the ART group and not in the spontaneous conception group.

Similar results were found in another study (Repokari et al., 2006), in which women who conceived via ART were found to have fewer depressive symptoms than the spontaneous conception group, while at 1 year postpartum there were no differences between the two groups. During the transition, spontaneous conception mothers experienced an increase of anxiety symptoms whereas the ART mothers did not. In this study, men were also included. Overall, the fathers through ART reported fewer mental health symptoms than did the spontaneous conception fathers. In addition, social and child-related stressors were found to have negative mental health impact on the spontaneous control couples whereas no impact was found among the ART couples. In a different study, self-esteem did not differ between parents who had conceived through IVF and those who conceived spontaneously (Cox, Glazebrook, Sheard, Ndukwe, & Oates, 2006). All women displayed levels of self-esteem in the normal range.

In a recent Israeli study (Harf-Kashdaei & Kaitz, 2007), no differences were found again between women who conceived through ART and spontaneous conception mothers. The ART mothers did score lower on negative affect and higher on measures of positive mood regarding baby, self and spouse; ART mothers' feelings about their spouse were related to whether he was the sole source of the fertility problem.

Theoretical discussion has focused on the overall and lasting effects of treatment on the previously infertile woman. Olshansky (2003) proposed a theory that infertile new mothers had an increased vulnerability to depression. The basis for this theoretical proposal was the synthesis of a series of grounded theory studies of infertility and pregnancy experiences of women parenting after infertility using a relational cultural theory. In grounded theory studies, the goal is to let the data drive the theory rather than starting the research with a hypothesis. Olshansky and Sereeka (2005) proposed the theory that, due to repeated and sustained interferences with significant relationships over the course of their infertility, previously infertile new mothers were more susceptible to depression. They proposed that a "divided self," wherein a woman presents an outer compliant self while experiencing anger and marital dissatisfaction, is a predictor of postpartum depression in women who delivered following infertility treatment.

Traditional research has not supported the Olshansky and Serieka theory. In a recent Hungarian study (Csatordai et al., 2007), the authors found that infertility was not significant for vulnerability to depression. Another study from the United Kingdom (Brockington, Macdonald, & Wainscott, 2006) considered anxiety rather than depression for vulnerability during pregnancy. Anxiety disorders were found to be more frequent than depression for pregnant women, and the most common theme was fear of fetal death; this fear was associated with a history of reproductive losses or infertility.

Many other factors may influence expectant mothers' feelings and reactions but not result in negative or dysfunctional responses. For example, concerns about multiple births as well as issues related to having children at an older age may contribute to the experience of pregnancy and the postpartum transition. These issues have been addressed in several studies, both as an artifact of the research—for example, finding that women who experience infertility are on average older than women who conceive spontaneously—and as a confound of the research—for example, more multiple pregnancies occur as a result of treatment and raising multiples has significantly different demands than parenting a singleton. This was demonstrated in this 2005 study, in which mothers who conceived through ART were found to be older and to have increased cesarean and multiple birth rates than those women who conceived spontaneously (Fisher, Hammarberg, & Baker, 2005). These factors led the authors to conclude that women who conceived through fertility treatment appear to have an associated risk of an increased rate of early parenting difficulties and thus may require additional support.

The opposite was found in a recent Australian study (McMahon, Gibson, Allen, & Saunders, 2007); the authors concluded that there was not any problematic adjustment to parenting in older couples but the study was limited by a small sample size. In a different study (Steiner & Paulson, 2007), mothers over age 50 were also not found to have increased parenting stress or reduced parenting capacity because of physical or mental ability.

Infertility treatment significantly increases the risk of having twins or higher-order multiple pregnancies and research has begun to explore the impact of infertility and being a parent of a multiple birth. In a British study (Glazebrook, Sheard, Cox, Oates, & Ndukwe, 2004), the authors found that mothers of multiples through ART did not have poorer mental health than mothers of singletons conceived through ART. The opposite was found in a French study of parents of twins (Olivennes et al., 2005), in which parents of ART-conceived twins were matched with parents who conceived singletons via ART: parents with twins conceived via ART had greater parenting and child development difficulties than those who conceived singletons via ART.

ISSUES OF PREGNANCY AND POSTPARTUM

There are many social cues about what women and men should expect during pregnancy. From the humorous scenario of the pregnant woman needing pickles and ice cream in the middle of the night and the harried partner running out to find them, to the emotionally charged clichéd scene of the expectant parents bonding profoundly with the developing baby in the mother's gently swelling belly, women and men are offloaded with information about what to expect when they are expecting. For those women and men who have had an extended period of time to anticipate pregnancy because of infertility treatment, these expectations can grow to be even greater. The desire and wish for the pregnancy and parenting experience may be built on a significant emotional as well as financial investment.

Overall, the literature indicates that women who have gone through IVF do not differ from women who have spontaneously conceived during pregnancy. However, the studies have been small in number and no studies have looked at the women who have gone through other types of infertility treatment. As usual, the men have been rarely studied. As mentioned previously, there are preliminary data that suggest that assisted conception is associated with significantly increased rates of early parenting difficulties, but the data are very limited.

Yet there is a distinction between establishing that there are major differences between women who conceived spontaneously and those through treatment and understanding the potential myriad of feelings and reactions to pregnancy after infertility. One of the most often heard remarks by women who have left their infertility practices and moved on to obstetrical care is the discomfort going from an environment where there is intense monitoring to the OB office where there is only monthly monitoring. Imagine that you are getting almost daily feedback and reassurance that your pregnancy is fine and the fetus is developing appropriately and then going to your obstetrician. Your obstetrician will complete the visit with assurances that all is well and then will schedule you for your next appointment in a month's time.

For women and men who have grown accustomed to failure or to receiving bad news, the next 4 weeks without any monitoring may loom very long indeed. As one patient remarked, "Next month? I want to be in the next day. Who knows what could happen? How would she (the OB) know if anything is going wrong? Don't get me wrong. I'm happy to be 'normal' and be with the other pregnant women. But they don't know what I know about what can go wrong." Many infertility patients express ambivalence between wanting to be like everyone else and wanting special consideration for their "precious" and sometimes precariously felt pregnancy.

Reassurance through physical changes may offer some relief. Breast tenderness, nausea, or fatigue may offer some tangible reassurance to the newly pregnant woman. But these symptoms may resolve relatively quickly and leave the expectant parent in limbo again without confirmation that the pregnancy is progressing. The second trimester, which brings the physical changes of increased belly size and then movement that can be felt by both partners, can greatly alleviate anxiety and provide ongoing reassurance to the expectant parents.

The establishment of a pregnancy and visits to the obstetrician's office is not the only transition. Many patients have developed support networks within the infertility network. Listservs, chat rooms, and patient support groups such as The American Fertility Association (www.theafa.org) and Resolve (www.resolve.org) have created a very real support network. Once a woman is pregnant, she has effectively "crossed over" to the fertile world and her previous support system frequently fails to provide her needed support due to the issues her pregnancy stirs up in them. Women and men get caught in a "no man's land," feeling apart from the other expectant parents and no longer belonging to their old infertility networks. One patient summarized this by remarking, "I'm neither normal nor infertile now." Internet chat rooms or listservs may bridge the gap, but the newly expectant parent may need to establish entirely new supports.

Early Pregnancy: No "Gerber" Baby Experience

Early pregnancy can be physically demanding. Morning sickness (otherwise known as all-day or any-time-of-the-day sickness), fatigue, cramping, and emotional lability are all part of the pregnancy landscape. Many patients express the belief that they have no right to complain about any of their experiences of pregnancy. This can be reinforced by friends and family members who tell them, "Well, you wanted this. Look at what you did to get pregnant! You better not complain!" Once again, the infertility intrudes to make them separate from those who were able to conceive spontaneously. Guilt toward any negative thought or reaction can be palpable, and expectant parents following infertility may either try to repress these thoughts or feelings or may not seek out any support. The partner of the pregnant woman may also find that the issues and demands that infertility placed upon the relationship may not spontaneously disappear with the pregnancy.

Partners may also find that their hopes and fantasies about what pregnancy would be like may be quite different from reality. Additionally, some relationships become strained because of the impact infertility may have had on their sexual intimacy. Timed intercourse or prescribed periods of abstinence (i.e., no sexual activity during retrieval and transfer times in an IVF cycle) may take their toll on the couple's sex life. One male partner exclaimed, "It's one extreme or another. First I had to have sex on demand when she was ovulating. Sex was a chore and had nothing to do with having fun. Now she doesn't want me near her and I'm not so sure how confident I feel about having sex right now. I'm afraid I'll hurt something."

Early pregnancy may not restore sexual intimacy; indeed, illness and fatigue may strain or disrupt sexual intimacy; fear of hurting the developing fetus may also intrude on the relationship. Emotional availability may also be limited by physical pregnancy symptoms or fatigue and the ability to move on and be closer in the relationship. Simply put, the pregnancy experience may not be as anticipated.

Conversely, some women and their partners get reassurance from the morning sickness and other signs of pregnancy, as it affirms that the pregnancy is ongoing. When these symptoms abate, anxiety can rise without those reassurances. For example, breast tenderness abates as the pregnancy goes on and some expectant parents express sadness in losing this tangible signal of the ongoing pregnancy. It is a long wait until these parents will feel the baby move. For many, until that baby moves, there is still some disbelief that the pregnancy is real.

Older Mothers

As a result of oocyte donation, motherhood at or beyond the edge of the typical reproductive age has become increasingly common. The 2001 birth rates for women 35–39, 40–44, and 45–49 were 30%, 47%, and 190%, as compared with 1990, and there were 239 births to women age 50 and older. Additionally, 1 out of 20 births to women age 40–49 and 1 out of 5 births to women over 45 years of age was a multiple pregnancy (Martin, Hamilton, & Ventura, 2001). Consider the myriad of issues that may arise from being an older parent. From factors such as age of retirement to energy level to obstetrical risks to desire, the older parent must consider how his or her individual circumstances contribute to their desire to parent. It is not a given that an older parent will be less involved, active, or loving. Indeed, with age may come certain advantages such as maturity and economic stability that may elude younger parents.

Yet pregnancy at an older age may invite attention that was unintentional and unwanted. Certainly, if the mother's own gametes are used, very real concerns about the health of the child may increase. Decisions about prenatal testing, termination, and care of a special needs child must be considered. Older mothers, in particular, may find themselves subject to negative public opinion. There appears to remain a strong social bias against the older mother as compared with the older father. This probably reflects the prime importance public opinion places upon the central and more traditional concept of the mother.

After delivery, the older parent may need to process her feelings should others assume her to be the grandparent. Adding to the experience may be a decreased informal social support network. Many friends and family members are often in the same age range as the new parent, and, consequently, may have significantly older children. New parents who are older may be more challenged by the transition to parenthood because they do not have the social supports of others experiencing similar challenges of early parenthood. While they are struggling with choosing preschools or childcare, their friends may be struggling with choosing colleges and taking on college loans.

Added to the challenge of disconnect from peers is the potential for bias or disapproval of choosing to parent later in life. The new mother (and father) may feel isolated or may simply lack the informal information exchange with others to provide a normative comparison base for the feelings and needs of new parents. One new mother stated, "I don't know if all new moms are this tired. I'm 45 years old and usually have tons of energy. But I'm exhausted every day—I'm lucky to have a shower. My friends are all talking about parents' day at their kids' colleges. I'm trying to figure out what diapers leak the least. I feel so alone sometimes."

Postpartum Issues

Infertility may contribute to a woman's depression prior to conception. Depression may remit once the stressor of the infertility is resolved. However, if the depression is independent of the infertility or the issues have become intertwined with preexisting issues, the depression may persist into pregnancy. Awareness of the vulnerability of women with depression during pregnancy to develop postpartum depression is very important in the infertility population. No studies are currently published that specifically address whether there is an increased risk rate of postpartum depression for women who experienced infertility.

Other postpartum issues may arise that may be specific to, or are exacerbated by, having had infertility experience. Vaginal delivery and/or breastfeeding may take on more significance in that it may become associated with the woman's self-esteem. Having failed at being able to achieve a pregnancy without assistance, she may have her expectations raised that delivery and breastfeeding should be unassisted. In other words, women who have experienced infertility may have heightened expectations that breastfeeding should be a task that they can accomplish easily and well. Feelings of inadequacy, failure, or difference can be reawakened if a woman feels that she has failed at breastfeeding or by having a cesarean section. As one woman explained after failing to breastfeed after conceiving her daughter via egg donation, "I failed at getting pregnant. I failed at having my own genetic child. Now I'm failing as a woman in doing something that should come naturally. I counted on breastfeeding to be the one area where I could be just like everyone else."

Multiple Pregnancies

As mentioned earlier in the literature, a multiple pregnancy may induce unique experiences to the pregnancy and postpartum transition. The multiple pregnancy risk for an individual or couple depends on a number of factors, including the age of the woman providing the eggs and the number of developing eggs or the number of embryos transferred. The American Society for Reproductive Medicine, the professional organization for the assisted reproductive technologies, offers practice guidelines for medical professionals about most aspects of the ARTs. Guidelines for practice for mental health professionals are also available (www.asrm.org).

A multiple pregnancy often translates into a higher-risk pregnancy because of various factors, including twin-to-twin transfusion and monochorionicity, and some data suggest that ART-conceived twin pregnancies may have more complications than spontaneously conceived twins (Daniel et al., 2000). Women and men who have just gone through demanding treatment following lengthy attempts and failures may be ill prepared to transition to a higher-risk pregnancy. Although many prospective parents may be initially thrilled with the idea of an "instant family," the demands and risks of a multiple pregnancy may counterbalance the initial excitement. Add the very real additional risks of prematurity and all its attending complications and the prospect of triplets or more can be overwhelming.

One option for multiple pregnancy management is to perform a selective reduction, which involves the selective termination of one or more of the developing fetuses, usually at the end of the first trimester. Pregnancy after fetal reduction is not well studied, and one of the potential issues for parents is coping with the decision to terminate.

For those parents who conceive and manage a multiple pregnancy, some of the issues that arise may involve the perceived higher risks of the pregnancy. Expectant mothers may find that they are monitored more closely and are put on restricted activity more often. As noted previously, the increased monitoring may be reassuring to many while others may find that the experience of more frequent monitoring makes their experience different from their friends or other family members.

The birth of twins also involves a different parenting experience for new parents. The demands of two newborns may make the much-anticipated and desired experience of parenthood very different from the fantasized one. The possibility of disappointment in their own expectations of their parenting ability is greater when parents cope with multiple newborns. One new mother of twins stated, "When I brought my twins home from the hospital I was overwhelmed at the thought of being left alone with them. No one ever prepared me for the constant demands of two babies. I felt I was a failure—two babies crying and not sleeping—and I hadn't taken a course or read a book about what to do. I kept dreaming of sitting in a rocking chair singing quietly to my baby. Instead it was a three-ring circus and I was the clown and not the ringmaster."

The fantasy Gerber baby needs to be replaced with the reality of the "good enough baby." The Gerber baby is the model in which prospective parents invest their dreams and hopes throughout treatment. The "good enough baby" is the one that is based in reality—the baby who cries, fusses, eats, sleeps, smiles, and plays, and never in the right order. The old joke of the first-time parents who ask the maternity nurse "And what time should we wake the baby up in the morning?" may apply even more strongly to those parents who have had longer than 9 months to develop dreams and expectations of new parenthood.

Third-Party Parenting

Building a family sometimes requires the assistance of a third party who provides either gametes (eggs or sperm or embryo) or gestation (a gestational carrier or gestational surrogate). These family-building options have resulted in a steady increase in the number of births from egg donation, sperm donation, and gestational carriers over the last decade (http://www.cdc.gov/art/).

When there is genetic inequity in a pregnancy, that is, one parent is genetically related and the other is not, there are many issues and feelings that may arise. The pregnancy may represent great excitement at the prospect of parenthood as well as great anticipation about how the nongenetic parent may feel or react. For example, when a heterosexual couple uses sperm donation, the increasing visibility of the pregnancy may awaken or reawaken feelings for the male partner about his masculinity and inability to impregnate his wife. For same-sex female couples, the pregnancy may bring about a greater openness about their identification as a lesbian couple. For single mothers by choice, the pregnancy will also make public their choice to parent without a partner and create the need to manage the public reaction. Some single mothers by choice will encounter negative attitudes about deliberately denying a child the possibility of having a father and the advancing pregnancy will demand that she process her own feelings about both parenting without a partner and her child's potential feelings about growing up without a father.

In a couple, the nongenetic parent in the relationship must mourn the loss of his or her genetic child. For some this begins during the pregnancy, for others after delivery, and for many others, this mourning begins long before the pregnancy is established. Heretofore, the infertility may have been more shared, whereas during the pregnancy and early parenthood the journey may diverge. The genetic parent may have his or her own feelings about having that genetic connection. One expectant mother whose husband could not contribute genetically to the child said poignantly, "I feel badly that I will be able to see my characteristics in this child and my husband won't. It doesn't feel fair and I worry that he will resent me." The genetic parent can describe this burden as almost like a "survivor's guilt," in which the feelings have to be processed about her guilt at being happy to have the genetic connection when her partner cannot.

One task each parent, genetic or nongenetic, must assume is whether to disclose the use of the donor in the child's conception. The transition to new parenthood may be more strikingly isolating when a donor is used—regardless of how open or private the new parents may be. Although mental health professionals have advocated for full disclosure, each parent must process his or her feelings and make his or her own decision. When parents choose not to disclose the child's donor origins, the pregnancy may bear the burden of a disconnection between the public reaction and the private uncertainty about their feelings or the grief of the loss of the genetic connection. Certainly, after the baby is born, the parents must cope with the assumption and reactions of others, including the often-queried "and who does the baby look like?"

A complication of the transition to parenthood when using a gamete donor may be that the new parents do not have a reference point for some of their feelings and reactions. Part of the challenge of parenthood is managing the negative feelings along with the positive. The demanding schedules, sleepless nights, and other newborn challenges can lead to feelings of fatigue and irritability, which are often not the emotions new parents expect or have been led to expect. For a parent who does not have a genetic connection, there may be uncertainty about whether these feelings are attributed to the lack of genetic connectedness or to "normal" new parent feelings. One father of a son through donor sperm said wistfully, "I'll always wonder if I would have felt differently if my sperm were used. I don't think I would love my son more, I just wonder if I would love him differently."

SUMMARY

Women and men who have experienced infertility prior to pregnancy can bring the challenges and feelings of that time to their pregnancy and postpartum experience. Having navigated the roller coaster ride of cycle failures and success, these women and men are particularly primed for expectations about how and what pregnancy, delivery, and postpartum may be like. The literature suggests that there are no pathological differences between individuals/couples that conceive through the ARTs and those who conceive spontaneously. Yet, understanding the qualitative experiences and perceptions of these women and men is critical for interventions and support.

Special consideration needs to be given to individuals and couples who build their families with the assistance of a sperm donor, egg donor, or gestational carrier/surrogate. Single mothers by choice may also have their unique challenges during pregnancy and postpartum. Compassion, caring, and concern should accompany the prospective parents who have experienced infertility into their pregnancy and postpartum experience in order to understand and aid their unique issues on their journey to parenthood.

REFERENCES

Brockington, I. F., Macdonald, E., & Wainscott, G. (2006). Anxiety, obsessions and morbid preoccupations in pregnancy and pueperium. *Archives of Women's Mental Health, 9,* 229–331.

Covington, S., & Burns, L. H. (2006). *Infertility counseling: A comprehensive handbook for clinicians* (2nd ed.). New York: Cambridge University Press.

Cox, S. J., Glazebrook, C., Sheard, C., Ndukwe, G., & Oates, M. (2006). Maternal self-esteem after successful treatment for infertility. *Fertility and Sterility, 85,* 84–89.

Csatordai, S., Kozinsky, Z., Devosa, I., Toth, E., Krajcsi, A., Sefcski, T., & Pal, A. (2007). Obstetric and sociodemographic risk of vulnerability to postnatal depression. *Patient Education Counseling, 67,* 84–92.

Daniel, Y., Ochshorn, Y., Fait, G., Geva, E., Bar-Am, A., & Lessing, J. B. (2000). Analysis of 104 twin pregnancies conceived with assisted reproductive technologies and 193 spontaneously conceived twin pregnancies. *Fertility and Sterility, 74,* 683–689.

Fisher, J. R., Hammarberg, K., & Baker, H. W. (2005). Assisted conception is a risk factor for postnatal mood disturbance and early parenting difficulties. *Fertility and Sterility, 84,* 426–430.

Glazebrook, C., Sheard, C., Cox, S., Oates, M., & Ndukwe, G. (2004). Parenting stress in first-time mothers of twins and triplets conceived after in vitro fertilization. *Fertility and Sterility, 81,* 505–511.

Harf-Kashdaei, E., & Kaitz, M. (2007). Antenatal moods regarding self, baby, and spouse among women who conceived by in vitro fertilization. *Fertility and Sterility, 87,* 1306–1313.

Klock, S. C., & Greenfeld, D. A. (2000). Psychological status of in vitro fertilization patients during pregnancy: A longitudinal study. *Fertility and Sterility, 73,* 1159–1164.

Martin, J. A., Hamilton, B. E., & Ventura, J. J. (2001) Births: Pregnancy data for 2000. *National Vital Statistics Report, 49,* 1–20.

McMahon, C. A., Gibson, F. L., Allen, J. L., & Saunders, D. (2007). Psychosocial adjustment during pregnancy for older couples conceiving through assisted reproductive technology. *Human Reproduction, 22,* 1168–1174.

Olivennes, F., Golombok, S., Ramogida, C., Rust, J., & Follow-Up Team. (2005). Behavioral and cognitive development as well as family functioning of twins conceived by assisted reproduction: Findings from a large population study. *Fertility and Sterility, 84,* 725–733.

Olshansky, E. (2003). A theoretical explanation for previously infertile mothers' vulnerability to depression. *Journal of Nursing Scholarship, 35,* 263–268.

Olshansky, E., & Sereika, S. (2005). The transition from pregnancy to postpartum in previously infertile women: A focus on depression. *Archives of Psychiatric Nursing, 19,* 273–280.

Repokari, L., et al. (2005). The impact of successful assisted reproduction treatment on female and male mental health during transition to parenthood: A prospective controlled study. *Human Reproduction, 20*(11), 3238–3247.

Repokari, L., et al. (2006). Ante- and perinatal factors and child characteristics predicting parenting experience among formerly infertile couples during the child's first year: A controlled study. *Journal of Family Psychology, 20,* 670–679.

Robin, P. (1993). *How to be a successful fertility patient.* New York: William Morrow.

Steiner, A. Z., & Paulson, R. J. (2007). Motherhood after age 50: An evaluation of parenting stress and physical functioning. *Fertility and Sterility, 87,* 1327–1332.

PART III

Professional Perspectives

9

Perinatal Mood Disorders: An Obstetrician's Perspective

ALEXANDRA C. SPADOLA

Caring for the majority of pregnant women in the United States, obstetricians have a special responsibility to recognize and obtain treatment for patients with perinatal mood disorders. Many women of reproductive age identify their obstetrician/gynecologist as their primary physician. This unique relationship may last decades and for some it will be associated with childbirth, one of the most profound and life-altering experiences for any woman. From the obstetrician's viewpoint, mood disorders are not only a source of suffering for the patient, but a potential barrier to partnering with the patient in her pregnancy care. Maternal or fetal "high-risk" conditions may increase maternal stress and exacerbate symptoms of depression and/or anxiety. And among low-income populations, the prevalence of mood disorders appears to be even greater than in low-risk populations (Howell, Mora, Horowitz, & Leventhal, 2005; Rich-Edwards et al., 2006). Additionally, depression is associated with domestic violence and maternal risk-taking behaviors (Zuckerman, Amaro, Bauchner, & Cabral, 1989). Depression and maternal stress appear to increase the incidence of abnormal perinatal outcomes, such as intrauterine growth restriction and preterm birth (Cooper et al., 1996; Hobel, Dunkel-Schetter, Roesch, Castro, & Arora, 1999), and adversely impact maternal-infant bonding, as well as fetal and infant behaviors (Bonari et al., 2004; Davis et al., 2007).

Worldwide, the recognition of postpartum depression is growing; however, studies report a majority of affected women are untreated or undertreated for this condition (Marcus, Flynn, Blow, & Barry, 2003). This chapter explores the routine obstetrician-patient relationship, the issues in treating women with a history of mood disorders, and the barriers faced by both physicians and patients. The obstacles obstetricians face in detecting and obtaining care for affected women include lack of consensus on effective screening methods, low awareness of the potential affects on fetal development and birth outcomes of antenatal mood disorders and maternal stress, and uncertainty about the safety of psychotropic medications during pregnancy and lactation. The current medical model of pregnancy care may exacerbate the underrecognition of illness. Untreated mood disorders can affect compliance with medical visits and with treatment of other maternal and fetal conditions. Affordable and accessible mental health care can be challenging in many communities. Recognition of existing barriers, physician and patient education, and team preparedness may lead to better care.

CASE REPORTS

Case 1

M. was a 39-year-old gravida 2 para 0010 with a twin pregnancy conceived by in vitro fertilization. Previously, she experienced episodes of major depressive disorder and panic attacks, both of which were in remission with medication and supportive therapy. She had been on sertraline for 4 years. Her previous pregnancy was terminated in the second trimester when the fetus was found to have a lethal birth defect. Along with her prenatal care, she followed throughout the pregnancy with a psychotherapist and a psychiatrist. She delivered the twins vaginally after spontaneous onset of labor. Postpartum, she hired a baby nurse, but still found it overwhelming to attend weekly therapy sessions in the first months.

Case 2

T. was a 36-year-old gravida 6 para 4014 with history of depression with psychotic features and poorly controlled type II diabetes mellitus with a history of short birth interval and prior postpartum psychosis in which she experienced intrusive thoughts of stabbing her newborn son. During pregnancy, her mood was stable on citalopram, ziprasidone, and clonazepam with monthly psychiatric consults and weekly visits with a therapist. She was admitted several times during pregnancy for poor glycemic control and felt "hopeless" while in the hospital, although she denied suicidal and homicidal ideation. She experienced an emergent cesarean delivery after preterm premature rupture of membranes at 32 weeks. She remained in the hospital for 1 week postpartum on a voluntary admission to the psychiatric unit due to her prior history. However, she was discharged with a home assistant and follow-up with outpatient psychiatric care feeling that she was "misunderstood" by the medical and psychiatric team.

ROUTINE OBSTETRICAL CARE AND SCREENING

An obstetrician's work includes screening, referring, and comanaging affected patients with mental health professionals during and after pregnancy. Routinely, patients initiate care in the first trimester of pregnancy. The American College of Obstetricians and Gynecologists (ACOG) suggests monthly visits until the third trimester, twice monthly until term, and weekly in the patient's last month before delivery around her estimated due date. The postpartum visit occurs 4 to 6 weeks following delivery. Common obstetrical complications such as gestational diabetes, chronic hypertension, and prior preterm birth will increase the frequency of care.

At the initial visit, it is appropriate to begin by asking whether the pregnancy was planned and/or desired. Approximately half of all pregnancies in the United States are unintended (Finer & Henshaw, 2006). Women may experience feelings of guilt or resentment about this "accident" even if the pregnancy is subsequently desired. By routinely asking these questions in an open and nonjudgemental fashion the obstetrician signals that the doctor's office is a place where conflicted emotions about pregnancy can be voiced. The patient's responses may help the clinician understand how she is coping and how she is integrating the pregnancy into her life. ACOG also recognizes the physician's important role in reviewing the patient's options in early pregnancy.

If the patient is multiparous, obtaining the obstetric history can be a great way for the obstetrician to gain understanding and develop trust. Whether the patient has experienced recurrent pregnancy losses, days of difficult prodromal labor, or an emergent cesarean delivery for nonreassuring fetal heart rate tracing, her narratives of pregnancy and birth provide insight into a patient's emotions and perceptions about her previous obstetrical experiences and screens for trauma. At one first prenatal visit, a patient cupped her ears and sang loudly while her husband recounted the events of their last child's difficult delivery. Trauma and unresolved grief may surface with a new pregnancy. In M.'s case, her prior history of a fetus with a birth defect was an obstacle to enjoying the many ultrasound exams for her twin pregnancy. Discussions of past events can initiate dialogue about feelings and adjustment in the current pregnancy.

The ACOG prenatal form includes an array of psychosocial screening questions. In addition to a prior history of mental illness, poor social/environmental factors and risk-taking behaviors are red flags for a patient at risk for depression in pregnancy or postpartum (Beck, 2002). History of sexual assault and eating disorders can be additional sources of difficulty during gestation. Physical transformations and changing roles are challenging for many women, but may be more so in these vulnerable populations. For M., the extra weight gain with a twin pregnancy was an area of anxiety. T. found the strict diabetic diet difficult to adhere to because snacking had always been a way to relieve stress.

After the initial intake, routine follow-up obstetrical visits are commonly allotted 15-minute slots on a busy provider's schedule. These are considered well-woman visits. For the majority of patients, screening exams and blood work do not uncover disease, but rather exclude pathology. Obstetricians lend authority to the patient's sense that they are "doing well." Ideally, these are reassuring visits where the doctor takes the opportunity to address the patient's concerns and questions. Visits routinely include opportunities for education on safety, toxic habits, as well as preparation for the birth and newborn period. Referral to appropriate reading material and Web sites can provide patients with additional information.

Weekly visits for the term patient allow the obstetrician time to reinforce the need for self-care during the postpartum period as the energies of the household are directed toward care of the newborn. Patients are informed about the high incidence of postpartum blues, up to 85% in first pregnancies (O'Hara & Swain, 1996). They should be reminded of the ways in which sleep depravation can exaggerate feelings of hopelessness and despair and that those 1 in 5 women with mild postpartum mood instability will progress to symptoms of postpartum depression (Suri & Burt, 1997). When they are not in a supportive relationship, patients can be encouraged to seek assistance from family and friends in caring for older children or doing household chores. Social support resources can often be found within the community. Many cultural and family organizations have groups focusing on new mother and infant care. Breastfeeding support meetings can be a great resource for women who are nursing and provide an ongoing sense of community.

CARE FOR WOMEN WITH A HISTORY OF MOOD DISORDERS

For women with prior mood disorders planning pregnancy, preconception counseling may be useful for insight and reassurance. Patients may find it useful to discuss risks and treatment plans with both a psychiatrist and an obstetrician. If the woman has suffered from exacerbations of mood disorders in her past pregnancy, a preconception visit may be particularly helpful to strategize for the future and potentially reduce maternal anxiety. The consultation content may include antenatal medical therapies, more intensive nonpharmacologic interventions, or a focus on prophylactic measures in the postpartum period.

When women with mood disorders are identified at the initial prenatal visit, a psychiatric consultation then becomes part of their prenatal care plan. Discussion of the woman's experiences in prior pregnancies is essential in screening for complications in the index pregnancy. Both peripartum depression (O'Hara & Swain, 1996) and postpartum psychosis (Jones & Craddock, 2001) have recurrences of up to 50%. Having the patient's permission to discuss her care with her mental health provider(s) may be helpful going forward. Better communication between T.'s providers may have helped the obstetric team understand the relationship between her compliance with her diabetic care and her psychiatric illness. Her mood symptoms were exacerbated with hospitalization and alternatives to inpatient management might have been explored.

Often the patient seeks opinions regarding treatment in pregnancy and during lactation from all her providers. Patients will self-discontinue medications due to concerns about harmful fetal effects. Others are encouraged to stop medications by well-intended health care providers, family, or friends. In M.'s case the emotional work of dealing with infertility engendered strong feelings that she needed to continue medical therapy in pregnancy, despite the couple's concerns regarding teratogenicity. T. also knew her baseline symptoms worsened off medication and felt supported by her medical team in the decision to stay on her effective treatment regimen.

Patients expect obstetricians to be knowledgeable about the safety profiles of antidepressant and mood stabilizing drugs. ACOG advises that all discussions of medical treatment for mental illness in pregnancy include an assessment of the risks and benefits of pharmacologic therapy. Medical treatment is dictated by the severity of symptoms and is best assessed by a psychiatrist comfortable with treating pregnancy patients. The literature surrounding the risks of pharmacologic treatment during pregnancy is growing, but suffers from a lack of well-designed trials. The majority of data originates from retrospective, observational studies that may not distinguish between drugs within therapeutic classes. In 2006, ACOG committee opinion echoed an FDA warning regarding paroxetine and increased risk for cardiac defects (ACOG, 2006b). Two large recent case control studies on serotonin reuptake inhibitor (SSRI) exposure in the first trimester were reassuring in that most congenital defects were not increased and that absolute risks of defects remained small (Alwan, Reefhuis, Rasmussen, Olney, & Friedman, 2007; Louik, Lin, Werler, Hernandez-Diaz, & Mitchell, 2007). Motherisk and Reprotox are two online resources that provide links or summaries of data about drug safety in pregnancy. Among various psychotherapeutic options, only intrapersonal therapy (IPT) has been demonstrated in a pilot study to be as effective as SSRIs in treating depression (Spinelli & Endicott, 2003).

The primary goal for the obstetrician, as illustrated by the case studies, is to connect the patient with a mental health professional that can address the patient's psychiatric needs and develop a plan for the pregnancy and puerperium. Depending on the patient's needs and schedule with her mental health provider, the obstetrician may see the patient more frequently than with routine care.

SYMPTOMATIC ILLNESS IN PREGNANCY AND POSTPARTUM

Women with active symptoms of depression or mania need immediate attention from providers. Office employees fielding patient phone calls need instruction on how to handle this category of call and the importance of prioritizing these messages. Every practice should have protocols for calls from patients with urgent psychiatric symptoms. Preparation entails knowledge of local emergency room psychiatric services, hotlines providing psychiatric triage, and psychiatric providers available for consult. Optimally, covering physicians should have access to patient records.

Obstetricians are comfortable with inpatient observation for many obstetrical complications, but may be less certain regarding the criteria for hospitalization during acute psychiatric illness. Treatment of acute symptoms may include education and reassurance, supportive psychotherapy, psychotropic medications, and, less commonly, electroconvulsive therapy (ECT). Depending on gestational age, inpatient fetal monitoring may be indicated for this particular modality. Obstetricians should always exclude medical etiologies of symptoms such as thyroid dysfunction. In one study, a third of women seeking psychiatric care for depression in the peripartum period had a comorbid axis I disorder, commonly anxiety disorders, or substance abuse (Battle, Zlotnick, Miller, Pearlstein, & Howard, 2006). With severe disease, hospitalization may prevent self-harm, and, in the postpartum period, harm to the newborn, although this does not mean that all programs require separation of the mother-infant pair. In patient T's case, she was able to visit her premature newborn in the neonatal intensive care unit while she was hospitalized in the psychiatric ward, but she did feel that her inpatient care limited her ability to be with her child and this was a source of distress.

BREASTFEEDING

Breastfeeding improves a number of maternal, neonatal, and early childhood health outcomes, and obstetricians often encourage their patients' decision to do so. The American Association of Pediatricians recommends exclusive breastfeeding for the first 6 months and continuing through the first year. For mothers, breastfeeding can be a powerful method to connect with and provide for a new infant. Breastfeeding may help improve maternal stress responses (Carter & Altemus, 1997), and formula feeding was noted in higher numbers of women presenting with psychiatric illness postpartum, although this may have multiple explanations (Battle et al., 2006). Women on psychotropic medication in the postpartum period should be educated about what is known and unknown about the neonatal effects of transference to breast milk. All SSRIs are excreted in the breast milk and the lowest effective dose should be used. While no significant adverse events have been demonstrated in exposed offspring, long-term neurobehavioral outcome data does not exist. Preferentially avoiding the SSRIs with greatest exposure in breast milk such as fluoxetine and citalopram may work for some, but not all patients (Burt, 2006). Mood stabilizers have less data about newborn effects and the AAP does not recommend their use. Avoidance of breastfeeding in premature infants with decreased drug metabolism is also recommended. For bipolar women for whom sleep disturbance may be a trigger for mood instability, infant feeding can be shared with others to decrease risks for the mother (Burt, 2006).

OBSTACLES FOR THE PATIENT

Women may face multiple barriers to obtaining treatment for mood disorders, including inadequate insurance coverage or financial support, lack of providers, and difficulty securing childcare or social support needed to comply with visits (Brown, 1989). The societal stigma of mental illness makes it more challenging for some women to seek out and accept treatment. Women may anticipate pregnancy to be joyous and provide a new sense of purpose, making significant mood symptoms unexpected and disappointing. A woman experiencing depression during pregnancy may feel further isolation from partners or family members as her lack of outward expressions of contentment causes confusion or resentment. Realistically complex portrayals of pregnant women in the media are uncommon, but images of the happy pregnant consumer abound. The cultural emphasis, which equates good parenting with consumption of goods, can be an additional stressor for economically disadvantaged women and families.

Ideally, the patient feels comfortable in the clinician's office and feels empowered as a partner in the health process. For some patients, however, there may be fear regarding disclosure of mood symptoms. Patients who have idealized the figure of the obstetrician may feel they are disappointing their doctor by admitting to difficult emotions or decreased ability to function in daily life. Some patients are silenced by the desire to keep the pregnancy event from being "tainted" by prior mental illness. Women express the wish to "start fresh" in taking on the new role of mother. Using nonjudgmental language and trying to normalize a therapeutic relationship with a social worker or psychologist can be useful.

Maternal and fetal complications in pregnancy add to patient stress and may increase symptoms of depression (Hedegaard, Henriksen,

Sabroe, & Secher, 1993). There can be significant anxiety about being placed in this category by the physician, and the patient may need to grieve for loss of the "normal" prenatal experience. It can be helpful to discuss these feelings with the patient. If patients are restricted from working or placed on modified bed rest, they should be advised about the risks of depression and the adverse effect on mental well-being (Maloni, Park, Anthony, & Musil, 2004). Poor perinatal outcomes, especially fetal and neonatal loss, increase risk of depression. A study measuring depressive symptoms a year after the second trimester pregnancy termination for fetal anomalies found 43% continued to report significant emotional distress (Davies, Gledhill, McFadyen, Whitlow, & Economides, 2005).

The prenatal care model in which women are seen frequently as birth approaches, but not for a month to 6 weeks after delivery, may contribute to a sense of isolation in women experiencing depression and anxiety during the immediate postpartum period. While patients are in contact with the newborn's pediatrician, this may be a new relationship and one that by necessity focuses less on their own health needs and psychosocial well-being as an individual. When depression develops in the postpartum period after an unremarkable pregnancy, the patient may feel she cannot reach out to her obstetrician, that the doctor has done his or her job and now this is the patient's time to "handle it." The reluctance to ask for help may be exacerbated by symptomatology and by familial and cultural perceptions of mental illness.

OBSTACLES FOR THE OBSTETRICIAN

Obstetricians face several barriers for the recognition and effective treatment of perinatal mood disorders. First, obstetricians may be less informed about the high prevalence of antepartum depression, its influence on postpartum depression, and treatment modalities. In a survey of 282 obstetrician-gynecologists, only 32% agreed with the statement, "I feel I've had the appropriate training to treat depression" (LaRocco-Cockburn, Melville, Bell, & Katon, 2003). Physicians may perceive time constraints as an obstacle to screening all patients as well as those with risk factors. It was found that 81% of generalists who were surveyed reported asking their own questions regarding mood instead of using a validated screening tool (LaRocco-Cockburn et al., 2003). The multiquestion Edinburgh Postnatal Depression Scale (EDPS), which has been validated for antenatal screening and supported in evidence-based reviews (Gaynes et al., 2005), might take up the entire allotted time for a routine visit. Based on evidence-based reviews, ACOG (2006a) recommends an abbreviated screening method utilizing the following two questions:

1. Over the past 2 weeks, have you ever felt down, depressed, or hopeless?
2. Over the past 2 weeks, have you felt little interest or pleasure in doing things?

In this way mood becomes a vital sign that is taken with each visit; both the patient and doctor become accustomed to this type of inquiry. However, the efficacy of these questions has not been as well studied as EDPS for detecting depression.

Traditionally, physicians have not prioritized addressing psychosocial risk factors linked to poor obstetrical and neonatal outcomes. Domestic violence, alcohol abuse, tobacco, and illicit drug use are associated with depression (ACOG, 2006a). Suicide among pregnant women often occurs in the context of partner violence and sexual assault (Shadigian & Bauer, 2005). One study of various level providers suggested that asking about depression may open communication about these other topics and increase trust and understanding between patient and provider (Herzig et al., 2006). Furthermore, one study demonstrated that patient satisfaction was improved when more time during the visit was spent on psychosocial issues rather than biomedical topics (Bertakis, Roter, & Putnam, 1991).

Another obstacle to identifying affected patients may be the array of somatic complaints that can present during gestation. A list of the most common pregnancy-associated physical conditions includes nausea and vomiting, sleep disturbances, urinary frequency, pelvic girdle and low back pain, constipation, heartburn, lower extremity swelling and cramping, shortness of breath, headaches, and discomfort with sexual intercourse. While these symptoms often do not signify major pathology, skilled obstetricians avoid sending the message that "minor complaints" are not important. Many of the above discomforts have remedies that, if not entirely, at least treat or alleviate symptoms in ways that can greatly enhance quality of life. In particular, measures such as maternal positioning, use of support pillows, and decrease in evening oral intake may improve length and quality of sleep with positive effects on daily physical and mental functioning. When a patient's reactions to pregnancy symptoms are persistently moderate or severe, further exploration of symptoms of depression is warranted.

Finally, the full array of medical and nonpharmacologic referral options for treatment of mood disorders in pregnancy may not be available to all provider practices. Obstetricians may be uncertain as to how to develop a strong network of mental health professionals. Some communities lack sufficient resources for affordable counseling and psychosocial support (i.e., postpartum doula services) serving underinsured patients. Organizations like Postpartum Support International may be able to assist individual physicians in finding local specialists. The Internet has also become a useful tool for accessing information regarding community services. Finally, patient follow-up after a diagnosis has been made to ensure ongoing care and determine responses to interventions is as important as recognizing illness.

SUMMARY

Mood disorders occur most commonly in the postpartum period, but can also present throughout pregnancy when patients have their most frequent contact with obstetricians. Women with a history of mood disorders are at high risk for relapses both during pregnancy and postnatally. Affected pregnancies are at higher risk for adverse maternal and obstetrical outcomes. Successful treatment for patients can assuage suffering as well as prevent neonatal and childhood sequelae of maternal depression (Grace, Evinder, & Stewart, 2003). Obstetricians may be less informed about these important associations and feel unprepared for positive screening results. The structure and timing of visits during and after pregnancy may result in fewer women being treated effectively. By using brief questions about mood and energy level, the obstetrician may see how mood may be thought of as a vital sign at routine obstetric encounters. Screening can be brief and still be effective, and follow-up with affected patients following referral is important.

The dynamic that the obstetrician has with a patient has the potential to be more intimate and profound than other doctor-patient relationships. Obstetricians are in a unique position to recognize pregnant and postpartum patients suffering from mood disorders and should be prepared with referral strategies to mental health professionals.

Psychotherapy and pharmacologic treatments can be effective to alleviate symptoms in both pregnant and lactating women. The risks of therapy may be outweighed by the risks of untreated depression. Obstetricians can be advocates for women's mental health, and, optimally, function as the point person for a team of providers taking care of the woman during and following pregnancy.

REFERENCES

ACOG Committee Opinion No. 343: Psychosocial risk factors: Perinatal screening and intervention. (2006a). *Obstetrics & Gynecology, 108*(2), 469–477.

ACOG Committee Opinion No. 354: Treatment with selective serotonin reuptake inhibitors during pregnancy. (2006b). *Obstetrics & Gynecology, 108*(6), 1601–1603.

Alwan, S., Reefhuis, J., Rasmussen, S. A., Olney, R. S., & Friedman, J. M. (2007). Use of selective serotonin-reuptake inhibitors in pregnancy and the risk of birth defects. *New England Journal of Medicine, 356*(26), 2684–2692.

Battle, C. L., Zlotnick, C., Miller, I. W., Pearlstein, T., & Howard, M. (2006). Clinical characteristics of perinatal psychiatric patients: A chart review study. *Journal of Nervous and Mental Disease, 194*(5), 369–377.

Beck, C. T. (2002). Revision of the postpartum depression predictors inventory. *Journal of Obstetric, Gynecologic, and Neonatal Nursing, 31,* 394–402.

Bertakis, K. D., Roter, D., & Putnam, S. M. (1991). The relationship of physician medical interview style to patient satisfaction. *Journal of Family Practice, 32,* 175–181.

Bonari, L., Pinto, N., Ahn, E., Einarson, A., Steiner, M., & Koren, G. (2004). Perinatal risks of untreated depression during pregnancy. *Canadian Journal of Psychiatry, 49,* 726–735.

Brown, S. S. (1989). Drawing women into prenatal care. *Family Planning Perspective, 21,* 71–83.

Burt, V. K. (2006). Mood disorders in women: Focus on the postpartum. *Womens Health Obstetrics-Gynecology Edition, 6*(2), 12–19.

Carter, C. S., & Altemus, M. (1997). Integrative functions of lactational hormones in social behavior and stress management. *Annals of the New York Academy Sciences, 807,* 164–174.

Copper, R. L., Goldenberg, R. L., Das, A., Elder, N., Swain, M., Norman, G., et al. (1996). The preterm prediction study: Maternal stress is associated with spontaneous preterm birth at less than thirty-five weeks' gestation. National Institute of Child Health and Human Development Maternal-Fetal Medicine Units Network. *American Journal of Obstetrics and Gynecology, 175*(5), 1286–1292.

Davies, V., Gledhill, J., McFadyen, A., Whitlow, B., & Economides, D. (2005). Psychological outcome in women undergoing termination of pregnancy for ultrasound-detected fetal anomaly in the first and second trimesters: A pilot study. *Ultrasound in Obstetrics Gynecology, 25*(4), 389–392.

Davis, E. J., Glynn, L. M., Schetter, C. D., Hobel, C., Chicz-Demet, A., & Sandman, C. A. (2007). Prenatal exposure to maternal depression and cortisol influences infant temperament. *Journal of American Academy of Child & Adolescent Psychiatry, 46*(6), 737–746.

Finer, L. B., & Henshaw, S. K. (2006). Disparities in rates of unintended pregnancy in the United States, 1994 and 2001. *Perspectives on Sexual and Reproductive Health, 38*(2), 90–96.

Gaynes, B. N., Gavin, N., Meltzer-Brody, S., Lohr, K. N., Swinson, T., Gartlehner, G., et al. (2005). Perinatal depression: Prevalence, screening accuracy, and screening outcomes. Evidence Report/Technology Assessment No. 119. Agency for Healthcare Research and Quality. Retrieved August 15, 2007, from www.ahrq.gov/clinic/epcsums/peridepsum.htm

Grace, S. L., Evinder, A., & Stewart, D. E. (2003). The effect of postpartum depression on child cognitive development and behavior: A review and critical analysis of the literature. *Archives of Women's Mental Health, 6,* 263–264.

Hedegaard, M., Henriksen, T. B., Sabroe, S., & Secher, N. J. (1993). Psychological distress in pregnancy and preterm delivery. *BMJ, 307,* 234–239.

Herzig, K., Danley, D., Jackson, R., Petersen, R., Chamberlain, L., & Gerbert, B. (2006). Seizing the 9-month moment: Addressing behavioral risks in prenatal patients. *Patient Education and Counseling, 61,* 228–235.

Hobel, C. J., Dunkel-Schetter, C., Roesch, S. C., Castro, L. C., & Arora C. P. (1999). Maternal plasma corticotropin-releasing hormone associated with stress at 20 weeks' gestation in pregnancies ending in preterm delivery. *American Journal of Obstetrics and Gynecology, 180,* S257–S263.

Howell, E. A., Mora, P. A., Horowitz, C. R., & Leventhal, H. (2005). Racial and ethnic differences in factors associated with early postpartum depressive symptoms. *Obstetrics & Gynecology, 105*(6), 1442–1450.

Jones, I., & Craddock, N. (2001). Candidate gene studies of bipolar disorder. *Annals of Medicine, 33*(4), 248–256.

LaRocco-Cockburn, A., Melville, J., Bell, M., & Katon, W. (2003). Depression screening attitudes and practices among obstetrician-gynecologists. *Obstetrics & Gynecology, 101*(5), 892–897.

Louik, C., Lin, A. E., Werler, M. M., Hernandez-Diaz, S., & Mitchell, A. A. (2007). First-trimester use of selective serotonin reuptake inhibitors and the risk of birth defects. *New England Journal of Medicine, 356*(26), 2675–2683.

Maloni, J. A., Park, S., Anthony, M. K., & Musil, C. M. (2004). Measurement of antepartum depressive symptoms during high-risk pregnancy. *Research in Nursing & Health, 28,* 16–26.

Marcus, S. M., Flynn, H. A., Blow, F. C., & Barry, K. L. (2003). Depressive symptoms among pregnant women screened in obstetrics settings. *Journal of Women's Health, 12*(4), 373–380.

O'Hara, M. W., & Swain, A. M. (1996). Rates and risk of postpartum depression: A meta-analysis. *International Review of Psychiatry, 8,* 37–54.

Rich-Edwards, J. W., Kleinman, K., Abrams, A., Harlow, B. L., McLaughlin, T. J., Joffe, H., et al.(2006). Sociodemographic predictors of antenatal and postpartum depressive symptoms among women in a medical group practice. *Journal of Epidemiology and Community Health, 60*(3), 221–227.

Shadigian, E. M., & Bauer, S. T. (2005). Pregnancy-associated death: A qualitative systematic review of homicide and suicide. *Obstetrical & Gynecological Survey, 60*(3), 183–190.

Spinelli, M. G., & Endicott, J. (2003). Controlled clinical trial of interpersonal psychotherapy versus parenting education program for depressed pregnant women. *American Journal of Psychiatry, 160*(3), 555–562.

Suri, R., & Burt, V. K. (1997). The assessment and treatment of postpartum psychiatric disorders. *Journal of Practical Psychiatry and Behavioral Health, 3,* 67–77.

Zuckerman, B., Amaro, H., Bauchner H., & Cabral, H. (1989). Depressive symptoms during pregnancy: Relationship to poor health behaviors. *American Journal of Reproductive Health, 160,* 1107–1111.

10 The Pediatrician's Role in Identifying Postpartum Mood Disorders

MARY ANN LOFRUMENTO, MD, FAAP

Pediatricians, who provide the care for newborn infants, encounter mothers in the postpartum period more frequently than any other health care provider. The mother's physician, usually the obstetrician, will see her at approximately 4 to 6 weeks postpartum, and, if there are no ongoing problems, will not see her again until the next annual visit or unless a medical problem arises. Pediatricians, on the other hand, will see the baby, and hopefully, the mother, for at least six visits at 2 to 4 weeks, and then at intervals of 2, 4, 6, 9, and 12 months. In addition to office visits, there are often multiple phone contacts during a baby's first year, especially by mothers of firstborn babies, as well as interactions with various staff members. Even the prenatal visit can be an opportunity for screening and identifying mothers with PPMD. If a mother has other children, an ongoing relationship has already been established with the pediatrician, who can compare her pre- and postnatal mood and behavior with what was seen previously.

These factors give pediatricians a unique opportunity to recognize postpartum mood disorders and provide both information and referrals when needed. However, this cannot occur unless pediatricians educate themselves and their office staff to recognize the often subtle presentations of this disorder, establish a universal screening method for all new mothers, and create an action plan for follow-up that is easily implemented.

WHO IS OUR PATIENT?

Although infants are the primary patients of pediatricians, babies cannot be cared for in isolation. The American Academy of Pediatrics Task Force on the Family (2003) has stressed the importance of "family-oriented" pediatric care to improve family outcomes. The "health and well-being of children is inextricably linked to their parents' physical, emotional, and social health" (Wertlieb, 2003). If a mother suffers from any disorder on the spectrum of PPMD, there may be negative effects on the health and well-being of the baby (see also chapter 3 "Effects of Maternal Postpartum Depression on the Infant and Older Siblings"). Therefore, a pediatrician must consider both the baby and mother as patients.

A growing body of evidence points to the negative impact of maternal postnatal depression on children of all ages (Grace, Evindar, & Stewart, 2003; Murray & Cooper, 1997; Murray, Fiori-Cowley, Hooper, & Cooper, 1996). Particularly vulnerable are infants and toddlers who can show signs of withdrawn behavior as young as 3 months of age when exposed to depressed mothers (Cicchetti, Rogosch, Toth, & Spagnola, 1997; Weinberg & Tronick, 1998).

The effects of untreated postpartum mood disorders, especially depression, can be long lasting. Infants of severely depressed mothers are at risk for child abuse, neglect, and, in cases of postpartum psychosis, infanticide (Beck, 1998; Cadzow, Armstrong, & Fraser, 1999). Even in milder cases, infants and toddlers of depressed mothers may exhibit sleep and feeding difficulties, be more withdrawn, and have increased periods of fussiness and crying (Weinberg & Tronick, 1998). Recent studies have also shown that maternal depression has an effect on preventative care practices, including use of an infant car seat or the utilization of regular pediatric care services (Mandl, Tronick, Brennan, Alpert, & Homer, 1999; McCarthy et al., 2000; McLennan & Kotelchuck, 2000; Minkovitz et al., 2005). As they grow older, children exposed to maternal depression in infancy may have cognitive, social, and behavioral problems even into the school age years (Sinclair & Murray, 1998). All of these studies should alert pediatricians to the urgent need to identify depressed mothers and have a plan to refer them for treatment.

THE IMPORTANCE OF ATTACHMENT

Secure attachment to a mother during infancy is vital to healthy emotional development. Pediatricians see this everyday in pediatric practice: the magic moment when a newborn infant is feeding and can only focus the distance between his and his mother's eyes. The mutual gaze is the first social connection and a baby will become very attuned to the facial expressions of his mother. Touch is almost as important, as a mother comforts her baby with a soothing rocking motion when needed. A baby develops trust when his cries of hunger, pain, or restlessness are met quickly. These seemingly minor interactions, as a baby develops in the first 3 months of life, are vital to a normal healthy attachment to his mother.

Case Study 10.1

Mrs. Jones and her 2-week-old are here for their first visit. She sits in a chair in your examination room, her eyes looking away from her newborn infant who is beginning to fuss as he lies in his infant seat on the floor next to her. She answers your questions but only minimally responds to the baby's cry. After greeting her and talking about the birth and how the baby is doing, you ask to see the baby. At first she doesn't seem to acknowledge your request. It takes her a minute to bring the baby to the exam table, but then she sits down again and leaves you with the baby.

In the case above, the mother has had difficulty making that crucial attachment to her newborn. Equally problematic, when a mother is depressed or anxious, it can be communicated to her baby through her gaze, her hold, and her response to the infant's discomfit. If a mother is depressed or withdrawn, she may not respond to the baby's cues in a timely way. When feeding her infant, her eyes may be more vacant or even averted away from the baby's eyes. An anxious mother may be too intense and may hold a baby too tightly or rock a bit too hard as she copes with her own anxiety. Infants exposed to maternal depression and anxiety are at risk of developing insecure attachment patterns that can last throughout their lives and have effects on all subsequent relationships (Cicchetti, Rogosch, & Toth, 1988; Weinberg & Tronick, 1998).

WHAT DOES A MOOD DISORDER LOOK LIKE?

Studies have indicated that with the exception of severely depressed and psychotic patients, mothers with PPMD may not be obvious. And they may present to pediatricians and the pediatric office staff with a variety of symptoms. Symptoms of depression ranging from mild to severe are the most common. However, looking for only the classic symptoms of depression, pediatricians may miss those mothers who present with anxiety, obsessive-compulsive behavior and/or obsessive thinking, panic disorder, and even various degrees of hypomania. All of these mothers are suffering from different forms of a postpartum mood disorder and may present to the pediatric office in several different ways.

Regardless of their symptoms, it is not uncommon for mothers to try to hide their depression, anxiety, or intrusive thoughts of harming the baby or themselves for fear of having the baby taken away. Because mothers with PPMD may minimize or hide their symptoms, pediatricians need to look carefully for clues.

Case Study 10.2

> Ms. Smith brings her 2-month old baby in for her well-child check up. She appears very tired and admits that she hasn't been sleeping very well. She holds the baby in her arms and tries to smile, but you notice that she seems to lack energy. You ask how she is feeling and she says "Fine. She's a really good baby." She goes on to say how well the baby is feeding and sleeping and how everyone says how lucky she is that the baby is so easy. You notice she is not really smiling as she says this and her affect seems a bit flat. "I'm just really tired, but I'm sure I'll feel better soon."

For mothers like Ms. Smith, it is the cognitive dissonance between her saying she is happy, yet not showing she enjoys her new baby that is a clue. When asked about how she feels about being a new mother, a mom suffering from depression may answer, "It's wonderful," but with a very flat affect and a look that does not seem to agree with the statement. Talking about what others are saying about the baby, rather than expressing her own feelings, is another clue.

Case Study 10.3

Mrs. Harris is a new mother with a 4-week-old baby. At her 2-week visit, she expressed concern that she was not producing enough breast milk and that the baby was not gaining enough weight. She has called the office and spoken with your nurse almost daily for the past 2 weeks and has insisted on bringing the baby in for another weight check. When she comes in she appears very anxious and asks repeatedly how she can tell how much breast milk she is producing. You weigh the baby and reassure her that the baby is gaining adequate weight, but she still insists that her milk is not enough.

As in the case above, an additional clue can be frequent phone calls to the doctors, nurses, and other staff members as well as frequent appointments to have the baby seen. The topics of concern may be serious or very mundane. It is not uncommon for new mothers to be anxious about their babies or insecure about their abilities as a mother; however, in these cases, it is the intensity of the concern that should be a clue. A common thread might be an overanxious nature and obsessive thoughts, such as clinging to the idea that something is wrong with the baby even when the evidence points to a healthy child.

Case Study 10.4

Mrs. Kelly has been your patient for many years and has two other children who are 3 and 5 years old. She brings her baby in for the 4-month check up and you notice that she seems much more fatigued and irritable than you have ever observed before. She snaps at her 5-year-old and breaks into tears. You have the nurse take her children outside and she confides in you that she is having trouble coping and has had repeated thoughts about just leaving the baby somewhere. "I can't stop thinking about leaving him somewhere, where someone else could care for him better. I'm such a horrible mother for thinking this, but I just can't stop the thoughts."

In most cases, obsessive and intrusive thoughts are secret and a mother may be very frightened to admit them to anyone, even her trusted pediatrician. Heneghan, Mercer, and Deleone, (2004) have shown that even if a woman feels comfortable and safe confiding in her doctor, she may not reveal these thoughts and will suffer in silence rather than risk being exposed as a "horrible mother." Screening tests can be helpful, as well as educating women that this type of obsessive thinking can occur postpartum. But there is no substitute for a pediatrician being aware and sensitive to the clues.

OPPORTUNITIES IN PEDIATRIC PRACTICE

The Prenatal Visit

Prenatal visits provide an opportunity for both obtaining information about a mother's risk factors for PPMD as well as observing a mother's prenatal mood. Although this visit is often a chance for the mother and father to interview a pediatrician about their practice, it can also be a chance for the doctor to get to know the parents. Information about PPMD can be given out with general information about baby care and breastfeeding. This may encourage a mother to open up to her pediatrician if she should experience any of these symptoms in the future. After the baby's birth, if a mother's mood or behavior is markedly different from her prenatal visit, this can be a warning sign.

After Delivery

In the hospital, pediatricians see new mothers during the first 2 to 3 days postpartum. It is not uncommon to have a mother experience the "baby blues." The combination of postpartum hormones and postdelivery exhaustion are most likely responsible for these feelings of sadness. These baby blues are a very common occurrence in the first 2 weeks postpartum and reassurance is all that may be needed at this time. Since most women feel better in a few days, telling a mother it is okay to have these feelings and that they will pass in a week or two can be appropriate. However, the presence of the baby blues, especially if they are severe, may be a warning sign that this woman may experience PPMD within a few weeks (Hannah, Adams, Lee, Glover, & Sandler, 1992). This is an opportunity to let the mother know that if she is not feeling better after 2 weeks that she should let her pediatrician or her obstetrician know. Although information pamphlets about postpartum mood disorders are given out to new mothers at many hospitals today, this brief discussion may be what she remembers if she is not feeling better soon.

Equally of concern is the mother who experiences euphoria or mild hypomania after delivery. Studies have shown that these mothers may also be at increased risk for depression a few weeks postpartum (Glover, Liddle, Taylor, Adams, & Sandler, 1994; Hannah et al., 1992). Since these mothers feel "wonderful," they will not be as receptive to talking about depression, but the pediatrician can make a note and be extra observant at the first two well-child visits.

The Postnatal Visit

"How are *you* feeling?" This simple question to the mother is vital at the first postnatal visit. Usually at 2 to 4 weeks after the birth of a baby, mothers are tired and even a bit overwhelmed by their new responsibilities. Most mothers will welcome the empathetic concern about how they are doing at a time when all the focus is on the new baby. They may also, however, be afraid to open up completely, even if they have a preexisting relationship with their pediatrician (Heneghan, Mercer, & Deleone, 2004). More important even than asking the question is listening carefully to the answer and observing the mother's face. If the answer is a quick "I'm doing fine" but the facial expression says otherwise, ask more detailed questions such as "How are you sleeping?" "Who is helping you with the baby?" "Are you worried about anything in particular about the baby?" Listening to the mother, observing her affect and her interaction with the baby are opportunities for identifying mothers who may be struggling with very uncomfortable feelings. Asking the questions can be the easy part. The challenge for pediatricians is to be prepared if these questions of concern bring an emotional answer.

The First-Year Visits

Pediatricians enjoy not only the growth and development of their young patients, but also the developing relationship with the mothers of these children, who are so much a part of the pediatric practice experience. Therefore, pediatricians have a unique opportunity to experience mothers as they go through the postpartum period and beyond. Being on the lookout for changes in a mother's mood or a sudden increase in worries or concerns about the baby's well-being is another opportunity for the pediatrician to identify those mothers with PPMD.

During the first year of life, there are multiple visits to the pediatrician, but the most important for identifying PPMD are the first three: 2-weeks, 2-months, and 4-months. Symptoms may not appear for 2 to 6 weeks postpartum and usually peak at about 3 months (Stowe, Hostetter, & Newport, 2005). It is during this critical period that symptoms of PPMD generally worsen. The challenge for the pediatrician is being able to distinguish between the normal new mother, who after weeks of sleeplessness, fatigue, and adjustment to being a parent, appears overwhelmed and exhausted, and the mother who is having true symptoms of PPMD (Heneghan, et al., 2007).

The 4-month visit is very important because, by this time, unless a baby has had severe colic, feeding difficulties, or a medical problem, most mothers begin to appear less exhausted, less anxious, and even a bit more confident about their new role. If at this visit, a mother exhibits any of the symptoms of depression, especially a somewhat flat affect or an intense preoccupation about the health of the baby or herself, it may be a signal that she has a PPMD.

An Established Relationship

PPMD can also affect mothers who are having their second, third, or fourth child, even if they have not had a previous history of PPMD after earlier births. The ongoing relationship and the level of trust between a mother and her pediatrician is another wonderful opportunity. A relationship is already established and most likely the pediatrician has a good sense of a mother's personality, mood, and the level of her anxiety. Her pediatrician has observed how she copes with stressful situations, such as a baby's illness, and can recognize a sudden change in her mood, her ability to cope, or her reported feelings of being overwhelmed by caring for her children. In fact, many members of the office staff may know this mother and might notice changes as well.

Even with a long-standing relationship, it may still be difficult for a mother to discuss her feelings of depression, sadness, or anxiety. In fact, she may be more uncomfortable because of her fear of appearing less competent in the eyes of her children's physician (Heneghan et al., 2004; Heneghan et al., 2007). Being sensitive and aware of changes in a mother after the birth of a second or third child is also important. Pediatricians may need to overcome their own uncomfortable feelings about discussing this sensitive topic with someone they have known for a long time.

The Phone Calls

Phone calls to the office provide pediatricians with another opportunity to identify those mothers who may be suffering from depression, obsessive thinking, or anxiety. Since many of these calls are handled by the pediatric nursing staff, it is vital that all the staff members be educated in the signs and symptoms of PPMD. Multiple calls about a baby's well-being may be a clue. These calls might be about feeding problems, especially concerns about not being able to nurse or that a baby is not getting enough breast milk, or concerns about the baby's weight. Or the calls may be about the baby's breathing pattern or concerns about choking. Many new mothers exhibit anxious fears about their new babies. The difference will be in the intensity of the concerns, the frequency of the calls, and the persistence of worry even after reassurance from the doctors and nurses.

Although the new baby may be the focus of the obsessive thinking, it can extend to other children in the family or even to the home itself. For example, a mother with a newborn suddenly becomes overwhelmed with anxiety and is convinced that her 4-year-old has Lyme disease, or a mother with several children who becomes convinced that her house is infested with mold, despite testing that proves otherwise.

Mothers suffering from obsessional fears and worries can often be identified by receptionists and nurses who receive the phone calls or schedule the visits. However, if the office staff is not educated about PPMD, these mothers may be labeled annoying and their concerns minimized: "Oh no, not Mrs. Jones again, I just spoke with her." The key is in recognizing that Mrs. Jones may be suffering from obsessive thoughts or intense anxiety.

To Screen or Not to Screen

Multiple studies have now shown the value of maternal screening. In one study, 50% of women with clinically significant symptoms of depression remained undetected by clinicians (Chaudron, 2003). The use of short questionnaires such as the Edinburgh Postnatal Depression Scale (EPDS) (Cox, Holden, & Sagovsky, 1987), Postpartum Checklist (Beck, 1995), or the Postpartum Depression Screening Scale (Beck & Gable, 2000) to screen mothers of newborns has been shown to significantly improve the identification of mothers with PPMD (Beck & Gable, 2000; Boyd, Le, & Somberg, 2005; Gjerdingen & Yawn, 2007). Chaudron, Szilagyi, Kitzman, Wadkins, & Conwell (2004) demonstrated that screening at well-child visits was both feasible and effective. In a perfect pediatric world, screening should be ideally done at each of the 2-week, 2-month, 4-month, and 12-month visits. In some states, such as New Jersey and Illinois, these screening tools are now mandated for pediatricians and obstetricians (at least at the first postpartum visits) and go hand in hand with educational programs aimed at informing members of the health care community about postpartum mood disorders.

Freeman et al. (2005) revealed that the use of these screening tools in a pediatric office or during well-child care visits identified 11%–13% of mothers who would not have been identified with clinical observation alone. Other studies have found that the use of screening questionnaires at well-baby visits is both feasible and accepted by both mothers and staff (Buist et al., 2006; Gemmill, Leigh, Ericksen, & Milgrom, 2006). By universally screening all mothers during the first year of life, identification of at-risk mothers improved from 1.6% to 8.5% (Chaudron et al., 2004), and from 29% to 40% in another study (Heneghan, Silver, & Stein, 2000). To be successful, screening must be simple, as well as easy to administer and score. However, the limitations of a screening tool must be understood. A positive screen does not necessarily mean that a mother definitely has a mood disorder (Gilbody, House, & Sheldon, 2005). A positive screen must be followed by further discussion and possible referral to another specialist if needed for further evaluation.

OBSTACLES AND CHALLENGES FOR THE PEDIATRICIAN

Obstacles to Identification

Although pediatricians have a unique opportunity to identify mothers suffering from or at-risk for PPMD, several obstacles exist in the pediatric practice (Horwitz et al., 2007). In a national survey of pediatricians, 57% felt they were responsible for identifying mothers who are depressed in the postpartum period, yet only 32% expressed confidence in their ability to diagnose PPMD (Olson et al., 2002). In another survey, less than one-third of the pediatricians questioned felt they could recognize the symptoms (Wiley, Burke, Gill, & Law, 2004). Therefore, the first obstacle for pediatricians to overcome is education in all aspects of postpartum mood disorders, including signs and symptoms as well as the risk factors in a mother's history.

The second obstacle is a shortage of time for visits (Horwitz et al., 2007). The average pediatrician spends approximately 10 to 15 minutes doing a well-baby check-up. Well-child visits are often booked back to back with other check-ups or sick visits. Depending on the type of practice, there might not be a second doctor to cover other patients if there is a problem and a doctor needs more time. Doctors who are in a hurry may not truly listen to the mother's needs, or they may feel too swamped to deal with mental health issues. Some pediatricians, already pressured for time, may be afraid to "open up a can of worms." There is not a great deal of room and flexibility in most doctors' schedules to allow an involved emotional discussion with a mother who may open up about her feelings, even for crisis management. Both a shortage of time and feelings of inadequacy can lead to playing down the mother's symptoms in the mistaken belief that this will go away with time.

For members of the office staff, the obstacles are not just a lack of knowledge about PPMD and therefore not recognizing the symptoms, but also not knowing how to approach the doctor with concerns, and perhaps being afraid of overstepping boundaries. Therefore, in addition to the need for education, a climate that encourages a team approach and open communication between staff and pediatricians must be established. It is the responsibility of the senior pediatricians in the office to do this in order to ensure the trickle-down effect of open communication.

Obstacles to Referrals

Having identified a mother as at-risk for PPMD, through clinical judgment or a screening tool, some pediatricians might still feel uncomfortable discussing this with someone who isn't really their patient. But the Academy of Pediatrics has made it clear that pediatricians are responsible for family-centered care. As with a mother who has a chronic illness or cancer, pediatricians cannot ignore the effects on the children and must offer support for her care. Asking a mother if she has discussed how she is feeling with her spouse, partner, or her obstetrician is a simple way of beginning the dialogue. The next step might be to offer to contact a family member, the mother's obstetrician, or her primary care doctor or a mental health professional.

Referral to a mental health professional, however, can also pose a challenge for the pediatrician. There may be a lack of adequate providers in the community, and many managed care companies place restrictions on referrals that come directly from physicians. While it might take more effort on the part of the staff, organizing and reviewing, in advance, a list of referrals in the area for therapists, especially those who specialize in perinatal mood disorders, and the plans they participate in, will be helpful to have when needed.

Another challenge can be resistance on the part of the mother to both the diagnosis and referral. As much as the pediatrician might want to help, the mother is not under obligation to seek help. And unless, in your opinion, either the baby or mother is at serious risk, the pediatrician is not under obligation to do much more than inform and provide information regarding available resources in the community, although every effort should be made to involve a family member or the mother's physician. In this situation, ongoing contact between the pediatrician and the mother is crucial to make sure both mother and baby are doing well.

TAKING ACTION AND OVERCOMING OBSTACLES

Education Is the First Step

The first step for any pediatrician is to become knowledgeable about postpartum mood disorders. This includes the risk factors, the signs and symptoms of all the possible presentations, treatment options, and, most important, for pediatricians, the effects on infants and children. Taking a continuing medical education (CME) course, reading literature, and taking advantage of the resources of organizations such as Postpartum Support International or local mental health experts in the field can all provide an important knowledge base for pediatricians. Some states, such as New Jersey, provide a tool kit of educational and referral materials for pediatric practices prepared by the state chapter of the American Academy of Pediatrics.

However, education cannot stop with the physician. In any pediatric office there are contacts with multiple members of the pediatric team. Therefore, the entire office, especially the nursing staff, must be educated about PPMD. As already mentioned, the mother who "overutilizes" the office staff and the doctors, or appears very anxious or needy, might be labeled as annoying, rather than depressed. But if the nurses, receptionists, even the back office billing and insurance staff, are educated about PPMD through handouts, a discussion with one of the doctors or a guest speaker, it improves the chances of identifying those mothers who may have one. One solution for the time-challenged doctor is to assign this task to a head nurse or office manager who could then prepare a program for other members of the staff.

Creation of an Action Plan

Once the education of the doctors and support staff has been accomplished, the next step is to create a plan that can be carried out easily within the busiest of office settings (see sample Action Plan). A meeting to create a workable plan should include at least one of the doctors, the head nurse, and the office manager. This ensures that all members of the team are involved and can contribute their ideas and solutions to potential obstacles. The action plan should be tailored to the specifics of each practice and the environment in which the practice resides. The simpler the action plan, the more likely it will be successful in identifying and referring women at risk or suffering from PPMD.

Information sheets that list the signs and symptoms of the spectrum of postpartum mood disorders should be included. The plan should outline the office policy regarding the screening of all mothers in the first year of life and should be available in a binder accessible to all staff. The exact visits in which screening will take place should be listed. The screening tool chosen by the doctors should be mentioned and a sample placed in the binder. If screening questionnaires are scored, the scores that would be considered positive should be noted. A consultation sheet to record the screening results for the mother should also be included.

The plan should include actions to be taken based on the severity of the mother's symptoms. For example, a mother who appears to have postpartum psychosis would be a medical emergency with notification of other family members and referral for emergency psychiatric care. Likewise, a mother who might be diagnosed with severe depression and thought to be at risk of harming herself or her infant might need an immediate referral. However, for mothers with milder forms of depression, anxiety, or obsessional thinking, information should be given explaining PPMD and the mother counseled about the possibility that she may be suffering from one of these postpartum conditions. Emphasis should be on the importance of treatment for both herself and her baby.

It should be emphasized that it is not the responsibility of the pediatrician to diagnose depression or other mood disorders in the mother. The responsibility is to screen, and if a mood disorder is suspected, to refer to other clinicians for diagnosis and treatment.

A practice may devise several categories for referral based on a combination of screening score and doctor's assessment. The first step is to refer the mother back to her primary care doctor or obstetrician who can directly provide treatment or referral. The pediatrician should offer to call the mother's doctor.

In addition, it is helpful to provide a list of available mental health professionals who have some expertise in caring for mothers with postpartum depression and other mood disorders. This list should be included in the action plan. A list of the managed care plans that each practitioner participates in should be attached. If the pediatrician has informed the mother of his or her concerns, and if a mother asks for a direct referral to a mental health provider, a selected member of the office staff can be designated to provide this mother with a list of these providers.

It is always prudent for the pediatrician to document all of this. Chaudron et al. (2007) recommend having a separate area for this documentation, such as a consultation sheet, since this information is regarding the mother's health and not the baby's and should not be a part of the baby's permanent medical record.

In addition to the Action Plan binder made for the staff, premade folders can be prepared in advance to give to mothers. The folders should include informational handouts on postpartum mood disorders; a list of related support groups, Web sites, books, and hotline phone numbers (if available in your area); and an additional list of mental health professionals in your area who treat mothers with PPMD.

Overcoming Legal and Privacy Concerns

Because of the Health Insurance Portability and Accountability Act (HIPAA) passed by Congress in 1996, privacy concerns present another challenge (Chaudron, Szilagyi, Campbell, Mounts, & McInerny, 2007). This remains a gray area for pediatricians because HIPAA applies to doctor-patient relationships, and for pediatricians, this refers to children, who are their primary patients, not their mothers. Pediatricians might be concerned about sharing information about the mother with family members or other physicians.

Ideally, a mother would ask the pediatrician to call a family member, her obstetrician, or even a mental health professional, if this was needed. But what if a mother is resistant or refuses permission for her pediatrician to discuss this with anyone? What can the pediatrician, concerned about both mother and baby, do? Depending on how concerned the pediatrician is about both mother and baby, the next step could be simply following up with the mother in a few days or notifying the father of the baby, assuming there are no custody issues. Because there are no obstacles to communication between health providers, another step could be to notify the mother's obstetrician or primary care doctor, who can then take the next steps to help the mother. A pediatrician would have to weigh these steps carefully because taking them could jeopardize the all-important relationship between pediatrician and mother.

However, if a pediatrician suspects that a mother is suicidal, homicidal, severely manic, or psychotic, or when there is physical evidence of the effects of the mother's mood disorder on the baby, such as failure to thrive or obvious evidence of neglect, the answer is actually uncomplicated. Pediatricians have a responsibility to protect the infant and any other children. In this type of case, pediatricians can call a family member, child protective services, or even the police.

Follow-Up Is Critical

Several studies have shown that, even after women with PPMD are identified through screening, they may not actually get referred to a mental health professional (Gjerdingen & Yawn, 2007). In emergency situations, follow-up must be done immediately and documented in the child's chart. For nonemergency situations, follow-up should not be longer than a week after the visit. Although in some practices, a member of the nursing or office staff could follow up on patients to see if contact with the mother's personal doctor or a mental health professional has occurred, it is ultimately the responsibility of the pediatrician to make sure that the follow-up has occurred. This can be accomplished with a simple phone call to the mother or to the mother's physician.

It is often difficult for mothers with a PPMD to seek help. There are many steps to take at a time when they may be feeling quite overwhelmed. Family members or friends may minimize the situation and advise them to "just wait it out." The encouragement and follow-up from a trusted professional can have great impact on whether a mother will get the help she needs.

SUMMARY

The welfare of babies is the responsibility of the pediatrician and for the welfare of these most vulnerable patients, pediatricians need to do everything possible to ensure that a mother is not suffering from a significant postpartum mood disorder or psychosis. To achieve this goal, pediatricians need the commitment to work toward a solution within their own practice settings. There may be challenges and obstacles to overcome, but through a combination of education, awareness, the creation of a workable action plan, and follow-up, pediatricians can play a vital role in helping mothers with postpartum mood disorders.

Sample of an Action Plan for a Pediatric Office

Office staff binder contains:

- Handouts that outline the different types of postpartum mood disorders and symptoms
- EPSD screening sheets
- Written policy encouraging any member of the office staff to speak to the doctor(s) if they suspect that a mother may have a mood disorder postpartum
- A sheet outlining the procedures for screening and schedule of when patients will be screened, that is, 2 weeks, 2 months
- Consultation sheet to record mother's screening results or doctor's notes

Procedure for screening:

- Receptionist places screening sheet in chart.
- Nurse gives to mother in exam room and explains the office policy (or state requirement) that all new mothers are screened for postpartum mood disorders; asks mother if she has any questions.
- Sheet is scored by nurse.
- Doctor is notified for scores of 10 or above.
- If patient answers 1, 2, or 3 to question 10, the doctor should be notified as soon as possible before he or she sees the mother.
- All sheets should be kept in the infant's chart.

Steps for referral (based on screening results or clinical evaluation):

If a mother's score is 10–19 and the doctor feels that she has mild to moderate symptoms of depression, anxiety, obsessional thinking, or panic attacks:

- Doctor informs mother of his or her concerns.
- Doctor informs mother of the importance of treatment for herself and for the baby (other children).
- Folder with information is given to mother.

- Doctor offers to call family members or mother's doctor.
- Document in consultation sheet.

If the mother's screening score is 20–30 and if the doctor feels that the symptoms are more severe, but that the mother is not an immediate danger to herself or to her baby:

- Immediately contact the mother's obstetrician or primary care doctor.
- Optionally, contact the father of the baby.
- Document in consultation sheet.

If the doctor feels that the mother is a danger to herself or the baby, or has symptoms of severe depression, mania, or psychosis:

- Immediate referral to mental health provider, hospital, or crisis hotline
- Notification of the mother's obstetrician or primary care physician
- Mother is not to leave with baby alone.
- Insist that family members be called.
- Document in consultation sheet.

Follow-up procedures

- All patients should be followed up within 2 weeks.
- Follow-up should be done by designated office staff, nurse, or physician.
- Document follow-up in consultation sheet.

REFERENCES

American Academy of Pediatrics Task Force on the Family. (2003). Report of the task force on the family. *Pediatrics, 111,* 1541–1571.

Beck, C. (1995). Screening methods for postpartum depression. *Journal of Obstetric Gynecologic & Neonatal Nursing, 24,* 308–312.

Beck, C. (1998). The effects of postpartum depression on child development: A meta-analysis. *Archives of Psychiatric Nursing, 12,* 12–20.

Beck, C. T., & Gable, R. K. (2000). Postpartum depression screening scale: Development and psychometric testing. *Nursing Research, 49,* 272–282.

Boyd, R. C, Le, H. N., & Somberg, R. (2005). Review of screening instruments for postpartum depression. *Archives of Women's Mental Health, 8,* 141–153.

Buist, A., Condon, J., Brooks, J., Speelman, J., Milgrom, B., Hayes, D., et al. (2006). Acceptability of routine screening for perinatal depression. *Journal of Affective Disorders, 93,* 233–237.

Cadzow, S., Armstrong, K., & Fraser, J. (1999). Stressed parents with infants: Reassessing physical abuse risk factors. *Child Abuse and Neglect, 23,* 845–853.

Chaudron, L. H. (2003). Postpartum depression: What pediatricians need to know. *Pediatrics in Review, 24,* 154–161.

Chaudron, L. H., Szilagyi, P. G., Campbell, A. T., Mounts, K. O., & McInerny, T. K. (2007). Legal and ethical considerations: Risks and benefits of postpartum depression screening at well-child visits. *Pediatrics, 119,* 123–128.

Chaudron, L. H., Szilagyi, P. G., Kitzman, H. J., Wadkins, H. I., & Conwell, Y. (2004). Detection of postpartum depressive symptoms by screening at well-child visits. *Pediatrics, 113,* 551–558.

Cicchetti, D., Rogosch, F., & Toth, S. L. (1988). Maternal depressive disorder and contextual risk: Contributions to the development of attachment insecurity and behavioral problems in toddlerhood. *Developmental Psychopatholgy, 10,* 283–300.

Cicchetti, D., Rogosch, F., Toth, S., & Spagnola, M. (1997). Affect, cognition and the emergence of self-knowledge in the toddler offspring of depressed mothers. *Journal of Experimental Child Psychology, 67,* 338–362.

Cox, J. L., Holden, J. M., & Sagovsky, R. (1987). Detection of postnatal depression: Development of the 10-item Edinburg Postnatal Depression Scale. *British Journal of Psychiatry, 150,* 782–786.

Freeman, M. P., Wright, R., Watchman, M., Wahl, R. A., Sisk, D. J., & Fraleigh, L., et al. (2005). Postpartum depression assessments at well-baby visits: Screening feasibility, prevalence, and risk factors. *Journal of Women's Health, 14,* 929–935.

Gemmill, A. W., Leigh, B., Ericksen, J., Milgrom, J. (2006). A survey of the clinical acceptability of screening for postnatal depression in depressed and non-depressed women. *BMC Public Health, 6,* 211.

Gilbody, S., House, A. O., & Sheldon, T. A. (2005). Screening and case finding instruments for depression. *The Cochrane Database of Systematic Reviews, 4,* Art No CD002792.pub2.

Gjerdingen, D. K., & Yawn, B. P. (2007). Postpartum depression screening: Importance, methods, barriers, and recommendations for practice. *Journal of the American Board of Family Medicine, 20,* 280–288.

Glover, V., Liddle, P., Taylor, A., Adams, D., & Sandler, M. (1994). Mild hypomania (the highs) can be a feature of the first postpartum week: Association with later depression. *British Journal of Psychiatry, 164,* 517–521.

Grace, S. L., Evindar, A., & Stewart, D. E. (2003). The effect of postpartum depression on child cognitive development and behavior: A review and critical analysis of the literature. *Archives of Women's Mental Health, 6,* 263–274.

Hannah, P., Adams, D., Lee, A., Glover, V., & Sandler, M. (1992). Links between early postpartum mood and postnatal depression *British Journal of Psychiatry, 160,* 777–780.

Heneghan, A. M., Chaudron, L., Storfer-Isser, A., Park, E. R., Kelleher, K. J., Stein, R., et al. (2007). Factors associated with identification and management of maternal depression by pediatricians. *Pediatrics, 119,* 444–454.

Heneghan, A. M., Mercer, M. B., & Deleone, N. L. (2004). Will mothers discuss parenting stress and depressive symptoms with their child's pediatrician? *Pediatrics, 113,* 460–467.

Heneghan, A. M., Silver, E. J., & Stein, R. E. (2000). Do pediatricians recognize mothers with depressive symptoms? *Pediatrics, 106,* 1367–1373.

Horwitz, S., Kelleher, K., Stein, R., Storfer-Isser, A., Youngstrom, E., Park, E., et al. (2007). Barriers to the identification and management of psychosocial issues in children and maternal depression. *Pediatrics, 119,* e208–e218.

Mandl, K., Tronick, E., Brennan, T., Alpert, H., & Homer, C. J. (1999). Infant health care use and maternal depression. *Archives of Pediatric and Adolescent Medicine, 153,* 808–814.

McCarthy, P., Freudigman, K., Cicchetti, D., Mayes, L., Benitez, J. L., Salloum, S., et al. (2000). The mother-child interaction and clinical judgement during acute pediatric illnesses. *Journal of Pediatrics, 136,* 809–817.

McLennan, J. D., & Kotelchuck, M. (2000). Parental prevention practices for young children in the context of maternal depression. *Pediatrics, 105,* 1090–1095.

Minkovitz, C. S., Strobino, D., Scharfstein, D., Hou, W., Miller, T., Mistry, K. B., et al. (2005). Maternal depressive symptoms and children's receipt of health care in the first 3 years of life. *Pediatrics, 115,* 306–314.

Murray, L., & Cooper, P. J. (1997). Postpartum depression and child development. *Psychology of Medicine, 27,* 253–260.

Murray, L., Fiori-Cowley, A., Hooper, R., & Cooper, P. (1996). The impact of postnatal depression and associated adversity on early mother-infant interactions and later infant outcome. *Child Development, 67,* 2512–2526.

Olson, A. L., Kemper, K. J., Kelleher, K. J., Hammond, C. S., Zuckerman, B. S., & Dietrich, A. J. (2002). Primary care pediatricians' roles and perceived responsibilities in the identification and management of maternal depression. *Pediatrics, 110,* 1169–1176.

Sinclair, D., & Murray, L. (1998). Effects of postnatal depression on children's adjustment to school. *British Journal of Psychiatry, 172,* 58–63.

Stowe, Z. N., Hostetter, A. L., & Newport, D. J. (2005). The onset of postpartum depression: Implications for clinical screening in obstetrical and primary care. *American Journal of Obstetrics and Gynecology, 192,* 522–526.

Weinberg, M. K., & Tronick, E. Z. (1998). Emotional characteristics of infants associated with maternal depression and anxiety. *Pediatrics, 102,* 1298–1303.

Wertleib, D. (2003). Converging trends in family research and pediatrics: Recent findings for the American Academy of Pediatrics Task Force on the Family. *Pediatrics, 111,* 1572–1587.

Wiley, C. C., Burke, G. S., Gill, P. A., & Law, N. E. (2004). Pediatricians' views of postpartum depression: A self-administered survey. *Archives of Women's Mental Health, 7,* 231–236.

11 The Nurses' Vantage Point

CHERYL TATANO BECK

Caring is the essence and unifying focus of nursing (Leininger & McFarland, 2006). It is the central dominant attribute of our discipline of nursing. The main points covered in this chapter include the NURSE Program Model of Care, nurses' caring for women suffering from postpartum mood and anxiety disorders, nurses' role in screening for postpartum depression, and posttraumatic stress disorder due to childbirth.

The power of caring lies in nurses making a difference in the lives they touch. Swanson (1999) conducted a meta-analysis of 130 published studies on caring. Positive consequences of patients experiencing nurses' caring included increased self-esteem and dignity, increased healing, and trusting relationships.

Nurses' caring is the foundation for creating a healing environment. Caring includes listening to patients, making one's presence felt, connecting with the spirit of the patient, and expressing emotions (Watson, 2006). Caring is an ethical guide to nurses' clinical practice.

Culturally based nursing care is a powerful means to maximize wellness, prevent illness, decrease cultural stresses, and enhance the quality of patients' cultural life (Leininger, 2007). Armed with culturally based knowledge, for instance, of postpartum mood and anxiety disorders, nurses can meet the needs of mothers in a rapidly growing multicultural world.

THE NURSE PROGRAM MODEL OF CARE

Sichel and Driscoll (1999) developed the NURSE program, which is a general plan of care for mothers experiencing a postpartum mood and/or anxiety disorder. This model includes five aspects of care that are crucial for healing. These aspects include Nourishment and Needs, Understanding, Rest and Relaxation, Spirituality, and Exercise (Driscoll, 2005).

In Nourishment and Needs, the focus is not only on food for the body, but also food for the mind—nutrition, vitamins, fluids, and medications (Beck & Driscoll, 2006). Nurses should ask mothers what they eat every day and also the amounts. Most often women concentrate on what their infants are eating and forget about their own nutritional needs. Adequate amounts of protein are essential for the mother in order to heal her body after delivery and for producing milk if she is breastfeeding. Vitamins, calcium, and omega-3 fatty acids are also important. Nourishment for the mind refers to medications if the mother needs these to treat her mood and/or anxiety disorder. Nurses need to explore with mothers what their needs are and how to negotiate how these can be obtained for her, for example, help with her older children.

In Understanding, the second aspect of the NURSE program, Sichel and Driscoll (1999) emphasize that psychotherapy is a key element in the treatment of postpartum mood and anxiety disorders. It is critical for a mother to have someone she trusts and feels safe with and someone whom she can share freely how she is feeling since the birth of her baby. Postpartum depression support groups are extremely helpful for women. Nurses can provide women with information on groups in their local area. They can also recommend books and Web sites on postpartum mood and anxiety disorders to assist women and their families to begin to understand their mental illness.

Rest and Relaxation is the third aspect of the NURSE plan. Sichel and Driscoll (1999) call for sleep to help restore a mother's brain biochemically and physiologically. Nurses can work with a mother to develop a sleep hygiene program where she goes to bed and wakes up at a regular time. This often involves the nurse bringing in the mother's family to help (Beck & Driscoll, 2006). Encouraging mothers to plan for rest and relaxation during the day is important. Relaxation breathing, yoga, and meditation can be suggested.

Spirituality involves helping a mother to experience what brings her joy in her life and connects her to a higher power (Beck & Driscoll, 2006).

Nurses can help new mothers explore things such as solitude, music, gardening, journaling, or connected relationships. Sichel and Driscoll (1999) stress that spirituality is not just considered organized religion, although religion may be important to a mother to help fulfill her spiritual needs.

Exercise, the final aspect in the NURSE program, is important to help secrete endorphins, which are mood enhancers. Nurses can help mothers plan an exercise regime appropriate for the number of weeks postpartum they are. Beck and Driscoll (2006) provide case studies using the NURSE program of care for each of the postpartum mood and anxiety disorders.

NURSES' CARING

What is it that mothers suffering from postpartum depression perceive as caring actions by nurses? In her qualitative study, Beck (1995) posed this question to 10 women who had experienced postpartum depression. Analysis of these interviews revealed the seven themes that describe the essence of nurses' caring for women who are grappling with mood disorder (see Table 11.1):

1. Having sufficient knowledge about postpartum depression to make a quick, correct diagnosis is viewed as an essential aspect of caring.
2. Using astute observation and intuition leads to an awareness that something might be wrong with the mother.
3. Nurses provide hope that the mothers' living nightmares will end.
4. A nurse's readily sharing valuable time was perceived as caring.
5. Caring involved making the appropriate referrals so the mother was started on the right path to recovery.
6. Caring involved the nurse making an extra effort to provide continuity of care for the mother.
7. Understanding what the mother was experiencing provided much needed comfort.

Each of the seven essential components of nurses' caring has implications for nurses who come in contact with new mothers. The results of this study will help alert and sensitize nurses to what the postpartum depressed mothers themselves perceive as nurses' caring.

Table 11.1

CARING THEME CLUSTERS WITH EXAMPLES OF SUBSUMED SIGNIFICANT STATEMENTS

Theme 1. Having sufficient knowledge about postpartum depression to make a quick, correct diagnosis is viewed as an essential aspect of caring.

- Now the tears are coming, and in 10 minutes she knew what was wrong with me. . . . I feel so fortunate.
- When I stopped by my nurse-midwife's office, all she had to do is ask one or two questions and the floodgates opened and then it became very obvious to her what was going on.
- Caring is knowing about postpartum depression because most really don't know about it, so you don't get diagnosed, especially if it hits you late like it hit me.

Theme 2. Using astute observation and intuition leads to an awareness that something might be wrong with the mother.

- I do remember a nurse coming into my room after things had really started to deteriorate. She seemed to be very aware that something could be going on with me that wasn't totally great.
- I've never really had any problems like PMS or anything. So I wasn't prepared for this, I would have thought I was going crazy. Lucky for me the nurse sensed something was wrong and prepared me. She said, "When you go home you may not feel that good."
- The nurse was good because she picked up I was upset on the second day in the hospital, and I had never said anything to her about these feelings.

Theme 3. Nurses provide hope that the mothers' living nightmares will end.

- It was so important that the nurse let me know that this would go away because I thought it would never go away.
- The nurse let me know that I was not alone, that there were other mothers who went through what I was going through and recovered.
- She told me I was sick and that it was an illness that could be treated.

Theme 4. A nurse's readily sharing valuable time was perceived as caring.

- I cried in my nurse-midwife's office for well over an hour. She sat with me and never made me feel like I was wasting her valuable time.
- The nurse from my obstetrician's office took the time to call my husband the next day to see if I was okay.

Table 11.1

CARING THEME CLUSTERS WITH EXAMPLES OF SUBSUMED SIGNIFICANT STATEMENTS (CONTINUED)

- I did not have an appointment with my nurse practitioner, but I stopped into the reception area and asked if she would have a couple of minutes for me. She came right out to see me even though I wasn't scheduled for an appointment.

Theme 5. Caring involved making the appropriate referrals so the mother was started on the right path to recovery.

- The nurse referred me to someone who understood about postpartum depression and wound up being my therapist for the next 9 months.
- About 4 weeks after the baby was born, I was finally getting desperate and I felt like I was going to pop. So I called my obstetrician and I talked to the nurse there, and thank God, she referred me to be evaluated.
- She referred me to a postpartum depression support group, and the network they are offering is absolutely fabulous.

Theme 6. Caring involved the nurse making an extra effort to provide continuity of care for the mother.

- I remember taking a shower because I knew I was going to have to go back in the hospital again. I was crying as hard as I could in the shower thinking that someone was going to admit me. Who was going to take care of the baby? At that point, the nurse from my obstetrician's office called me to ask how I was. I didn't feel so alone then.
- One of my labor and delivery nurses came to visit me on the postpartum floor, to see how I was doing, and noticed I was different and something was wrong.
- The nurse said this is my name. You can call me when I am next here if you experience any further problems.

Theme 7. Understanding what the mother was experiencing provided much needed comfort.

- She understood it was an illness and it was not my fault.
- One nurse understood what a real bad time I was going through. The rest of the nurses did not understand about postpartum depression. They thought I was just having a down time, the baby blues.
- The nurse did not pass judgment. She tried to understand what I was experiencing.

From "Perceptions of Nurses' Caring by Mothers Experiencing Postpartum Depression," by C. T. Beck, 1995, *Journal of Obstetric, Gynecologic, and Neonatal Nursing, 24,* p. 823.

In 1984 McCord reported that "a striking aspect of postpartum depression is how covertly it is suffered" (p. 244). Sadly, almost 25 years later, this statement is still true. As one woman in Beck's study shared, "I was petrified to ask for help. I didn't know what it was. I was petrified to speak out."

Nurses have a responsibility to keep abreast of current research not only on postpartum depression, but also on other postpartum mood and anxiety disorders. The more mothers shared with nurses, the more nurses became astute in their ability to identify if something was not right, and whether the mother was suffering from postpartum depression. Additional knowledge vital to caring was information on resources in their local communities for treating postpartum mood and anxiety disorders. If armed with this knowledge, nurses can immediately refer mothers to get appropriate help. Knowledge of local postpartum depression support groups is essential. Nurses quickly making these critical referrals were perceived as caring by the women suffering from this devastating mood disorder.

In the midst of nurses' hectic schedules, mothers are appreciative of nurses readily sharing their time. Often, women reveal that they had never intended to cry, but once they realize how caring a nurse is being and that their call for help was heard, the floodgates open. Nurses need to be cognizant of their nonverbal behaviors and try to provide new mothers with an unhurried and caring atmosphere where they will feel safe to reveal their painful thoughts and feelings. These are emotions that they may have been feeling ashamed and guilty about for having since the birth of their babies.

In our society, where motherhood is idealized and equated to total happiness, mothers struggle with postpartum depression. They believe that family, friends, or health care providers cannot truly understand how devastating their mood disorder is. For these mothers to encounter a nurse who understands what they are experiencing is comforting and viewed as caring.

Loss of control is the basic problem women experience with postpartum depression: loss of control over their thoughts, emotions, and all aspects of their lives. Mothers go through a four-stage process called "Teetering on the Edge" to cope with and resolve this basic problem (see Figure 11.1; Beck, 1993). Each stage has specific implications for nursing practice. The first stage, called Encountering Terror, is where women are hit with an array of distressing symptoms: horrifying anxiety, relentless obsessive thinking, and enveloping fogginess. It is critical that

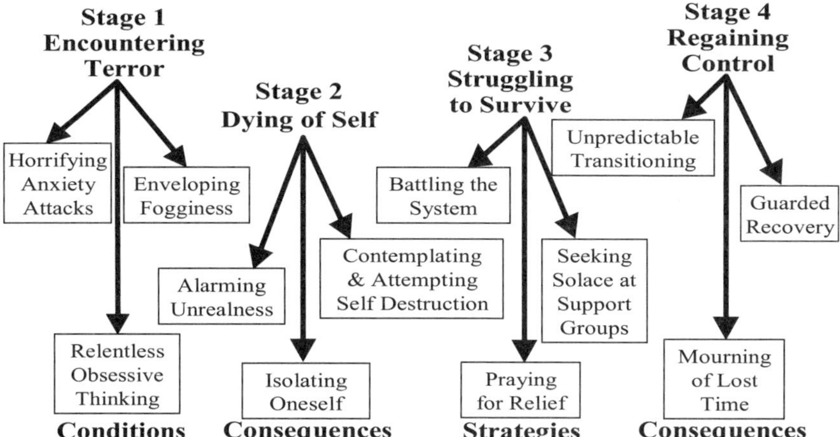

Figure 11.1 The four-stage process of Teetering on the Edge.

From "Teetering on the Edge: A Substantive Theory of Postpartum Depression," by C. T. Beck, 1993, *Nursing Research, 42*, p. 43. Copyright 1993 by Lippincott, Williams, & Wilkins. Reprinted with permission.

nurses are aware of the constellation of symptoms women may experience with this mood disorder, such as anxiety. Women may describe to nurses how anxious they have become since the birth of their baby. Feeling like their skin is literally crawling is a phrase women may use to describe their anxiety. If clinicians are not aware that, for some women, anxiety may be much more of a problem than the sadness or depression, the clinician may fail to identify that a mother may be experiencing postpartum depression. Women also frequently describe that they feel like there are cobwebs in their brains or that the fog is rolling in their brain. These images portray the mental confusion they are grappling with.

The second stage, Dying of Self, comprises Alarming Unrealness, Isolating Oneself, and Contemplating and Attempting to end their own lives. In Alarming Unrealness, mothers feel like their normal selves are gone. They do not feel real. They feel like robots who are just acting. This is a distinctive symptom of postpartum depression that nurses need to explore with mothers. At this point in their depression, women tend to isolate themselves because they believe no one really understands the depth of the living nightmare they are going through. Obviously, the most serious aspect of this second stage is suicidal ideation. Women carry a suffocating guilt over their perception of being failures as mothers and of their thoughts of harming their infants, which can lead to suicidal thoughts.

In stage 3, Struggling to Survive, women use differing strategies to try and cope with their postpartum depression: battling the health care system, prayer for relief, and seeking solace at support groups. The strategy of battling the system has important implications for nursing. When mothers finally get the courage to open up and admit to clinicians how they have been feeling since delivery, often women feel like they are patronized and their symptoms are minimized. Women are often told to just hang in there because what they are experiencing is the maternity blues and will go away on its own. These health professionals fail mothers in their initial call for help.

In the fourth and final stage of Teetering on the Edge, women start regaining control of their lives. The stage involves unpredictable transitioning, mourning lost time, and guarded recovery. During the unpredictable transitioning, women feel erratic as they feel their depression lift. There are "good days" and "bad days" and women wake up in the morning unable to predict which type of day it will be. Nurses need to provide anticipatory guidance to mothers during this unpredictable transitioning.

Mourning lost time has tremendous implications for nursing practices. Once mothers have recovered from postpartum depression, nurses need to be alert to the fact that these women still need help. Now that the mothers are no longer struggling to get through each day, they begin to mourn the lost time with their infants that the postpartum depression stole. Women will feel that they would never be able to recapture those times. Nurses need to become involved in grief work with these women.

Nurses need to remain vigilant about observing mother-infant interactions when women are suffering from postpartum depression. This troubled dyad may be in need of nursing's help (Beck, 1996). When postpartum depressed mothers are "teetering on the edge," they often fail to respond to their infants' cues. Women may erect an invisible wall between themselves and their infants to emotionally separate themselves from their infants. We know that mothers are primarily the major source of stimulation, which their infants need to develop normally. Nursing interactions that can be initiated to help this struggling dyad include teaching mothers massage therapy for infants to increase the tactical stimulation they need. Mothers can also be taught interaction coaching to increase their sensitivity to their infants' cues (Field, 1992).

Family-centered care is one of the hallmarks of the profession of nursing. The patient is not the only focus of nurses, so is the patient's family. Women suffering from postpartum depression are not the only ones of concern for nurses. The infant and the mother's partner are also under the purview of nursing care.

Partners of women with postpartum depression are at a significantly increased risk for experiencing psychological symptoms and disturbances, such as depression, compared to partners of nondepressed mothers (Roberts, Bushnell, Collings, & Purdie, 2006).

Even after controlling mothers' postpartum depressions, Ramchandani and colleagues (2005) found that elevated depressive symptoms in fathers during this time period are significantly related to adverse emotional and behavioral outcomes in children between the ages of 3 to 5, especially in boys. Evidence mounts from research that alerted nurses should also focus attention on partners of postpartum depressed women. Screening of partners for depression in the postpartum period may be necessary not only for the partners' quality of life, but also to help ensure appropriate development of their children. Partners of postpartum depressed women admit to feeling overwhelmed, isolated, frustrated, and stigmatized (Davey, Dziurawiec, & O'Brien-Malone, 2006). These men, who participated in a focus group with other partners of women with postpartum depression, valued this opportunity to share their experiences with others who were "in the same boat" and to learn different coping strategies. Karen R. Kleiman's *The Postpartum Husband: Practical Solutions for Living with Postpartum Depression* contains practical suggestions for men with postpartum depressed partners (2000).

Patient and family teaching are vital aspects of nursing care for women suffering from postpartum mood and/or anxiety disorder. Women and their family members can search for information on the Internet. However, nurses should warn mothers that the quality and accuracy of information about these disorders on the Web is quite varied. Summers and Logsdon (2005) reviewed the content of 34 Web sites that included materials on postpartum depression. They reported that only five of these Web sites provided more than 75% correct responses to defining depressive symptoms, what to do if a woman has suicidal thoughts, treatment, and sources of information for consumers.

Nurses have a responsibility to keep up to date on Web sites that provide information on postpartum mood and anxiety disorders. Mothers need guidance to navigate through the maze of Web sites so they will know which ones are providing the correct information. An excellent resource for women, their families, and clinicians is Postpartum Support International's Web site (www.postpartum.net). In addition, there is a Web site devoted to helping men whose partners are suffering from postpartum depression (www.postpartumdads.org).

Postpartum depression is no longer considered confined to Western/industrialized countries. It is a universal phenomenon (Affonso, De, Horowitz, & Mayberry, 2000; Goldbort, 2006). In order to provide culturally competitive care, nurses need to become aware of the different ways women from specific cultures experience postpartum depression and what type of symptoms they may present with. In this chapter it is not possible to cover all cultural perspectives, but two will be focused on: Korean and Muslim women.

Koreans tend to express their emotional problems in somatic terms as symptoms (Kim & Buist, 2005). In Confucian society, a sign of well-bred upbringing and a high level of education is a person's ability to repress their emotions. Expressing one's emotions in somatic symptoms is a more acceptable way of expressing distressing feelings. Korean mothers will often share symptoms, such as headaches, chills, numbness, and dizziness, with their nurses when they are trying to express their emotional problems.

Muslim women experiencing postpartum depression have a different problem to contend with. According to Islamic medicine, illness occurs when an individual has moved away from the will of Allah (Fonte & Horton-Deutsch, 2005). Because of this cultural belief, Muslim mothers suffering from postpartum depression may be hesitant to admit they have a mental health problem. Nurses need to be respectful that Muslim women may wish to include prayer and meditation to help them connect with Allah.

POSTPARTUM DEPRESSION SCREENING

The help-seeking barriers for women suffering with postpartum depression have important implication for nurses working with new mothers. Reasons why women do not proactively seek help include lack of knowledge about this mood disorder, fear of disclosing their feelings, and belief in myths of motherhood (Dennis & Chung-Lee, 2006).

How can nurses facilitate help-seeking behaviors of mothers experiencing postpartum depression? Nurses are in the forefront of care and can either promote or hinder women seeking treatment. If mothers' feelings and symptoms are minimized by nurses or other clinicians, women may be reluctant to seek treatment. Nurses need to provide a trusting, caring environment where open dialogue can flourish. Women must feel comfortable when approaching nurses about their postpartum depressive symptoms. Decreasing the stigma attached to this mood disorder is critical so that women will not experience fear, shame, or embarrassment when sharing their distressing thoughts and feelings. By dispelling destructive myths of motherhood, nurses can give women permission to express any negative feelings they are having since the birth of their infants. Nurses can also explain to new mothers that childbirth can be viewed from a framework of grief and loss (Driscoll, 1990). Women can experience a series of losses due to childbirth: loss of energy, relationships, roles, lifestyle, and self.

Studies are revealing that women experiencing postpartum depression use health care services more frequently than mothers who are not depressed (Dennis, 2004; Webster et al., 2001). Health services frequently used included medical walk-in clinics, emergency departments, family physicians, and public health nurses. Increase in health service use by new mothers can provide an important clue to nurses. Perhaps these women are suffering from postpartum depression. These women are prime candidates to screen for this crippling mood disorder.

POSTTRAUMATIC STRESS DISORDER DUE TO CHILDBIRTH

Up to 6% of women develop PTSD secondary to childbirth (Creedy, Shochet, & Horsfall, 2000). The rate of women reporting traumatic births, however, is a much higher percentage. Recently, for example, reported prevalence of birth trauma was 32% (Maggioni, Margola, & Filippi, 2006). What is it about labor and delivery that could result in women perceiving their childbirth as so traumatic? In her research, Beck (2004a) reported four core components that described women's experiences of birth trauma, their perceived lack of caring and communication by labor and delivery staff, unsafe care, and an overshadowing of their trauma by a focus on the delivery outcome.

Labor and delivery nurses are in an ideal position to help prevent birth trauma by ensuring that women feel respected and cared for and by keeping the lines of communication open. On the postpartum unit, nurses can actively engage women in a dialogue about their birthing process so that they do not feel like their experiences are not valued.

In Matthews and Callister's study (2004), mothers revealed that nurses played a pivotal role in preserving their dignity during childbirth.

Women shared that nurses' presence, encouragement, continuity of care, respect, and making them feel valued as individuals were critical to the nursing care that promoted their dignity. Crompton (2003) stressed that, in labor and delivery, every woman needs to be gently cared for and treated as though she were a survivor of a previous traumatic experience.

Nurses should have a proactive role in preventing PTSD due to childbirth by being vigilant in observing mothers during the postpartum period for early trauma-related symptoms such as a dazed appearance, appearing withdrawn, temporary amnesia, anxiety, decreased consciousness, and appearing disoriented and depressed (Church & Scanlan, 2002).

During admission to labor and delivery, it is important for nurses to take a careful history regarding any specific fears women may have about giving birth, such as fear of an epidural. Once identified, nurses can take special care regarding these fears. If the woman is a multipara, nurses need to explore with her what her perceptions of her previous births are. Does she perceive these births as traumatic?

If a woman has been a victim of previous trauma, nurses need to be aware of symptoms that may be indicative of this earlier trauma so that special care can be given. Some of these symptoms include an intense need for control during labor and delivery, a very detailed birth plan, extreme fear and lack of trust, flashbacks, dissociation, and extreme modesty (Crompton, 1996).

The best intervention to prevent PTSD secondary to childbirth is to prevent birth trauma in the first place. Nurses' knowledge of risk factors for PTSD due to traumatic births is important so that they can be alert to these high-risk women. Some of these predictors include high levels of medical intervention and dissatisfaction with care received during labor and delivery (Creedy et al., 2000) as well as a history of psychiatric counseling (Wijma, Soderquist, & Wijma, 1997). Just as with postpartum depression, part of the nurses' role with PTSD due to childbirth is screening. Instruments are available for their use such as the Perinatal PTSD Questionnaire (Callahan, Borja, & Hynan, 2006).

Valuable information not only for mothers but also for nurses and other health care providers on birth trauma and its resulting PTSD can be found at Trauma and Birth Stress' (TABS) Web site (www.tabs.org.nz). TABS is a charitable trust located in New Zealand with a mission to provide information and support to women who have experienced a traumatic birth.

Researchers are beginning to focus attention on the long-term effects of birth trauma and its resulting PTSD. Beck (2006) reported that some mothers are tormented by the yearly anniversary of their traumatic childbirth. Clinicians and family failed to rescue these women. Just as what had happened the day of the traumatic delivery, mothers' distressing experiences were not valued and were pushed into the background as the celebration of the child's birthday took center stage. To survive the actual day of the anniversary, mothers often shared that they scheduled their child's birthday on a different day. Once the actual birthday was over, mothers were in a fragile state, as they needed to recuperate and heal those freshly reopened wounds (Beck, 2006).

Nurses need to be able to differentiate postpartum depression from other postpartum mood and anxiety disorders. Critical to achieving this is knowledge of symptoms related to each of these specific disorders. What are the predominant symptoms mothers may present with when suffering from PTSD due to birth trauma? In studying 38 mothers diagnosed with PTSD due to their traumatic births, Beck (2004b) reported five themes that captured the essence of their experience. Flashbacks and nightmares of the traumatic birth plagued mothers during the day and also at night. As one woman, who had a failed vacuum extraction followed by a forceps delivery, revealed, "I had nightmares of my delivery doctor as a rapist, coming knocking on my door. I also believed when my son was born that the doctor had ripped his head off. These two images were what affected my existence" (Beck, 2004b, p. 219). Women with PTSD also experienced a disturbing numbness and detachment to others, even to their infants.

Mothers shared that they were obsessed with wanting to know what had gone so wrong with their childbirth. Anger, anxiety, and depression consumed the women's daily existence as they tried to care for their infants. One of the most disturbing themes that emerged from Beck's (2004b) qualitative study was how isolated women with PTSD secondary to birth trauma were from the world of motherhood. With PTSD, women try to avoid at all costs reminders of the traumatic event. In this case mothers are avoiding reminders of childbirth. One such trigger, with tremendous implications for mother-infant bonding, is the infant.

REFERENCES

Affonso, D. D., De, A. K., Horowitz, J. A., & Mayberry, L. (2000). An international study exploring levels of postpartum depressive symptomatology. *Journal of Psychosomatic Research, 29,* 207–216.

Beck, C. T. (1993). Teetering on the Edge: A substantive theory of postpartum depression. *Nursing Research, 42,* 42–48.

Beck, C. T. (1995). Perceptions of nurses' caring by mothers experiencing postpartum depression. *Journal of Obstetric, Gynecologic, and Neonatal Nursing, 24,* 819–825.

Beck, C. T. (1996). Postpartum depressed mothers' experiences interacting with their children. *Nursing Research, 45,* 98–104.

Beck, C. T. (2004a). Birth trauma: In the eye of the beholder. *Nursing Research, 53,* 28–35.

Beck, C. T. (2004b). Posttraumatic stress disorder due to childbirth: The aftermath. *Nursing Research, 53,* 216–224.

Beck, C. T. (2006). The anniversary of birth trauma: Failure to rescue. *Nursing Research, 55,* 381–390.

Beck, C. T., & Driscoll, J. W. (2006). *Postpartum mood and anxiety disorders: A clinician's guide.* Sudbury, MA: Jones and Bartlett.

Callahan, J. L., Birja, S. E., & Hynan, M. T. (2006). Modification of the Perinatal PTSD Questionnaire to enhance clinical utility. *Journal of Perinatology, 26,* 533–539.

Church, S., & Scanlan, M. (2002). Postraumatic stress disorder after childbirth: Do midwives play a preventative role? *The Practicing Midwife, 5,* 10–13.

Creedy, D. K., Shochet, I. M., & Horsfall, J. (2000). Childbirth and the development of acute trauma symptoms: Incidence and contributing factors. *Birth, 27,* 104–111.

Crompton, J. (1996). Post-traumatic stress disorder and childbirth: Part 2. *British Journal of Midwifery, 4,* 354–356, 373.

Crompton, J. (2003). Posttraumatic stress disorder and childbirth. *Childbirth Educators New Zealand Education Effects,* Summer, 25–31.

Davey, S. J., Dziurawiec, S., & O'Brien-Malone, A. (2006). Men's voices: Postnatal depression from the perspective of male partners. *Qualitative Health Research, 16,* 206–220.

Dennis, C-L. (2004). Influence of depressive symptomatology on maternal health service utilization and general health. *Archives of Women's Mental Health, 7,* 183–191.

Dennis, C-L., & Chung-Lee, L. (2006). Postpartum depression help-seeking barriers and maternal treatment preferences: A qualitative systematic review. *Birth, 33,* 323–331.

Driscoll, J. (1990). Maternal parenthood and the grief process. *Journal of Perinatal and Neonatal Nursing, 4,* 1–10.

Driscoll, J. W. (2005). Recognizing women's common mental health problems: The Earthquake Assessment Model. *Journal of Obstetric, Gynecologic, and Neonatal Nursing, 34,* 246–254.

Field, T. (1992). Infants of depressed mothers. *Development and Psychopathology, 4,* 49–66.

Fonte, J., & Horton-Deutsch, S. (2005). Treating postpartum depression in immigrant Muslim women. *Journal of the American Psychiatric Nurses Association, 11,* 39–44.

Goldbort, J. (2006). Transcultural analysis of postpartum depression. *MCN: American Journal of Maternal Child Nursing, 31,* 121–126.

Kim, J., & Buist, A. (2005). Postnatal depression: A Korean perspective. *Australasian Psychiatry, 13,* 68–71.

Kleiman, K. (2000). *The postpartum husband: Practical solutions for living with postpartum depression.* Philadelphia: Xlibris Corporation.

Leininger, M. (2007). Theoretical questions and concerns: Response from the theory of culture care diversity and universality perspective. *Nursing Science Quarterly, 20,* 9–15.

Leininger, M. M, & McFarland, M. R. (2006). *Culture care diversity and universality: A worldwide nursing theory* (2nd ed.). Sudbury, MA: Jones and Bartlett.

Maggioni, C., Margola, D., & Filippi, F. (2006). PTSD, risk factors, and expectations among women having a baby: A two-wave longitudinal study. *Journal of Psychosomatic Obstetrics & Gynecology, 27,* 81–90.

Matthews, R., & Callister, L. C. (2004). Childbearing women's perceptions of nursing care that promotes dignity. *Journal of Obstetric, Gynecologic, and Neonatal Nursing, 33,* 498–507.

McCord, G. (1984). Postpartum depression: Out of the closet—and then what? *Birth, 11,* 244–245.

Ramchandani, P., Stein, A., Evans, J., O'Connor, T. G., & The ALSPAC Study Team. (2005). Paternal depression in the postnatal period and child development: A prospective population study. *Lancet, 365,* 2201–2205.

Roberts, S. L., Bushnell, J. A., Collings, S. C., & Purdie, G. L. (2006). Psychological health of men with partners who have post-partum depression. *Australian and New Zealand Journal of Psychiatry, 40,* 704–711.

Sichel, D. A., & Driscoll, J. W. (1999). *Women's moods: What every woman must know about hormones, the brain, and emotional health.* New York: William Morrow.

Summers, A. L., & Logsdon, C. (2005). Web sites for postpartum depression. *MCN: The American Journal of Maternal Child Nursing, 30,* 88–94.

Swanson, K. M. (1999). What is known about caring in nursing science: A literary meta-analysis. In A. S. Hinshaw, S. L. Freethan, & J. L. F Shaver (Eds.), *Handbook of clinical nursing research* (pp. 31–60). Thousand Oaks, CA: Sage.

Watson, J. (2006). Caring theory as an ethical guide to administrative and clinical practices. *Nursing Administration Quality, 30,* 48–55.

Webster, J., Pritchard, M. A., Linnane, J. W., Roberts, J. A., Hinson, J. K., & Starrenburg, S. E. (2001). Postnatal depression: Use of health services and satisfaction with health-care providers. *Journal of Quality Clinical Practice, 21,* 144–148.

Wijma, K., Soderquist, M. A., & Wijma, B. (1997). Post-traumatic stress disorder after childbirth: A cross sectional study. *Journal of Anxiety Disorders, 11,* 587–597.

12

Mothers Who Suffer From Postpartum Illnesses and the Pitfalls of the Criminal Justice System

GEORGE PARNHAM

Over the last several years we have seen the media focus on the horrific details of instances where the life of a child is taken by the very person who gave life to that child: the mother. The attention generated for the most part ignores the mental health aspects of the mother who is impacted with a postpartum illness to some degree. The sensationalism of the tragedy drives the reporters in order to ratchet up ratings by attracting a greater share of the viewing public than their competition. This leads to a misunderstanding of, and, in many instances, a total dismissal of the illness that caused the tragic consequences to occur. Prosecutors more often than not reflect the attitude of the community when a young child is harmed, regardless of the illness of the mother. The authorities pursue a criminal prosecution without considering what actually caused the child's harm.

Thus, forensic experts hired by the state and federal governments look at the objective circumstances of the incident, paying lip service to the reality of the mother's mental illness and render opinions that the mother knew the wrongfulness of her actions at the time she hurt or killed her young child. Prisons across this land house mothers who labored under an unreal reality of a postpartum illness at the time of the act. In many cases, this mother did what she believed to be in her baby's best interest, yet serves a lengthy prison sentence with little or no mental health care. When reality eventually sets in, that is especially needed to get beyond the realization of taking the life of her child. This care behind bars is simply not available.

It is imperative that clinicians who treat a new mother and her baby (be they ob-gyns, maternity ward nurses, or pediatricians) be aware of the reality of postpartum illnesses and the legal consequences of such should any act put the mother in the spotlight of the criminal justice system. To meticulously document the acts and interactions between mothers and children and to gently probe the mental wellness of the mother will be of enormous benefit in the unfortunate future should something dreadful occur. This will better prepare the health care provider to educate judges and juries about the reality of the postpartum mother in order to have her actions judged through her eyes at the time of the act. To bring medicine back into the courtroom dynamics is the purpose of this chapter. It will also have the added benefit of protecting against the abuse of the insanity defense, vis-à-vis the use of a postpartum "defense" in cases where there truly is no evidence of a postpartum illness.

PROLOGUE

On June 20, 2001, at 942 Beachcomber in Houston, Texas, the unspeakable happened. Between approximately 9 A.M. and 10 A.M. on that Wednesday morning, Andrea Pia Yates, alone with her five children, Noah, John, Paul, Luke, and Mary, took the lives of each by drowning. After each died, she placed the child's body in the master bed, head on pillow. She could not retrieve the body of the oldest child, Noah, age 7, from the tub because of exhaustion. She then called 911 and calmly told the dispatcher to send the police, without telling the operator why she needed them. Finally, she stated "because my kids are here" (dispatch tape of Yates's 911 call, June 20, 2001, Houston Police Department Officer Knapp's testimony in Yates' trials).

When Officer Knapp of the Houston Police Department arrived, she met him at the front door, by now soaking wet and breathing heavily, and announced, "I just killed my kids." Knapp, disbelieving the words he heard, was directed down a water-soaked carpeted hallway to the master bedroom. When he pulled back the bedsheet, he saw what he initially thought were four sleeping children. Mary, the youngest, at 6 months of age at the time of her death, was resting on the arm of John, with his hand protectively intertwining her own—as if big brother were taking care of baby sister. After checking for vital signs, Office Knapp soon realized that Andrea was telling the truth.

When questioned at the residence, she clearly, in an unemotional monotone, provided correct answers to each question, which asked for statistical responses like names of children, dates of birth, name of husband, occupation, etc. She was as cooperative as a person under arrest could be. From law enforcement's view, the perfect "citizen accused."

Transported to the City of Houston Homicide Division, she calmly and without emotion provided Sgt. Eric Mehl with an accurate account of the statistical information, as well as the tragic events of that morning. And then Sgt. Mehl stumbled on the tell-all question: "*Why* did you drown your children?" For an agonizing 15 seconds, Andrea Yates was silent. Finally, the silence was interrupted by Mehl: "Were you mad at your children?" "No." "Were they being punished for something they had done?" "No" (Audio tape of Andrea Yates' confession to Sgt. Eric Mehl, June 20, 2001).

During the second Yates trial, Sgt. Mehl, an experienced and highly respected law enforcement officer, was asked the following question:

Mr. Parnham: "And when she was not answering that (the "why" question), what was she doing?

Sgt. Mehl: "Her lips quivered somewhat as if it was trying to come out, and it would not" (Testimony of Sgt. Eric Mehl about his observations of Andrea Yates during confession. June 26–27, 2006)

He realized he was only seeing half the picture; the missing piece of the puzzle that Sgt. Mehl did not see was the severe mental illness that drove Andrea Yates to do the incomprehensible—to take the lives of her children in order to save their souls. She did not answer his question because she could not. Years of postpartum illnesses, some bouts more severe than others, with medication regimens, had so impacted the frontal lobe of her brain that she simply could not "connect the dots." She was in the throes of a severe postpartum psychosis with all the cognitive effects, and she was about to face the penalty of death by execution for the charge of capital murder in the death penalty capital of the world—Houston, Harris County, Texas.[1]

---

[1] If Harris County were a state, it would rank third behind Texas and Florida in the number of executions.

MISSION STATEMENT

This chapter hopefully will provide some insight into when and how postpartum illnesses are treated by the criminal justice systems within this country. The various insanity standards will be addressed and attention paid to the inadequacy of the criminal law in dealing with acts of a gender-based mental illness.

The competency of forensic experts will be discussed as well as the impact of the 2006 Supreme Court case of *Clark v. Arizona* on the legal future of women's mental health issues. Infanticide, a defense in most civilized countries, absent the United States, is presented and discussed.

These insights into the real world of the courtroom are a direct result of an arduous and difficult learning process as a result of the Yates's trials.

On July 27, 2006, Andrea Pia Yates was found *not guilty by reason of insanity*. Although there is no verdict wording that includes reference to the type of mental illness a person suffered, there is no question that the jury determined that she was suffering from psychosis, postpartum, on the day she drowned her children. Todd Frank, foreman of the jury, confirmed this jury determination after the verdict was returned.[2]

The saga of Andrea Pia Yates and her journey through the judicial system presents, unfortunately, the atypical example of the manner in which mothers who commit acts while under the influence of postpartum illnesses are treated within the criminal justice system.

INSANITY STANDARDS

Obviously, it is important to have a grasp of the insanity definition applicable to each case. The case of M'Naghten (10 Cl. & Fin., at 210, 8 Eng. Rep., at 722 [1843]) is the foundation of all current insanity standards:

> The jurors ought to be told . . . that to establish a defense on the ground of insanity, it must be clearly proved that, at the time of the committing of the act, the party accused was laboring under such a defect of reason, from disease of

[2] Todd Frank's statement—Foreman of the Jury for Andrea Pia Yates's second trial—confirmed there was no question but that postpartum psychosis was responsible for the children's deaths in conversations with the author.

> the mind, as not to know the nature and quality of the act he was doing; or, if he did know it, that he did not know what he was doing was wrong.

M'Naghten basically consists of two prongs:

- *Cognitive:* mental illness preventing the actor from understanding or "knowing" the nature of the acts he or she was committing, and
- *Moral:* even if the actor did "know" the nature of the actions, he or she did not "know" what he or she was doing was wrong.

M'Naghten, in its various forms, had not been seriously tinkered with until the shooting of President Reagan and the acquittal of John Hinckley. A collective legislative backlash occurred to change the insanity standard, and, in some cases, to eliminate insanity as a defense altogether. The Insanity Defense Reform Act of 1984 changed the federal standard. Basically, the federal and state reforms eliminated the ability of the defendant to prove that he or she was unable to conform their conduct to the law.

As indicated, states' standards are diverse and depend on various factors and legal concepts, ignoring for the most part the reality of mental illness and its effect on the thought processes of the particular defendant. A state's right to determine its own way of dealing with the acts of mothers who suffer state to state from the identical mental illness is given priority over the illness itself.

As the Supreme Court pointed out in *Clark v. Arizona,* 126 S.Ct.2709 [2006]), there are four basic principles incorporated in the various states' standards (and federal standard) that deal with mental illness within the criminal justice systems. They are:

1. *Cognitive incapacity:* The severity of one's mental illness causes one not to appreciate the nature and quality of his or her action. (M'Naghten's first prong)
2. *Moral incapacity:* Did the severity of mental illness result in one not knowing his or her actions were wrong? (M'Naghten's second prong)
3. *Volitional incapacity:* Did the severe mental illness cause the actor not to be able to control his or her actions (a/k/a irresistible impulse)?
4. *Product of mental illness:* Simply put, were the actions of the defendant a product of mental illness?

Seventeen states and the federal government have both incorporated M'Naghten to some degree (the "cognition" plus the "morality" prong).[3]

Only one state, North Dakota, has a unique test, a modified version of M'Naghten, asking whether the defendant "lacks substantial capacity to comprehend the harmful nature or consequences of the conduct, or the conduct is the result of a loss or serious distortion of the individual's capacity to recognize reality."

One state, Alaska, has as its standard the first M'Naghten prong of cognition.

Ten states have only the second M'Naghten prong, that is, the moral incapacity test (*Clark v. Arizona,* 2006).[4]

The ALI, Model Penal Code, Section 4.01 (1) incorporates the following definition:

> A person is not responsible for criminal conduct if at the time of such conduct as a result of mental illness or defect he lacks substantial capacity either to appreciate the criminality (wrongfulness) of his conduct or to conform his conduct to the requirements of the law.

Fourteen jurisdictions have adopted a form of this standard.[5] Three states (Michigan, New Mexico, and Virginia) have as their standard a combination of volitional incapacity with the M'Naghten standard. One state, New Hampshire, has the "product of mental illness test." Lastly, four states (Idaho, Kansas, Montana, and Utah) have no insanity standard at all (*Clark v. Arizona,* 2006).

Also, there exists a "standard" incorporated for the most part as a "lesser included" pragmatic alternative to an insanity defense. That standard is "guilty and mentally ill." (The wording may vary from state to state in some form, i.e., "guilty except for mental illness," etc.) Generally, if the defense fails to produce sufficient evidence of insanity to meet its burden of proof (either by a preponderance of evidence or clear and convincing evidence) on any of the issues presented in the insanity definition, then the fact finder can return a verdict of "guilty but mentally ill." The defendant is then transported to a mental health facility until "better" and then is taken into "general population" to serve the sentence imposed.

---

[3] Alabama, California, Colorado, Florida, Iowa, Minnesota, Mississippi, Missouri, Nebraska, Nevada, New Jersey, New York, North Carolina, Oklahoma, Pennsylvania, Tennessee, and Washington.

[4] Arizona, Delaware, Indiana, Illinois, Louisiana, Maine, Ohio, South Carolina, South Dakota, and Texas.

[5] Arkansas, Connecticut, Georgia, Hawaii, Kentucky, Maryland, Massachusetts, Oregon, Rhode Island, Vermont, West Virginia, Wisconsin, Wyoming, and the District of Columbia.

To make applicable the various standards to the acts of a mentally ill mother and to persuade a jury of this reality is a daunting task indeed. At the onset, mothers who harm a newborn are treated for the most part without any consideration given to the mindset of that mother. This is not to say that there may exist objective circumstances that support a prosecution, that is, insurance motives, boyfriend involvement, etc. However, it is particularly disturbing to witness time and again the criminalization of the mentally ill acts of a suffering mother, and, in some of those instances, to be involved in a judicial process that could lead to her execution.

Why does this happen? In a civilization supposedly as advanced as ours, how can the authorities be so blind to the reality of postpartum illnesses as to ignore the obvious? Be it the mother who kills her child because she believes Satan is embodied in her infant[6] and then smothers herself to death, or the mom who kills her child and then jumps from a building to her own death. What is it that we don't understand—or perhaps choose not to understand? Can the political pressure of an outraged community not appreciating the issues of postpartum illnesses be the cause? Absolutely, in many instances; or perhaps the magnitude of what happened influences a state attorney's office of prosecutors, as in the Yates case, to seek the absolute penalty. But obviously, we as a society simply don't get it.

When a mother harms a child regardless of the reason why, the very definition of the symbol we hold most dear is turned upside down. What is more cherished than the image of Madonna and child? Immediately, thoughts of our connection with our own mother's love provide the basis of "How could this happen?" But a mother who suffers from postpartum psychosis lives in an unreal mental world of motherhood. In many instances, all of the maternal instincts remain: to nurture, to love, to protect from danger are kept intact. But the cruelest of all mental illnesses permits a mother to see danger when in reality, there is none. Within the psychotic world of Andrea Yates on June 20, 2001, in her real world, her children were doomed to the eternal fires of hell unless she stepped in to stop their downward spiral into Satan's clutches. Again, *she had to take their lives to save their souls.* And she goes a step further. She wants to go to death row to be executed so that Satan who singularly resided within the tabernacle of her body could be slain by the ruler, the chief executive of the State of Texas. With her execution, the world would be saved from "the evil one."

---

[6] E.g. Dr. Mine Ener, Professor at Villanava University. Died August 30, 2003, her daughter Raya Donagi died August 3, 2003.

Ironically, the severity of Andrea Yates's mental illness was never contested, as the State of Texas stipulated. Yet the state's ignorance of the implication of her mental illness on her actions is emphasized:

> Let the State be clear. The Appellant (Yates) is and was severely mentally ill. There is absolutely no legitimate question about that. The only question lies in whether the appellant should be held criminally responsible for killing her children. (State of Texas Appellate Brief, 1st Ct. App., Houston, Tx., Cause Nos. 01–02–00462-Cr, 01–02–00463-Cr., pg. 63)

POSTPARTUM ILLNESSES AND THE INSANITY STANDARD

The crux of the reality of the postpartum defense in the Yates cases and others is to explain through testimony of competent mental health experts that the word *know* as in "to know the wrongfulness of her actions" must be interpreted through her mind's eye at the time of the act that lands the mother in the courtroom chair of a criminal defendant. Unfortunately, no jury in this country is given a definition of what the word *know* means in an insanity definition. Jurors are at liberty to use Webster's dictionary as a basis for judging the mental processes of a mentally ill mother. Nor in most jurisdictions are juries provided a definition of what the word *wrong* in the standard means. Is it a "legal" wrong or a "moral" wrong that should apply to a mother who is doing what she believes to be in the best interest for her child? Surely, if one were to tap Andrea Yates on the shoulder in the midst of taking her child's life and ask, "Andrea, aren't you aware it is against the law to kill your child?" She would no doubt answer, "Yes, I'm aware of that. But don't you understand what I am doing is the only right thing for my child? I'm making sure they are going to heaven." It is legally unfair and unjust to judge the criminality of such a mother on the present insanity standards and factual circumstances of her conduct without taking into account the reality of her postpartum psychosis. It's not the logic of the "expert" who reviews objectively the facts of the offense that should count. It is the mindset of the mentally ill mother and what she "knows" in her unreal world of mental illness that should matter. To further properly judge the mother's actions "through her eyes" necessitates an understanding of postpartum illnesses.

CLARK V. ARIZONA

On June 29, 2006, the Supreme Court of the United States rendered its decision in *Clark, Supra.* Unfortunately, the majority opinion did little to underscore the reality of mental illness when judging the actions that placed Clark within the criminal justice system.

Eric Michael Clark had shot and killed a police officer in Flagstaff, Arizona. It was uncontested that Clark suffered from paranoid schizophrenia and was acutely psychotic around the time of the shooting. The defense was insanity.

The Arizona definition is mirrored after the "moral" prong of M'Naghten. The burden on the defendant is by clear and convincing evidence. In other words, the defense must prove that the mental illness resulted in the defendant not knowing what he or she was doing was wrong.

Second, the defense attacked the *mens rea* element of the offense, that is, he did not intend to kill a human being (it is uncontested that Clark believed that frequently aliens who were out to kill him were using the identity of government agents). Had Clark been successful in establishing reasonable doubt as to whether his mental illness prevented him from intentionally killing a police officer, Clark would have been successful even though the insanity defense was rejected by the Court. The problem lies in the trial court's prohibition of expert psychiatric testimony about Clark's mental illness on the issue of *mens rea.* The Court had no problem admitting "observation" evidence—what Clark said to others, what he did with the weapon (hide it), and in general his actions before and after the killing as witnessed by others.

On appeal, Clark complained that the trial court's denial of the use of evidence of mental illness in attacking the *mens rea* element was a denial of due process. The Supreme Court rejected this argument. The Court stressed the right of the states to establish their individual standard of insanity and admissibility of psychiatric evidence on the *mens rea* element of the offense. In effect, it sustained the lower court's prohibition of psychiatric testimony on the *mens rea* intent issue. (Interestingly, evidence of mental illness in the four states that do not have an insanity defense *is admissible* on the issue of *mens rea.*)

Unfortunately, the Court in its opinion goes out of its way to denigrate psychiatry and its ability to connect uncontested mental illness with the thought process of the defendant at the time of the act. The Court in prohibiting mental illness testimony emphasizes that dueling psychiatric experts can easily mislead the jury to the wrong verdict. *Clark* states (at pg. 10):

> Though mental disease evidence is certainly not condemned wholesale, the consequence of this professional ferment (the mental illness diagnoses and the debate over the "very contours of the mental disease itself") is a general caution in treating psychological classifications as predicates for excusing otherwise criminal conduct.

The majority in affirming the state court's decision accomplishes two perhaps unintentional goals: first, the quality of psychiatric testimony is placed in doubt, and second, the door is now wide open to the opinions of forensic experts, no longer in need of clinical experience because that element is suspect. As a result, the insanity defense in whatever form we know it is in danger of being undermined in courtrooms and perhaps abolished in states across this country.

Conversely, however, the Court, perhaps unwittingly and by inference, invited trial courts and psychiatry to raise the bar when the legal determination is made concerning who is qualified and who is not qualified to testify as an expert in matters dealing with women's mental health. The argument can be made that only those experts with a foundation in postpartum illnesses should be permitted to render an opinion as to whether the mother on trial either appreciated the nature and quality of the act she was committing or "knew" her conduct was "wrong." In Yates's second trial, an amicus brief supporting this proposition was filed with the trial court.

> Jurors are legally entitled to informed testimony from qualified experts. Mentally ill defendants must be judged not on the basis of speculation and conjecture, but on scientific fact and informed expert analysis. Therefore, Amici respectfully suggest specific criteria pursuant to *Kelly v. Texas,* 824 S.W.2d 568 (Tex.Crim.App.1992) as utilized in both *Sexton v. State,* 93 S.W.3d 96 (Tex.Crim.App.2002) and *E. I. DuPont de Nemours & Co., Inc., v. Robinson,* 923 S.W.2d 549 (Tex.1995), that apply to expert witnesses testifying to the mental state of mothers experiencing postpartum psychosis. Under the particular facts of this case, this standard requires that only mental health experts with significant experience in the area of postpartum psychosis be permitted to testify regarding whether Mrs. Yates knew that her conduct was wrong. (Memorandum of Law presented to the Yates trial court prepared by Fordham Law School)

Certainly, medical science has sufficiently progressed to document the reality of this gender-based, biologically based mental illness. To limit the expert's testimony to only those professionals with knowledge of postpartum illnesses and the effect on the cognition of the mother would answer the Supreme Court's concern that jurors are in danger of being misled by the controversial nature of psychiatric opinions from psychiatrists, who may not be qualified to testify about women's mental health issues. (Again, an excellent reference outlining the progression of medical science in the understanding of postpartum illnesses is contained in the Memorandum of Law prepared by Fordham Law School and joined by other Friends of the Court.)

The testimony of Dr. Park Dietz is a prime example from Yates's first trial. Dr. Dietz , the state's only forensic expert, acknowledged that he was not an expert in women's mental health, particularly in the area of postpartum, yet was permitted to testify, in effect, that Yates "knew" what she was doing was "wrong" at the time of the drowning of the children. (Testimony of Dr. Park Dietz, the State's forensic psychiatric expert, March 9, 2002.)

Perhaps a Bit of Legal Encouragement

In *Clark*, Justice Kennedy, joined by Justice Stevens and Justice Ginsburg, authored a ringing dissent. Not only does Justice Kennedy emphasize the reality of mental illness and the necessity of permitting this type of testimony to be presented to the fact finder, he further draws the distinction between the rational intent to commit a specific act and the reality of that act within the delusional world of a schizophrenic mind.

> The central theory of Clark's defense was that his schizophrenia made him delusional. He lived in a universe where the delusions were so dominant, the theory was that he had no intent to shoot a police officer or knowledge he was doing so. It is one thing to say he acted with intent or knowledge to pull the trigger. It is quite another to say he pulled the trigger to kill someone he knew to be a human being and a police officer. (*Clark, Supra*, at pg. 41)

And

> In sum, the rule forces the jury to decide guilt in a fictional world with undefined and unexplained behaviors but without mental illness. This rule has no rational justification and imposes a significant burden upon a straight-

forward defense: He did not commit the crime with which he was charged. (*Clark, Supra,* at pg. 47)

INFANTICIDE

Virtually every civilized country has long legally recognized the reality of postpartum illnesses and its effects, except for the United States. Generally, in those countries, women who harm a child within 12 months of the delivery of that child and suffer from an issue of postpartum dimensions receive immediate care with a statutory defense of "infanticide."[7]

In this country, these mothers are either sent to a penitentiary and/or death row unless a jury can be persuaded that they are not guilty by reason of insanity.

THE FAILURES

It is not an easy task to review from afar the reasons behind the tragedies of June 20, 2001, and the manner in which the justice system reacted to the mental illness of Andrea Yates. But we do review if for no other purpose than to answer the question, "why." Before the drowning of the children, all the signs were there, to be recognized by the professionals and the nonprofessionals alike. There is no question but that Andrea Pia Yates suffered from the severest form of a postpartum illness, postpartum psychosis. Her medical records are replete with references to and diagnoses of a postpartum illness. From the severity of her depression after the birth of Luke in 1999, to her documented thoughts about her fears that she might hurt the kids, or that they would all go to hell, or the physical effects of her mental illness—catatonic, mute, severe psychomotor retardation—all present.

---

[7] In England, Canada, Australia, New Zealand, and more than a dozen other countries, the importance of female biology as a cause for a child's death produced the infanticide law of 1948, which provided for a maximum 5-year sentence, as opposed to the maximum death penalty or life sentence for manslaughter and murder.

The Canadian statute reads: "A female person commits infanticide when by a willful act or omission, she causes the death of her newly born child, if at the time of the act or omission she was not fully recovered from the effects of giving birth to the child and by reason thereof or of the effect of lactation consequent on the birth of the child her mind is then disturbed."

This statute covers the time frame of 1 year from the child's birth (Canada Criminal Code, Section 233).

Her hospitalization on July 21, 1999, under the care of Dr. Starbranch, her psychiatrist, included the following observations: "Hadn't eaten in days. Bald spot on her scalp where she had been scratching . . ." And finally, a diagnosis of postpartum depression with psychosis (probable delusions). The admission by Dr. Starbranch that "any additional pregnancy will surely guarantee future psychotic depression" (evaluation by Dr. Eileen Starbranch, December 1999–March 2001), but she was prescribed the harsh antipsychotic, Haldol, and it worked!

By the time Andrea was admitted into Devereux on March 31, 2001, she was off Haldol and had given birth to her fifth child, Mary, the preceding December. Andrea physically presented the same symptoms to Dr. Albritton, her admitting psychiatrist at Devereux, as she had to Dr. Starbranch after the birth of Luke: catatonic, flat affect, severe psychomotor retardation, etc. Dr. Albritton attempted to get a medical history from Andrea and her husband. But Andrea couldn't talk and Rusty failed to inform Albritton about the effect of Haldol the year before. Andrea was subsequently admitted with the diagnosis of a major depressive disorder, postpartum onset (rule out psychotic features; admission notes of Andrea Yates at Devereux Texas Treatment Center, March 31, 2001). The insurance company, using its precoded determination that 11 to 13 days hospital stay should be sufficient to cure the problem, limited its financial obligations to this time period.

Enter Dr. Mohammed Saeed and that diagnosis was never changed. Throughout her two hospitalizations at Devereux (March 31, 2001–April 13, 2001 and May 4, 2001–May 14, 2001) that diagnosis never changed. There was no communication between Dr. Saeed and Dr. Starbranch during the entire time that Saeed was her psychiatrist (from March 31 through the day her children died). During the Devereux second stay after Mr. Yates informed Dr. Saeed that Andrea had previously been placed on Haldol and it was successful, a fax was sent to Dr. Starbranch's office for medical records but was never followed up on. Saeed, at the husband's request, placed Andrea temporarily on Haldol (Dr. Mohammed Saeed's admission notes concerning Andrea Yates, May 4, 2001).

On June 4, 2001, after Andrea had been discharged from Devereux, Dr. Saeed decided to take her off of Haldol. Astonishingly, the day she was discharged from Devereux, she was still on "suicide watch" (Devereux Hospital records, May 4, 2001).

On June 18, without the benefit of an antipsychotic, Rusty brought his wife to Dr. Saeed's office for an outpatient visit. Instead of administering an antipsychotic, Dr. Saeed gave an almost-catatonic Andrea Yates a pep talk: "You must begin to think 'happy thoughts,'" and she leaves his office with a slight modification in her antidepressant medications (testimony of Russell "Rusty" Yates, May 5, 2002). Two days later her children were dead.

THE MESSAGE

These matters are revisited for a twofold purpose—to limit future occurrences such as what happened to the children of Andrea Yates from happening again, and, should it occur, to assist the judicial system, judges, prosecutors, defense attorneys, and forensic experts in understanding the mental realism behind the act.

In October 2002, the Mental Health Association of Houston agreed with this author to sponsor an effort to establish a memorial for Noah, John, Paul, Luke, and Mary Yates. The Yates Children Memorial Fund was founded for the purpose of bringing education and awareness to the community about the reality and ravages of postpartum illnesses. Seminars on women's mental health, as well as the law relating to insanity and its inadequacy in addressing postpartum issues, have been presented to groups not only in the Houston area but across the country.

The message is simple—Prevention Through Awareness. After all, every child deserves to be raised by the one person upon whom that child relies for every need—its mother—and for that mother to be as free from mental illness as possible. If future lives are spared, the Yates children will not have died in vain.

SUMMARY

As this conclusion was being written, there was breaking news of a newborn found in a trash bin. One can't help but wonder about the ultimate question, "why." Certainly, other explanations exist besides a postpartum illness that contributes to or causes a mother to kill her child. But the importance of ferreting out the reasons, particularly, to answer this question, should never be underestimated. Surely, this mother, if she committed this act, will face criminal prosecution no matter her mindset. If postpartum illness in whatever degree contributed to the death of this child, it in all probability will be a factor not considered in the criminal justice resolution.

The lives of future generations depend on the education of the public in general and lawyers, prosecutors, judges, and juries in particular about the reality of postpartum issues and the legal understanding of the effect of the mind of the mother accused. The responsibility in large part for this education depends on the professional who evaluates and treats, and, unfortunately, sometimes testifies when tragedy strikes.

Treatment Options for Perinatal Mood Disorders

PART IV

13 To Medicate or Not: The Dilemma of Pregnancy and Psychiatric Illness

CATHERINE A. BIRNDORF AND ALEXANDRA C. SACKS

Historically, the question of managing psychiatric illness in pregnancy has been not *how* to treat, but *if* to treat at all. The literature has posed this problem as one where maternal and fetal health were at cross purposes: Should we medicate the mother and thus expose the fetus to the possibility of side effects, or not medicate, and expose the mother to risk of psychiatric disease (Allison, 2004)? Managing psychiatric illness in pregnancy creates a dilemma: how to treat illness in the mother without causing harm to the fetus.

The U.S. Department of Health and Human Services estimates that there are approximately 6 million pregnancies every year in the United States (Hamilton, Martin, & Ventura, 2005). Roughly 10%–20% of pregnant women suffer from depression during pregnancy (Marcus, Flynn, & Blow, 2003). National Comorbidity Survey (NCS) data have shown that the most likely time in a woman's life for depression is the childbearing years (Kessler, McGonagle, Swartz, Blazer, & Nelson, 1993). And, it seems that now more than ever, women with a history of psychopathology are considering pregnancy. Allison (2004) points out that advances in psychopharmacology are largely responsible for helping women with psychiatric history reach levels of functioning in which they are able to seriously consider pregnancy: "It is a cruel irony that the medication that made the dream of motherhood a possibility may now threaten it—by putting the mother or her unborn infant at risk."

Until recently, the effect of psychotropic drugs on the fetus has been poorly understood; therefore, pregnant women have traditionally been advised to avoid medications. Prior to the early 1990s, the Federal Drug Administration (FDA) medical trials did not include any women in their studies, based on the fear that they could be pregnant (Willis, 1997). Certainly, women in pregnancy were explicitly excluded from FDA trials. The feminist movement ushered in an era of including women in clinical trials, offering limited, but more, information on the reproductive safety of certain medications. Furthermore, the medical community started to view women more holistically, considering other systems in addition to reproductive health.

With this complex approach came considerations about women's mental health in the setting of pregnancy, a prevalent issue that had been neglected for decades. And with new deserved attention, a problem was born: how to protect the mother without harming the fetus. In 2003, the National Institute of Mental Health (NIMH) issued a call to arms to expand investigations of this arena, announcing its concern in the 108th Congress (NIMH, 2003). However, as this chapter will unpack, the dilemma persists, but the question is unfortunately more complicated still.

In light of current scientific knowledge that untreated mental illness itself can be harmful to a fetus, a new question must now be posed: How to manage psychiatric disease by causing the *least* harm to the mother and fetus alike? Current clinical knowledge puts mental health practitioners and patients between a rock and a hard place.

The historical exclusion of pregnant women from clinical trials and limited systematic data complicate current knowledge about psychotropic use in pregnancy. In addition, interference in collecting accurate data exists for a number of reasons. There is an overlap in the symptoms of pregnancy and major depression; for example, changes in appetite, sleep, concentration, and fatigue are found in both (Newport, Wilcox, & Stowe, 2001). Some physicians may be deterred by data showing that screening instruments such as the Beck Depression Inventory may overdiagnose depression because of this symptom overlap (Salamero, Marcos, Gutierrez, & Rebull, 1994). However, other studies have shown that without such screening, depression is often missed in obstetrical clinics (Powers, Zahorik, & Morrow, 1993).

Social forces may also be at play, including the prevailing myth that pregnancy is protective against psychiatric illness, and is somehow a naturally "happy" time in life. Raskin describes this phenomenon as a myth that is embedded in our society's deeper value system: "We are culturally invested in believing that pregnancy is a blissful time, that a pregnant women should be so overjoyed, feeling so personally blessed that she is happy, no matter what" (1997, p. 209). Needless to say, while some women may find pregnancy to be a period of relative calm, others will certainly experience it as a stressful time (Stowe, Hostetter, Newport, 2005). It is unknown whether these stresses are primarily physiological, due to hormonal changes, or the contribution of psychological changes as a woman faces motherhood. Nonetheless, the impact of these changes has been documented (Cohen et al., 2006).

While no woman is immune from psychiatric symptoms in the setting of pregnancy, certain risk factors have been identified to help predict problems in pregnancy, and thus may help target screening (Nonacs & Cohen, 2003). One group of these risk factors is those intrinsic to a woman's biology and psychology, including genetics, personal and family history of mental illness, and character traits. Other risk factors more indirectly affect a woman's environment in the setting of pregnancy, including behaviors such as unhealthy patterns of sleep, exercise, nutrition, and relaxation. Additionally, poor psychosocial supports, marital or family discord, low socioeconomic status, or recent stressful life events have also been identified. Feelings about the pregnancy itself, such as an unplanned or unwanted pregnancy, may also serve as a source of stress, thereby contributing to risk.

The reality of having to make a single management plan to suit two patients (mother and fetus) with different needs can be overwhelming for practitioners. Nonetheless, it is important not to respond to this intimidating challenge by lowering psychiatric standard of care. Traditionally, physicians have approached the treatment of medical illnesses, such as hypertension, with a lack of ambivalence that is seen with psychiatric illness. In part, this may be because the risks of these medical conditions have been seen as equivalent or greater to the potential risks of the medications themselves. It is accepted that untreated hypertension can lead to disastrous fetal effects. However, as will be outlined in subsequent sections in this chapter, untreated psychiatric disease itself appears to affect fetal outcomes. This fact must not be minimized by bias that psychiatric pathology in pregnancy is less dangerous than medical disease, and thus treatment-optional. One must not equate untreated illness with doing no harm. No decision is risk-free because untreated psychiatric illness and medication each carry their own problem of exposure (NIMH, 2003).

It is the health care practitioner's job to guide and counsel patients as they ultimately make this difficult decision for themselves, weighing the risks and benefits of psychiatric illness and medication. This must be determined by factoring in each woman's psychiatric disease profile (considering past psychiatric history at baseline as well as during past pregnancies, risk factors, coping skills, treatment adherence, etc.).

Additionally, medication history must be considered: Which drugs work best to treat this patient's illness? Are there nonpharmacological options that may be acceptable treatment alternatives? Are there drug alternatives that pose a lesser fetal risk that may be equally effective? Can medication dose be effectively reduced/tapered?

The last question is the patient's preference: How do she and her partner feel about taking psychopharmacologic agents? Many patients come to the consultation with a strong preference about medications in pregnancy. Informed consent is essential. Health practitioners must understand the patient's needs, risks, and value system in order to advise her with the most up-to-date information. Ultimately, at the core of the decision-making process will be the patient's individual psychiatric history, current mental status, and personal values/philosophy. Case studies at the end of the chapter will provide some examples of how to take on this approach.

LITERATURE REVIEW

Effects of Untreated Maternal Mood Disorders: Fetal

Antenatal: Untreated Depression

Untreated mental illness can have a multitude of effects on the developing fetus. Suicide and decision to terminate because of the intolerable effects of being off medication are obvious disastrous consequences (Coverdale, McCullough, & Chervenak, 1997). Risk of suicide overall in pregnant women may be lower than in nonpregnant women; however, certain factors are associated with increased suicide risk. An unwanted pregnancy, being abandoned by a partner, or having had a prior pregnancy loss/death of a child put a woman at greater risk (Lester & Beck, 1998).

Additionally, it appears that untreated depression can increase maternal behaviors that may be risky for the fetus: disordered eating (decreased appetite, decreased nutritional quality, binge eating with fluctuating blood sugar) can cause fetal malnutrition and dehydration (Halbreich & Kornstein, 2004). Furthermore, the likelihood of maternal use of harmful substances, such as drugs, alcohol, and cigarettes may be increased in the setting of untreated antenatal depression (Amaro, Fried, Cabral, & Zuckerman, 1990).

Untreated antenatal depression may have detrimental impact on obstetrical care itself. Untreated symptoms of anxiety may promote phobias, such as fear of leaving the house, thus preventing patients from keeping their obstetrical appointments (Hans, 1999). Decreased energy associated with untreated maternal depression may make it impossible for patients to get out of bed. Hopelessness may also prevent patients from making/keeping medical appointments and participating in their prenatal care (prenatal vitamins, etc.) (Lester & Beck, 1998).

The effects of untreated maternal depression on the fetus have been studied. It appears that these newborns are at increased risk for low birthweight/small for gestational age, low Apgar scores, delayed fetal heart rate responsivity, preterm birth, smaller head circumference, and developmental delay (Berle et al., 2005; Federenko & Wadhwa, 2004; Galler, Harrison, Ramsey, Forde, & Butler, 2000; Lou et al., 1994; Monk et al., 1999; Orr & Miller, 1995). Other studies have shown that newborns of mothers with untreated antenatal depression may cry more often and may be more difficult to console than the control group (Davis et al., 2007). Neuropsychiatric studies have also measured elevated cortisol and catecholamine levels and lower dopamine and serotonin levels in newborns of mothers with untreated antenatal depression when compared with controls (Diego et al., 2006; Lundy et al., 1999).

Antenatal: Untreated Anxiety

Untreated anxiety disorders have been associated with preterm labor, low birthweights, prolonged labor, higher rates of planned cesarean section, heightened startle response in infants, and increased infant inconsolability (Andersson, Sundstrom-Poromaa, Wulff, Astrom, & Bixo, 2004; Orr, Reiter, Blazer, & James, 2007; Teixeira, Fisk, & Glover, 1999; Werner et al., 2007). Untreated panic attacks in pregnancy may contribute to mild or more severe complications, such as placental abruption (Cohen, Rosenbaum, & Heller, 1989).

Antenatal: Untreated Bipolar Disorder

Untreated mania can cause high-risk behaviors, which may have dangerous effects for the fetus and the mother. Sexual behavior with high risk for sexually transmitted infections (STIs), harmful substance use, and likelihood of being involved in acts of violence may be increased. Decreased prenatal visits, as well as the inability to follow prenatal instructions, such as bed rest or gestational diabetes mellitus diet, have also been associated (Field et al., 2003; Van den Bergh, Mulder, Mennes, & Glover, 2005).

Mechanism of Action

The mechanism of how untreated antenatal illness affects the fetus is still being examined. Panic attacks provide a helpful physiological example: it is thought that the transient sympathetic nervous system arousal and hypertension occurring in panic attacks may cause a constriction in placental blood supply. This may be the mechanism for such effects as placental abruption (Cohen et al., 1989). Increased cortisol and catecholamine levels seen in other psychiatric diseases may also affect placental function by this mechanism of altering uterine blood flow and inducing uterine irritability (Glover, 1999). Additionally, it is thought that the dysregulation of the hypothalamic-pituitary-adrenal (HPA) axis, the source of these hormonal changes previously described, may also directly affect the fetus (Van den Bergh et al., 2005).

Corticotrophin-releasing hormone (CRH) is a hormone expressed in the placenta as well as the hypothalamus (Federenko & Wadhwa, 2004). There is a known relationship between maternal stress hormones of ACTH and cortisol and placental CRH (Weinstock, 2005). Studies have shown that women in preterm labor have increased CRH when compared to pregnant age-matched controls, suggesting that elevations in CRH seen in psychiatric diseases may affect the onset of spontaneous preterm labor (Wadhwa et al., 2004).

Antenatal Exposure: Postpartum Effects

Studies have also identified longer-term effects of untreated antenatal mood disorders that impact the infant and early childhood years, as well as affect larger family dynamics. Huizink found that increased maternal cortisol and ACTH in late pregnancy were associated with lower developmental scores and poor adaptation in infancy (Huizink, Robles de Medina, Mulder, Visser, & Buitelaar, 2003). In infants weighed at 2, 6, and 12 months with depressed mothers and psychologically healthy mothers, it was found that infants of depressed mothers had poorer weight gain, lower growth rates, and increased rates of diarrhea (Rahman, Iqbal, Bunn, Lovel, & Harrington, 2004).

Other possible effects of antenatal depression are behavioral. Rahman and colleagues found that mothers with antenatal untreated depression have more disability in the postnatal period, resulting in deficits in physical and emotional care as well as psychosocial stimulation of the infant (Rahman, Harrington, & Bunn, 2002). And, O'Connor found that untreated antenatal stress predisposes infants to behavioral disturbances at four years old (O'Connor, Heron, Golding, Beveridge, & Glover, 2002).

Untreated antenatal depression also significantly increases the likelihood of postpartum depression (O'Hara & Swain, 1996). In the general population, postpartum depression is not uncommon. In fact, postpartum mood disorders have been called the most common complication associated with childbirth (Robertson, Grace, Wallington, & Stewart, 2004). Postpartum blues, a transient condition 3–14 days postpartum not requiring treatment, has an 85% incidence. The more disabling treatment-requiring postpartum depression, occurring 4 weeks to 6 months postpartum, has a 10%–20% incidence (Medline Plus, 2007).

Postpartum psychosis, a medical emergency, is seen in .07% of the population at large, 0.04% of the population without psychiatric history, and 9.24% of women with prior prenatal psychiatric hospitalizations (Harlow et al., 2007). And, 70% of all cases of postpartum psychosis are patients with a history of bipolar or unipolar depression. The risk of suicide is increased 70-fold in the first year postpartum (Appleby, Mortensen, & Faragher, 1998). Although maternal infanticide is rare, it is much more prevalent in those with postpartum mood disorders (Spinelli, 2004).

It is important to note that postpartum mood disorders can also affect partners, with an estimated 10% of men being affected (Paulson, Dauber, & Leferman, 2006). When a mother has a chronic mental illness, she is not the only one who suffers; the partner, infant, other children, and entire family are affected by this familial disease. Even without the compounding effect of psychiatric disease, the first year postpartum is strongly associated with marital problems due to the extreme stress of early parenting (Wilson et al., 1996). Postpartum depression may subsequently pose risk for the women's parenting capability (Logsdon, Wisner, & Pinto-Foltz, 2006). Studies have shown a positive association between postpartum depression, inadequate parenting, and child abuse (Buist, 1998).

Studies of infants of mothers with postpartum depression have also shown an association with future behavioral consequences, including conduct disorder as well as more school problems such as truancy and dropping out (Azar, Paquette, Zoccolillo, Baltzer, & Tremblay, 2007). A study of untreated maternal anxiety postpartum in the ALSPAC community sample showed increased behavioral problems at 4 years of age (O'Connor et al., 2002).

Emotional problems have also been isolated in the children of mothers with untreated postpartum depression; impaired mother-infant interaction and attachment has been shown to affect later development, resulting in more emotional instability in these children as well as impaired relationships with peers (Weinberg & Tronick, 1998). Childhood depression itself has also been found in greater incidence in children of mothers with untreated depression. Weissman and colleagues found an 8% increase in rates of children's diagnosis of depression in mothers whose depression did not remit, with an 11% decrease in rates of children's diagnosis of depression in treated mothers (Weissman et al., 2006).

Effects of Untreated Maternal Mood Disorders: Maternal

For women, one consequence of not treating mood disorders may be increased virulence of psychiatric disease. Dr. Lee Cohen and his colleagues at the Center for Women's Mental Health have led a series of trials, which have shown that women with untreated antenatal psychiatric illness have a high rate of recurrence both during and after pregnancy. In women with major depressive disorder who discontinue antidepressant treatment proximate to conception, there is a 68% recurrence risk in comparison to 25% to those who maintained medical treatment (Cohen et al., 2006). Of the group with a recurring episode in pregnancy, 50% manifested symptoms of such severity that pharmacologic treatment had to be reintroduced (Cohen, Altshuler, Stowe, & Faraone, 2004). Viguera has shown that women with bipolar disorder who go untreated have a 50% relapse rate in pregnancy when compared to those who maintained medical treatment (Viguera et al., 2000).

Untreated postpartum depression may also affect the women's long-term psychiatric prognosis (Philipps & O'Hara, 1991). Though most women recover within a year, postpartum mood disorders may become chronic and refractory if left untreated.

Another consequence of not treating mood disorders is psychological. Women with untreated postpartum distress may feel shame about how their illness is preventing them from properly caring for their infant. They may worry about difficulty with bonding and attachment to their child, and fear for the harm being done by their limited caretaking. Mothers may also feel guilty about the impact of their symptoms on their partner and on other family members, such as other children. In light of social pressures to be happy with their new infant, many women keep their distress a secret (Morrissey, 2007).

How to Treat Antepartum Mood Disorders: A Stepwise Approach

The goals for managing psychiatric illness in pregnancy are 3-fold: minimize fetal exposure, limit risk of maternal psychiatric illness, and reduce risk of relapse. Raskin (1997) offers a rubric that may be helpful to reconcile this multitude of aims.

Step One in evaluation is to weigh the risks of untreated illness. This can be accomplished by taking a thorough past medical history that explores the severity of past psychiatric symptoms both at baseline and in past pregnancies, the past response to medications, and the past occurrences of relapse. Furthermore, the patient should be asked about how she would cope should relapse occur if taken off of her medications.

Step Two is to explore nonmedical alternatives to pharmacological treatment of psychiatric disease, such as therapy and other alternative interventions that will be discussed subsequently.

Step Three-A, if it is decided that the woman will stay on a medication, is choosing the best psychopharmacological alternative to the prior effective medication; this is that medication that will be both effective and have the safest profile in pregnancy. Alternatively, if it is decided that the woman will stop her medication, Step Three-B would be to plan when and how to stop the medication, including discussions about tapering and pregnancy planning.

Step 1: Weighing the Risks

After taking a thorough history, it is important to ask the patient herself about her feelings regarding medication. If a patient expresses a sense of surprise or even alarm at the suggestion of discontinuing medication, that is often meaningful information that medication is profoundly helpful, if not essential, for the patient. Again, it is important to regard these strong feelings with perspective: sometimes they are due to myths or erroneous assumptions about medication management, but other times they reveal helpful data. In reducing these biases and incorrect assumptions, it is essential to answer the patient's earliest questions. Clarifying what is scientifically known and unknown may help reduce the risk of bias impacting the patient's initial impressions. Oftentimes, patients need to express fears or concerns they have about how others (friends, family, partners) would judge them as an inadequate mother if they were to decide to stay on medications through pregnancy.

While each recommendation should be considered on an individualized basis, it may be helpful to think about severity of disease on a spectrum. At one end of the spectrum are women who have experienced mild to moderate psychiatric illness recently but are not currently symptomatic. These women can, generally, be advised to go through pregnancy without medication. However, these patients need to know that their risk of illness in pregnancy is higher than that of women with no past psychiatric history. This category of women may most benefit from psychotherapy to protect against, monitor for, and treat signs and symptoms should they arise.

The opposite end of the spectrum are women who have severe recurrent illness, have been hospitalized, or have had severe exacerbation when going off medications in the past. These patients should, on the whole, be advised to continue their medications, as their risk for relapse in pregnancy is very high with the discontinuation of medical management.

Most other women will fall in the "grey zone," somewhere in between these two extremes. These may be women with significant psychiatric history who are currently on medication and doing well. Alternately, these patients may be off medication, but only recently in remission or just mild to moderately symptomatic. These patients constitute a grey zone and comprise the most challenging group for consultation because there is no easy answer for their treatment plan. Management to stay on, discontinue, or change their medications in pregnancy must be made on a case-by-case basis, factoring in their personal values and individual ability to tolerate risk. Whatever the recommendation, these women must be treated and carefully followed. However, the decision to medicate or employ an alternative form of support such as psychotherapy must be individually assessed by the patient and health care provider.

Step 2: Nonmedical Alternatives

For those patients not taking medication in pregnancy but who need some form of support, it is often advisable to try alternative, nonpharmacologic management. For every pregnant woman, as physiology and psychology changes, the treatment plan must constantly be reevaluated for appropriateness.

Every pregnant woman should maximize her environment for good mental health and overall wellness. Professional counsel is important because patients are often more motivated to take care of themselves and fetus after hearing advice from a practitioner. The elimination of caffeine, nicotine, and alcohol are advised for a multitude of reasons. Despite obvious fetal risks, these substances can complicate psychiatric symptoms. Sleep deprivation has also been shown to exacerbate psychiatric symptoms (McEwen, 2006). Reduction of psychosocial stressors in a woman's environment can also be a very important intervention.

Therapy offers a dual opportunity for treatment as well as the regular monitoring of psychiatric symptoms. Regular obstetrical visits can also be a way to monitor for changes. If a woman who has discontinued medications is currently in therapy alone, it may be advisable to increase the frequency of visits to maximize support in this time of transition.

Many different types of therapy have been found to be successful to treat mood disorders in pregnancy. However, in pregnancy, short-term, symptom-focused therapies may be more appropriate than psychoanalytically based therapy. Dr. Margaret Spinelli at the College of Physicians and Surgeons of Columbia University has found that interpersonal psychotherapy is not only successful in resolving the symptoms of depression during pregnancy, it seems to protect women from postpartum depression later on, making it as effective as medication for many depressed pregnant women (Spinelli, 1997). Other forms of therapy such as cognitive behavioral therapy (CBT) may be good for anxiety, panic, agoraphobia, obsessive-compulsive disorder (OCD), and depression (Misri, Reebye, Corral, & Milis, 2004) (see chapter 14 "Comorbid Presentations in Perinatal Mental Health: Dialectical Behavior Therapy as a Treatment Model"). Short-term insight-oriented psychotherapy, supportive therapy, marital therapy, and group therapy also may be effective.

In addition to therapy, other alternative interventions may be helpful. Freeman has studied the use of Omega-3 essential fatty acids to treat depression in pregnancy and postpartum (Freeman et al., 2006) (see chapter 6 "Omega-3s, Exercise, and St. John's Wort: Three

Complementary and Alternative Treatments for Postpartum Depression"). The early data are promising but inconclusive about efficacy. While no recommended dose has been conclusively established, the usual recommendation is 300–500 mg daily. It is important to recommend sources that are free of excessive mercury to minimize fetal teratogenic risk of this substance.

Phototherapy, also known as light therapy, has also been used to treat antepartum depression (Epperson et al., 2004). Epperson et al. (2004) have shown promising pilot data. Patients should sit in front of a 10,000 lux light box each morning for 20–60 minutes. Certainly, if the woman is responsible for the care of an infant or small child, this modality may be practically difficult. Current data suggest that this is a safe modality that does not incur any UV light exposure (Lam, Buchanan, Mador, Corral, & Remick, 1992). One caveat is that it may be inappropriate for patients with bipolar disease, as it may uncover or exacerbate underlying disease.

Electroconvulsive therapy (ECT) has also been used to treat severe depression with suicidality or acute psychosis in pregnancy (Bozkurt et al., 2007). In the 300 case reports that have been reviewed in the literature over the past 50 years, some risks have been identified, mainly occurring at later stages of pregnancy, including four reports of premature labor (Miller, 1994). There has been one recent report of fetal infarct (Pinette, Santarpio, Wax, & Blackstone, 2007). However, there have not been any reports of premature rupture of membranes. Ultimately, ECT has been found to be safest for use during the early stages of pregnancy. This modality remains a reasonable treatment alternative for women who need a quick positive response (effects can be seen within 1 to 2 weeks of the start of treatment); want to avoid prolonged exposure to medications; or with illness refractory to conventional antidepressants. Modifications to the procedure guidelines that have been established for nonpregnant women should be followed (Miller, 1994).

Step 3-A: Best Pharmacological Choice

Before discussing the different psychopharmacological options for the treatment of psychiatric illness pregnancy, it is important to comment on the context of the information. The *Physicians' Desk Reference* (*PDR*), a compilation of FDA-approved drugs, is currently one of the primary resources. However, this database is highly imperfect for our purposes because, as stated before, women, and specifically pregnant women, have not been included in the majority of clinical control trials.

Furthermore, there are methodological flaws in the studies that do exist (Stowe, Calhoun, Ramsey, Sadek, & Newport, 2001). Most data are gathered retrospectively, from large databases of national-birth, drug-company, and insurance-company registries. It need not be said that prospective, randomized, double-blind placebo controlled (DBPC) trials are the gold standard. However, there are also ethical problems inherent in such trials for pregnant women.

Studies are further complicated by the fact that pregnant women have distinct physiology. Therefore, general knowledge about psychiatric drugs cannot necessarily be applied to pregnant women. Animal studies are the source of much information on the reproductive safety of drugs. The data are limited by the fact that not all medication effects can be generalized from one species to another.

No psychiatric drug has yet been approved by the FDA as being safe for use during pregnancy or lactation (see Table 13.1). This is despite the 30-some years of research that suggest that many psychiatric medications are relatively safe (Einarson, 2005).

We recommend that health practitioners view the FDA pregnancy categories as both helpful but maybe misleading, and thus should not solely guide treatment. Practitioners should not rely only on the letter category of risk, but additionally should consider the research findings for each drug. If a practitioner feels ill equipped to evaluate each drug independently, expert consultation may be necessary.

Class A is drugs in which controlled studies have shown no risk in human pregnancy. Examples of drugs currently included in this category are folic acid and thyroid hormone. Currently, no psychiatric medications are included in this category. Class B is drugs with "no evidence of risk in humans." In other words, "presumed safety based on animal studies" (Green, 2007). We stress that Class B drugs be used with caution because animal data are not always generalizeable to humans. Class C is drugs in which no human or animal studies have shown adverse effect, but "risk cannot be ruled out." Most psychiatric drugs fall into this category. We argue that Class C drugs may be preferable to Class B drugs because of what is known in both animal as well as human studies. Class D shows "positive evidence of risk," but use may be justifiable if benefits outweigh risks. Class X drugs are contraindicated in pregnancy because use outweighs any possible benefit.

Table 13.1

KEY TO FDA USE-IN-PREGNANCY RATINGS

The U.S. Food and Drug Administration's use-in-pregnancy rating system weighs the degree to which available information has ruled out risk to the fetus against the drug's potential benefit to the patient. The ratings, and their interpretation, are as follows:

CATEGORY	INTERPRETATION
A	**CONTROLLED STUDIES SHOW NO RISK.** Adequate, well-controlled studies in pregnant women have failed to demonstrate a risk to the fetus in any trimester of pregnancy.
B	**NO EVIDENCE OF RISK IN HUMANS.** Adequate, well-controlled studies in pregnant women have not shown increased risk of fetal abnormalities despite adverse findings in animals, or, in the absence of adequate human studies, animal studies show no fetal risk. The chance of fetal harm is remote, but remains a possibility.
C	**RISK CANNOT BE RULED OUT.** Adequate, well-controlled human studies are lacking, and animal studies have shown a risk to the fetus or are lacking as well. There is a chance of fetal harm if the drug is administered during pregnancy; but the potential benefits may outweigh the potential risk.
D	**POSITIVE EVIDENCE OF RISK.** Studies in humans, or investigational or post-marketing data, have demonstrated fetal risk. Nevertheless, potential benefits from the use of the drug may outweigh the potential risk. For example, the drug may be acceptable if needed in a life-threatening situation or serious disease for which safer drugs cannot be used or are ineffective.
X	**CONTRAINDICATED IN PREGNANCY.** Studies in animals or humans, or investigational or postmarketing reports, have demonstrated positive evidence of fetal abnormalities or risk which clearly outweighs any possible benefit to the patient.

From *Physicians' Desk Reference,* 2008, p. 215. Copyright 2007 by Thomson Healthcare, Inc. Reprinted with permission of Thomson Healthcare, Inc.

In considering the use of any psychotropic in pregnancy, one must discuss categories of risk. The first is pregnancy loss or miscarriage. Second is the true definition of *teratogenicity:* organ malformation. Third, the perinatal symptoms of neonatal toxicity or withdrawal. And fourth, behavioral teratogenicity (Altshuler et al., 1996).

There are other confounding variables that must be considered in assessing teratogenicity. Other prescription and nonprescription drugs that the mother is ingesting, nutrition, genetic influences, the effects of treated psychiatric illness, environmental toxins, maternal age, time of gestation, and stress are all possible confounders of health in pregnancy. These confounding factors must be controlled for when studying the effects of psychotropics in pregnancy.

Physiologic changes in pregnancy also complicate drug treatment in pregnancy. Drug doses may need to be increased in quantity in pregnancy. This is because the physiologic increase in total body water content in pregnancy may lower the drug serum concentration. Drug binding may also be reduced, as total protein content is lowered in pregnancy. Some drugs, like Lithium, are excreted more quickly due to the increased glomerular filtration rates in the kidney during pregnancy. Because in pregnancy a women's physiology is constantly changing, it is essential to carefully monitor drug levels, therapeutic response, side effects, and toxicity through the entire pregnancy (Wisner, Perel, & Wheeler, 1993). Surveillance must continue into the postpartum period, a time of rapid physiologic change, as doses may need to be decreased to prevent maternal toxicity (Menon, 2008).

When choosing a medication in pregnancy, the first line drug should be both efficacious and relatively safe. This often presents a clinical challenge if symptoms are not well controlled by the drug with the best safety profile. Therefore, medication management must be done on a case-by-case basis, considering each patient's psychiatric symptoms, response to individual medications, and tolerance to drug side effects. Examples of this multidimensional approach will be provided in the Case Studies section.

Another treatment challenge is that of polypharmacy: how to advise patients who are managed prepregnancy on multiple medications. Monotherapy is the preferable option because it offers a single exposure; polypharmacy in pregnancy has not been studied. It is ideal to find the best single agent for a patient and maximize its efficacy, rather than continue on multiple medications at lower doses.

Prepregnancy is the ideal time for making medication changes, such as streamlining to monotherapy. However, some patients may come for consultation already pregnant. If a pregnant patient is doing well psychiatrically on her prior medications, and if these psychotropics are relatively safe in the setting of pregnancy, this treatment should likely continue. The risk of changing or starting a new medication during pregnancy may

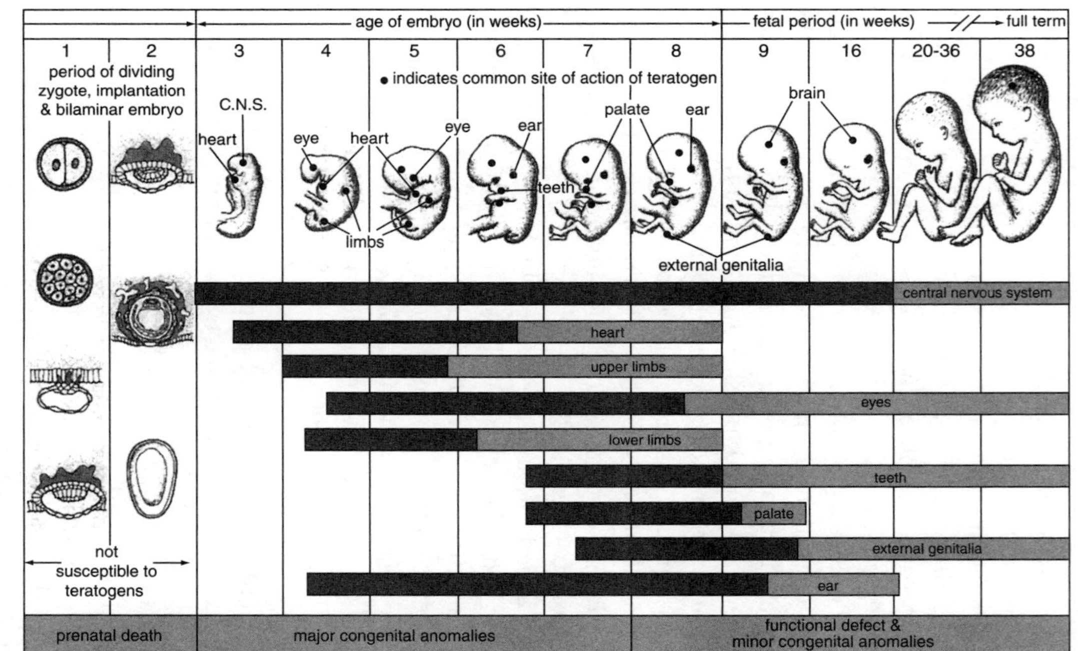

Figure 13.1 Schematic illustration of the critical periods in human development. During the first 2 weeks of life, the embryo is usually not susceptible to teratogens. During these preembryonic stages, a teratogen damages either all or most of the cells, resulting in death or damages, or only a few cells, allowing the conceptus to recover and the embryo to develop without birth defects.

Bar graphs in figure: *Black,* highly sensitive periods of development when major defects may be produced (e.g., absence of limbs). *Gray,* stages that are less sensitive to teratogens, when minor defects may be induced (e.g., hypoplastic thumbs).

Source: Reprinted from Moore KL, Persaud, TVN: *The Developing Human: Clinically Oriented Embryology.* Philadelphia, PA: W.B. Saunders, 1993, p. 156. Used with permission.

pose a greater danger to the woman and fetus than the medication side effects. However, if a pregnant patient is highly symptomatic, changing or starting a medication may be justifiable.

The information on specific drugs is constantly evolving, so the best advice for each clinician would be to follow the current literature for the most up-to-date information.

Step 3-B: Discontinuing Medication

Ideally, the decision to discontinue medication is made prepregnancy, before the woman decides to attempt to conceive. Timing of medication discontinuation is important. In an ideal world, a patient would discontinue her medication and become pregnant shortly thereafter, minimizing risk of relapse off of medication. However, because it can take months to conceive, staying on medication and becoming pregnant will incur early first trimester exposure. This risk may be worth taking if a woman wants to minimize time off of medication. This is all complicated by the fact that women usually find out that they are pregnant at the first day of their missed menses; this is when they are already 4 weeks pregnant (2 weeks postconception).

Raskin (1997) explains that she will give a patient the option to remain on her psychiatric medication while trying to conceive until the first day she misses her period. While this option would not provide for medication taper or discontinuation until 2 weeks after conception, Raskin says that we can accommodate for that by "nature's grace period." She explains that it takes 5 weeks for the blood system that transports maternal substances to the fetus to develop (see Figure 13.1).

CASE STUDIES

The following are case studies of patients who may be helpful prototypes for those you may encounter in your office. We have framed them in three groups: patients who may not need medication in pregnancy, patients who will likely need medication, and patients who fall in the "grey zone" between. Each case, however, should shed light on the subtlety inherent in this work. While generalities can be made, each patient must be evaluated on a case-by-case basis, factoring in not only what is clinically indicated (Step One) but also a plan that is compatible with the patient's values, lifestyle, and comfort.

Likely, No Medication Needed

D.B. is a 39-year-old married women with no past pregnancies who comes to your office for a prepregnancy consultation. In her early 30s, she had a mild depressive episode around the time of a job transition, and was started on Zoloft. The medication was therapeutic, and she continued to stay on Zoloft for the past 9 years with neither a recurrence of her depressive symptoms nor side effects. While she sought brief counseling 9 years ago during her depressive episode, she has not been in therapy since. Significant in her past medical history is childhood diabetes mellitus type I, diagnosed at age 10 and managed since that time with insulin.

Considering her advanced maternal age and history of diabetes, her obstetrician has told her that she would be a high-risk pregnancy. Considering her psychiatric disease is in remission and her high-risk pregnancy status, her obstetrician has advised her that she should discontinue her antidepressant medication as she attempts to conceive. After hearing this advice, she comes to you for a consultation. She understands her obstetrician's advice, but is frankly feeling overwhelmed about the idea of discontinuing her medications. A major source of her stress is her pregnancy risk, so she asks you about the risks of Zoloft and you discuss the potential risks of drug side effects as well as untreated depression. You present the data, and a reminder that some information remains unknown, leaving some of her questions unanswered. You also tell the patient that her prior episode was mild and remote enough that you would be comfortable tapering down her medication and meeting with her on a weekly basis to monitor symptoms and try psychotherapy for support.

Without hesitating, the patient tells you that she has a strong opinion on this matter. The risks that her obstetrician explained about diabetes and advanced maternal age are so much more impressive than the potential risks of Zoloft side effects that she feels that "it's not worth it" to discontinue her Zoloft at this stressful time. After confirming that the patient has informed consent, you make some appointments to regularly meet with her for symptom and medication management, and possible psychotherapy.

A.P. is a 27-year-old married women with no past pregnancies who is currently 4 weeks pregnant. She has had one episode of major depression 7 years ago while in college, after a breakup, and was treated with a short course of Prozac and brief therapy at the college counseling center. She is asymptomatic off medication and has not been in therapy for the past 5 years. Her sister had a severe episode of postpartum depression last year after giving birth to her first child, and this has caused A.P. to worry about a relapse of her own depression during or subsequent to this pregnancy. She comes to you asking if she should restart on Prozac in this pregnancy.

You discuss the risks of untreated illness versus the risks of medication on the fetus, and also note that you prefer not to start psychiatric medications in pregnancy for prophylaxis. However, you also explain that the patient is at a higher risk of postpartum depression due to her personal and family history.

In response to your comments, the patient sits and stares at you blankly. "It's so hard to know what the right decision would be," she says. "Please just tell me what you would do." You respond by telling her that you still need to gather more information, and ask the patient more about her social history, medical history, her past depressive episode and the related circumstances, how she copes in times of transition and stress, how she has coped around her period and birth control pills, her extensive family history, her current social supports, and her relationship to her partner.

After gathering this information, you provide the patient with some scenarios and ask her to tell you how she would react: if she had a relapse of her depression antepartum or postpartum; if her child had some sort of a complication, of unknown etiology, but possibly related to the medication exposure, or to the exposure of untreated illness. Essentially, your goal here is to help the patient articulate her personal values. Even though she has already asked you to make the decision for her, it is your job to help her make this decision for herself. From these scenarios, the patient decides, with your empathy and support, that she does not want to start Prozac at this point in the pregnancy.

You discuss alternative modes of treatment (Step Two), including prophylactic efforts. She agrees to start psychotherapy to both monitor for and manage any symptoms that should arise. You spend time educating the patient about the symptoms of depression and postpartum depression, specifically reminding her how they have presented for her in the past, and advise her to be vigilant about monitoring her mood and behavior and ask her loved ones to do the same. You give her the opportunity to return to your office with her partner, so that he can be on board to help her monitor her symptoms. And, you remind her that while she has decided to not start medication now, you can always revisit this issue later if symptoms arise.

C.F. is a 30-year-old married woman who is 6 weeks pregnant. She has never been pregnant before. She has no psychiatric history, has never been medicated or diagnosed with a psychiatric disorder. Her obstetrician sends her to you for a consult after learning that the patient has had a recent onset of insomnia. She has never experienced this before, but does describe herself as a "worry-wart." On further questioning about the insomnia, she explains that she has been unable to fall asleep because she is constantly worrying about her impending motherhood. She denies panic attacks, avoidance, and phobias, but admits to constant worrying about everything. She tells you that she has a complicated relationship with her own mother who divorced her father in childhood and has since spent most of her time with her younger stepchildren. History reveals that the patient has also had some emotional difficulty during times of transition in her life.

You discuss risks and benefits of untreated anxiety versus medication options in pregnancy. You review treatment options with the patient, advising her that her symptoms may very well be treated with alternative therapies before considering medication. You introduce the option of therapy, and she says that it's always been something she's wanted to try. You refer her to a therapist for psychotherapy, and agree to meet with the patient in the future if symptoms increase.

Likely, Medication Needed

L.T. is a 33-year-old married women coming in for a prepregnancy consultation. She has a history of severe recurrent depression since early adolescence and has been on multiple antidepressants for 17 years. Ten years ago her psychiatrist at that time discontinued her medications and she had to be hospitalized for suicidal ideation with a plan but no attempt. Since then, she has been stable on her medication, most recently Effexor, as well as weekly insight-oriented therapy. She has not been hospitalized since, but admits to having thoughts of hurting herself when she gets really down. She is planning on going off of her birth control and wants to get pregnant. You ask her some more questions about her history, give her some scenarios, consult about some medication alternatives, and explain risks and benefits related to treatment of depression in pregnancy. Before you can finish your questions, the patient interrupts you to say, "I don't know if this makes me a bad person, but I just know I can't live with what it feels like when I'm off of my medication."

You trust the patient's strong feelings and agree to medically manage her through the pregnancy. However, you explain to her that Effexor is an antidepressant that has less safety data in pregnancy, and you would rather try her on a medication that has more data in pregnancy. You agree to switch her medication and evaluate her stability before she goes off of her birth control, recommending that she try to conceive when she is psychiatrically stable on the new medication. If the alternative medication is nontherapeutic, you tell her that she could go back on Effexor for pregnancy if necessary.

R.L. is a 30-year-old woman who is coming to you for a prepregnancy consultation. She was diagnosed with bipolar disorder in late adolescence and has had multiple episodes of depression with psychotic features and acute mania, with four hospitalizations in the past 15 years. She has never been suicidal. R.L. was started on Lithium 14 years ago, and enjoyed a 2-year period in graduate school where she was tapered off of Lithium and was able to function without symptoms. After 2 years, however, her symptoms recurred and she immediately went back on the medication.

She comes to you with her husband after telling her obstetrician and psychiatrist that she wants to get pregnant and under no circumstances would expose her baby to the possible risk incurred from Lithium exposure that she read about on the Internet. Her obstetrician and psychiatrist are deeply concerned that, given her serious history, medication discontinuation may not be a good idea. She is confident that she knows her disease and can monitor her own symptoms with medical supervision. She explains that she understands that she might not make it through the entire pregnancy without a relapse, but wants to try and will agree to go back on her Lithium if that is what is medically advised.

After taking a thorough history, you advise the patient that, given her severe history, her likelihood of relapse is high. You advise that she stay on her Lithium, based on a risk/benefit analysis for both the patient as well as a future fetus. The patient listens, but then strongly responds, "If I don't at least try to go off of my medication and my child has a birth defect, I will feel like it's child abuse." Once again, you review the risks that are involved in not taking medication, and establish that the patient has informed consent.

From this conversation, you are convinced that regardless of what you recommend, this patient will not take any medication during her pregnancy unless she is in an emergency situation or forced. Rather than turn her away, you reason that it is better for you to monitor this patient aggressively for symptoms so that you will be able to restart medications when the likely time arises. Ultimately, you decide that you and the patient must agree to disagree and come up with a compromise plan together. "Do you accept the possibility that the next time we might see each other is in the hospital?" you ask the patient, and she nods yes. You document and discuss a personalized algorithm for the conditions under which the patient must start taking medications, should she relapse. You ask her to chart her mood symptoms daily, and ask her husband to also observe her for daily change. You maximize any and all alternative treatments.

The patient and her husband responsibly follow your algorithm and are punctual for every appointment you make. You slowly taper down the Lithium. Despite their impressive efforts, the patient relapses 1 week after discontinuation. You get a call from the emergency room to tell you that the patient has been admitted to inpatient psychiatry for a manic episode. The patient is started on Haldol in the inpatient unit as a safer alternative to Lithium for pregnancy or a woman trying to conceive. Though the patient's symptoms are responsive to Haldol, the patient cannot tolerate the side effects. She is restarted on Lithium at her prior dose. Ultimately, she agrees that it is best for her to continue trying to conceive while still on Lithium and stay on that medication should she become pregnant.

The "Grey Zone"

C.H. is a 35-year-old woman who was sent to you by her obstetrician for a prepregnancy consultation. She was diagnosed with bipolar disorder at age 18 and was briefly hospitalized for one manic episode, and has been stable on Lithium 900 mg daily without symptoms and hospitalizations for the past 17 years. She has been fully functional, working as a successful business executive. She explains to you that no one in her life except her parents, sister, and husband know about her bipolar diagnosis and this privacy is crucial to her. She fears that if she were to go off of her medication and relapse, thus exposing her psychiatric disease, it would risk her social status as well as her family's financial stability, as she is the "breadwinner."

You ask her more questions about her past psychiatric history and undergo a thorough discussion to learn more about her values, following Step

One of the consultation guidelines. After gathering this additional information, you advise the patient that her stable history for 17 years on such a low dose of Lithium suggests that her risk for relapse is low. You review that Lithum has been associated with a risk of cardiac malformation if used in the first trimester, and advise the patient to discontinue the medication during the first trimester or through the course of the pregnancy in full.

Considering her apprehension before, you are not surprised that the patient remains concerned. You reassure the patient that you and she will work closely to monitor her symptoms, so that at the first sign of any recurrence, she can be restarted on Lithium. You decide to frame your recommendation as a range of three options for how to taper the medications. Option one: you could try to taper off her Lithium before she conceives just to see how she does, ultimately discontinuing the medication. The patient could be monitored for recurrence by her husband and therapist. Option two: the patient could taper off of her Lithium, and you could restart a less teratogenic agent that has a better safety profile and will be therapeutic should she have symptoms. Option three: you could taper off her Lithium at a positive pregnancy test to minimize exposure during cardiac formation for the fetus and time off medication for the woman.

The patient decides to think about it, and returns for a follow-up visit with her husband. Her husband urges her to follow your advice and either taper off or try an alternative medication. Nonetheless, after a lengthy counseling session and establishing informed consent, the patient insists on staying on her Lithium. The patient quickly conceives. After close monitoring of her Lithium levels, and renal and thyroid functioning in pregnancy, the patient delivers a healthy baby boy.

S.T. is a 28-year-old woman who is 2 months pregnant and is referred to you from your hospital's obsessive-compulsive disorder clinic. In the clinic, she was counseled to start Zoloft, but has been sent to you to discuss the standard of care for management in pregnancy. She has always had some obsessive features, such as checking the locks of her doors several times before leaving the house, but has been able to maintain a good relationship with her husband and friends, and function well at work. However, since becoming pregnant, she has been staying up at night worrying about causing harm to her baby. She avoids social events in restaurants because she is concerned about food safety and infections. She only gets 3 hours of sleep each night because she is so distressed by visions of harming her unborn child.

You explain to the patient that while she would benefit from Zoloft or a similar drug during pregnancy, there are risks of exposure to the fetus. She adamantly states that there is no way she would ever take a medication in pregnancy. You go on to counsel that some of her behaviors like her disordered sleeping and eating could also cause harm to her fetus, in addition to herself. She expresses feeling overwhelmed, and asks you if there's anything that can be safely done. You counsel about alternative treatment modalities, and she agrees to start psychotherapy. With the patient's consent, you collaborate with her therapist to monitor for symptom exacerbation during the pregnancy.

L.R. is a 30-year-old single woman who has recently found out she is pregnant, unplanned. She has chronic bipolar disease with psychotic features, currently managed with Depakote, and has been hospitalized multiple times. She believes that she conceived 1 month ago during a manic episode that included sexually promiscuity and cocaine use. In addition, she has also been having difficulty at work, and fears that she is at risk for getting fired. She presents to you, overwhelmed, after a referral from her gynecological clinic. She is tearful and ambivalent, and says that while she does want to have children at some point in her life, she is not sure if this is the right time.

You ask the patient more questions about her history, lifestyle, and desires for this pregnancy. You explain to her that if she were to continue with her pregnancy and stay on psychiatric medications, there is a risk of being on Depakote because of its likely teratogenic effects. If she were psychiatrically stable enough, you could consider an alternative medication. If she continues on the Depakote, you would work with her obstetrician to assess any fetal teratogenicity. At this point in the conversation, she clearly articulates that her primary priority at the present time is to maintain her emotional stability and that she does not feel that she could experiment with her psychiatric medications. The patient decides to electively terminate the fetus. You tell the patient that you will support whatever personal decision she decides to make, and reassure her that you will communicate with her regular psychiatrist to monitor her closely through this time.

CONCLUSION

The goal of this chapter has been to provide guidance for the management of mood disorders in pregnancy. It is emphasized that no decision is risk-free, and each case must be considered individually with up-to-date data. The Case Studies section stresses that, while sometimes clinical indications seem clear or in the grey zone, there are many situations when patients come to you with their own opinions and plans. While standard of care must never be compromised, the health care practitioner must craft a treatment plan that the patient will reasonably follow. It is the health practitioner's job to educate and advise patients while considering their values. The NIMH call to arms for more research in this area, both on the exposure of medications, as well as that of untreated mental illness, must be aggressively pursued so scientific knowledge can help us better answer our patient's questions.

REFERENCES

Allison, S. K. (2004). Psychotropic medication in pregnancy: Ethical aspects and clinical management. *Journal of Perinatal and Neonatal Nursing, 18*(3), 194–205.

Altshuler, L. L., Cohen, L., Szuba, M. P., Burt, V. K., Gitlin, M., & Mintz, J. (1996). Pharmacologic management of psychiatric illness during pregnancy: Dilemmas and guidelines. *American Journal of Psychiatry, 153*(5), 592–606.

Amaro, H., Fried, L. E, Cabral, H., & Zuckerman, B. (1990). Violence during pregnancy and substance use. *American Journal of Public Health, 80*(5), 575–579.

Andersson, L., Sundstrom-Poromaa, I., Wulff, M., Astrom, M., & Bixo, M. (2004). Implications of antenatal depression and anxiety for obstetric outcome. *Obstetrics and Gynecology, 104*(3), 467–476.

Appleby, L., Mortensen, P. B., & Faragher, E. B. (1998). Suicide and other causes of mortality after post-partum psychiatric admission. *British Journal of Psychiatry, 173,* 209–211.

Azar, R., Paquette, D., Zoccolillo, M., Baltzer, F., & Tremblay, R. E. (2007). The association of major depression, conduct disorder, and maternal overcontrol with a failure to show a cortisol buffered response in 4-month-old infants of teenage mothers. *Biological Psychiatry, 62*(6), 573–579.

Berle, J. O., Mykletun, A., Daltveit, A. K., Rasmussen, S., Holsten, F., & Dahl, A. A. (2005). Neonatal outcomes in offspring of women with anxiety and depression during pregnancy: A linkage study from The Nord-Trondelag Health Study (HUNT) and Medical Birth Registry of Norway. *Archive of Women's Mental Health, 8*(3), 181–189.

Bozkurt, A., Karlidere, T., Isintas, M., Ozmenler, N. K., Ozsahin, A., & Yanarates, O. (2007). Acute and maintenance electroconvulsive therapy for treatment of psychotic depression in a pregnant patient. *Journal of Electroconvulsive Therapy, 23*(3), 185–187.

Buist, A. (1998). Childhood abuse, parenting and postpartum depression. *Australian and New Zealand Journal of Psychiatry, 32*(4), 479–487.

Cohen, L. S., Altshuler, L. L., Harlow, B. L., Nonacs, R., Newport, D. J., Viguera, A. C, et al. (2006). Relapse of major depression during pregnancy in women who maintain or discontinue antidepressant treatment. *Journal of the American Medical Association, 295*(5), 499–507.

Cohen, L. S., Altshuler, L. L., Stowe, Z. N., & Faraone, S. V. (2004). Reintroduction of antidepressant therapy across pregnancy in women who previously discontinued treatment: A preliminary retrospective study. *Psychotherapy and Psychosomatics, 73,* 255–258.

Cohen, L. S., Rosenbaum, J. F., & Heller, V. L. (1989). Panic attack-associated placental abruption: A case report. *Journal of Clinical Psychiatry, 50*(7), 266–267.

Coverdale, J. H., McCullough, L. B., & Chervenak, F. A. (1997). Sexually transmitted diseases and unwanted pregnancies in chronically ill psychiatric patients. *The Medical Journal of Australia, 166*(5), 231–232.

Davis, E. P., Glynn, L. M., Schetter, C. D., Hobel, C., Chicz-Demet, A., & Sandman, C. A. (2007). Prenatal exposure to maternal depression and cortisol influences infant temperament. *Journal of the American Academy of Child & Adolescent Psychiatry, 46*(6), 737–746.

Diego, M. A., Jones, N. A., Field, T., Hernandez-Reif, M., Schanberg, S., Kuhn, C., et al. (2006). Maternal psychological distress, prenatal cortisol, and fetal weight. *Psychosomatic Medicine, 68*(5), 747–753.

Einarson, A. (2005). The safety of psychotropic drug use during pregnancy: A review. *Psychosomatic Medicine, 7*(4), 3.

Epperson, C. N., Terman, M., Terman, J. S., Hanusa, B. H., Oren, D. A., & Peindl, K. S. (2004). Randomized clinical trial of bright light therapy for antepartum depression: Preliminary findings. *Journal of Clinical Psychiatry, 65*(3), 421–425.

Federenko, I. S., & Wadhwa, P. D. (2004). Women's mental health during pregnancy influences fetal and infant developmental and health outcomes. *CNS Spectrum, 9*(3), 198–206.

Field, T., Diego, M., Hernandez-Reif, M., Schanberg, S., Kuhn, C., Yando, R., & Bendell, D. (2003). Pregnancy anxiety and comorbid depression and anger: Effects on the fetus and neonate. *Depress Anxiety, 17*(3), 140–151.

Freeman, M. P., Hibbeln, J. R., Wisner, K. L., Davis, J. M., Mischoulon, D., & Peet, M. (2006). Omega-3 fatty acids: Evidence basis for treatment and future research in psychiatry. *Journal of Clinical Psychiatry, 67*(12), 1954–1967.

Galler, J. R., Harrison, R. H., Ramsey, F., Forde, V., & Butler, S. C. (2000). Maternal depressive symptoms affect infant cognitive development in Barbados. *Journal of Child Psychology and Psychiatry, 41*(6), 747–757.

Glover, V. (1999). Maternal stress or anxiety during pregnancy and the development of the baby. *Pract Midwife, 2*(5), 20–22.

Green, S. M. (2007). *Tarascon pocket pharmacopoeia: 2007 classic shirt-pocket edition.* Tarascon Publishing.

Halbreich, U., & Kornstein, S. G. (2004). Mental symptoms and disorders during pregnancy. *CNS Spectrum, 9*(3), 176.

Hamilton, B. E., Martin, J. A., & Ventura, S. J. (2005). *Births: Preliminary Data for 2005. Health E-Stats.* Retrieved November 21, 2006, from http://www.cdc.gov/nchs/products/pubs/pubd/hestats/prelimbirths05/prelimbirths05.html

Hans, S. L. (1999). Demographic and psychosocial characteristics of substance-abusing pregnant women. *Clin Perinatol, 26*(1), 55–74.

Harlow, B. L., Vitonis, A. F., Sparen, P., Cnattingius, S., Joffe, H., & Hultman, C. W. (2007). Incidence of hospitalization for postpartum psychotic and bipolar episodes in women with and without prior prepregnancy or prenatal psychiatric hospitalizations. *Archive of General Psychiatry, 64,* 42–48.

Huizink, A. C., Robles de Medina, P. G., Mulder, E. J., Visser, G. H., & Buitelaar, J. K. (2003). Stress during pregnancy is associated with developmental outcome in infancy. *Journal of Child Psychology and Psychiatry, 44*(6), 810–818.

Kessler, R. C., McGonagle, K. A., Swartz, M., Blazer, D. G., & Nelson, C. B. (1993). Sex and depression in the National Comorbidity Survey. *Journal of Affect Disorders, 29*(2–3), 85–96.

Lam, R. W., Buchanan, A., Mador, J. A., Corral, M. R., & Remick, R. A. (1992). The effects of ultraviolet-A wavelengths in light therapy for seasonal depression. *Journal of Affected Disorder, 24*(4), 237–243.

Lester, D., & Beck, A. T. (1998). Attempted suicide and pregnancy. *American Journal of Obstetrics and Gynecology, 158*(5), 1084–1085.

Logsdon, M. C., Wisner, K. L., & Pinto-Foltz, M. D. (2006). The impact of postpartum depression on mothering. *Journal of Obstetrics Gynecology and Neonatal Nursing, 35*(5), 652–658.

Lou, H. C., Hansen, D., Nordentoft, M., Pryds, O., Jensen, F., Nim, J., et al. (1994). Prenatal stressors of human life affect fetal brain development. *Developmental Medicine and Child Neurology, 36,* 826–832.

Lundy, B., Field, T., Nearing, G., Davalos, M., Pietro, P. A., Schanberg, S., et al. (1999). Prenatal depression effects on neonates. *Infant Behavior and Development, 22,* 119–129.

Marcus, S. M., Flynn, H. A., & Blow, F. C. (2003). Depressive symptoms among pregnant women screened in obstetrics settings. *Journal of Women's Health, 12,* 373–380.

McEwen, B. S. (2006). Sleep deprivation as a neurobiologic and physiologic stressor: Allostasis and allostatic load. *Metabolism, 55,* S20–S23.

Medline Plus. (2007). *Postpartum depression.* Retrieved November 13, 2007, from http://www.nlm.nih.gov/medlineplus/postpartumdepression.html

Menon, S. J. (2008). Psychotropic medication during pregnancy and lactation. *Archive of Gynecology and Obstetrics, 277*(1), 1–13.

Miller, L. J. (1994). Use of electroconvulsive therapy during pregnancy. *Hospital and Community Psychiatry, 45*(5), 444–450.

Misri, S., Reebye, P., Corral, M., & Milis, L. (2004). The use of paroxetine and cognitive-behavioral therapy in postpartum depression and anxiety: A randomized controlled trial. *Journal of Clinical Psychiatry, 65*(9), 1236–1241.

Monk, C., Fifer, W. P., Myers, M. M., Sloan, R. P., Trien, L., & Hurtado, A. (1999). Maternal stress responses and anxiety during pregnancy: Effects on fetal heart rate. *Developmental Psychobiology, 36,* 67–77.

Morrissey, M. V. (2007). Suffer no more in silence: Challenging the myths of women's mental health in childbearing. *International Journal of Psychiatric Nursing, 12*(2), 1429–1438.

National Institute of Mental Health. (2003). *Women's mental health in pregnancy and the postpartum period.* Retrieved October 10, 2007, from http://grants.nih.gov/grants/guide/pa-files/PA-03-135.html

Newport, D. J., Wilcox, M. M., & Stowe, Z. N. (2001). Antidepressants during pregnancy and lactation: Defining exposure and treatment issues. *Seminars in Perinatology, 25*(3), 177–190.

Nonacs, R., & Cohen, L. S. (2003). Assessment and treatment of depression during pregnancy: An update. *Psychiatric Clinics in North America, 26*(3), 547–562.

O'Connor, T. G., Heron, J., Golding, J., Beveridge, M., & Glover, V. (2002). Maternal antenatal anxiety and children's behavioural/emotional problems at 4 years: Report from the Avon Longitudinal Study of Parents and Children. *British Journal of Psychiatry, 180,* 502–508.

O'Hara, M., & Swain, A. (1996). Rates and risk of postpartum depression: A meta-analysis. *International Review of Psychiatry, 8,* 37–54.

Orr, S. T. & Miller, C. A. (1995). Maternal depressive symptoms and the risk of poor pregnancy outcome: Review of the literature and preliminary findings. *Epidemiology Review, 17*(1), 165–171.

Orr, S. T., Reiter, J. P., Blazer, D. G., & James, S. A. (2007). Maternal prenatal pregnancy-related anxiety and spontaneous preterm birth in Baltimore, Maryland. *Psychosomatic Medicine, 69*(6), 566–570.

Paulson, J. F., Dauber, S., & Leferman, J. A. (2006). Individual and combined effects of postpartum depression in mothers and fathers on parenting behavior. *Pediatrics, 118*(2), 659–668.

Philipps, L. H., & O'Hara, M. W. (1991). Prospective study of postpartum depression: 4½-year follow-up of women and children. *Journal Abnormal Psychology, 100*(2), 151–155.

Pinette, M. G., Santarpio, C., Wax, J. R., & Blackstone, J. (2007). Electroconvulsive therapy in pregnancy. *Obstetrics and Gynecology, 110*(2 Pt 2), 465–466.

Powers, Z. L., Zahorik, P., & Morrow, B. (1993). An evaluation of residents' recognition of depressive symptoms in obstetrical patients. *Journal of the Tennessee Medical Association, 86*(4), 147–149.

Rahman, A., Harrington, R., & Bunn, J. (2002). Can maternal depression increase infant risk of illness and growth impairment in developing countries? *Child Care Health Development, 28*(1), 51–56.

Rahman, A., Iqbal, Z., Bunn, J., Lovel, H., & Harrington, R. (2004). Impact of maternal depression on infant nutritional status and illness: A cohort study. *Archive of General Psychiatry, 61*(9), 946–952.

Raskin, V. (1997). *When words are not enough: The women's prescription for anxiety and depression.* New York: Broadway Books.

Robertson, E., Grace, S., Wallington, T., & Stewart, D. E. (2004). Antenatal risk factors for postpartum depression: A synthesis of recent literature. *General Hospital Psychiatry, 26*(4), 289–295.

Salamero, M., Marcos, T., Gutierrez, F., & Rebull, E. (1994). Factorial study of the BDI in pregnant women. *Psychological Medicine, 24*(4), 1031–1035.

Spinelli, M. G. (1997). Interpersonal psychotherapy for depressed antepartum women: A pilot study. *American Journal of Psychiatry, 154*(7), 1028–1030.

Spinelli, M. G. (2004). Maternal infanticide associated with mental illness: Prevention and the promise of saved lives. *American Journal of Psychiatry, 161*(9), 1548–1557.

Stowe, Z. N., Calhoun, K., Ramsey, C., Sadek, N., & Newport, D. J. (2001). Mood disorders during pregnancy and lactation: Defining issues of exposure and treatment. *CNS Spectrums, 6*(2), 150–166.

Stowe, Z. N., Hostetter, A. L., & Newport, D. J. (2005). The onset of postpartum depression: Implications for clinical screening in obstetrical and primary care. *American Journal of Obstetrics and Gynecology, 192*(2), 522–526.

Teixeira, J. M., Fisk, N. M., & Glover, V. (1999). Association between maternal anxiety in pregnancy and increased uterine artery resistance index: Cohort based study. *BMJ, 318*(7177), 153–157.

Van den Bergh, B. R., Mulder, E. J., Mennes, M., & Glover, V. (2005). Antenatal maternal anxiety and stress and the neurobehavioural development of the fetus and child: Links and possible mechanisms. *Neuroscience and Behavioral Reviews, 29*(2), 237–258.

Viguera, A. C., Nonacs, R., Cohen, L. S., Tondo, L., Murray, A., & Baldessarini, R. J. (2000). Risk of recurrence of bipolar disorder in pregnant and nonpregnant women after discontinuing lithium maintenance. *American Journal Psychiatry, 157*(2), 179–184.

Wadhwa, P. D., Garite, T. J., Porto, M., Glynn, L., Chicz-DeMet, A., Dunkel-Schetter, C., et al. (2004). Placental corticotropin-releasing hormone (CRH), spontaneous preterm birth, and fetal growth restriction: A prospective investigation. *American Journal of Obstetrics and Gynecology, 191*(4), 1063–1069.

Weinberg, M. K., & Tronick, E. Z. (1998). The impact of maternal psychiatric illness on infant development. *Journal of Clinical Psychiatry, 59*(2), 53–61.

Weinstock, M. (2005). The potential influence of maternal stress hormones on development and mental health of the offspring. *Brain, Behavior, and Immunology, 19*(4), 296–308.

Weissman, M. M., Pilowsky, D. J., Wickramaratne, P. J., Talati, A., Wisniewski, S. R., Fava, M., et al. (2006). Remissions in maternal depression and child psychopathology: A STAR*D-Child report. *Journal of the American Medical Association, 295*(12), 1389–1398.

Werner, E. A., Myers, M. M., Fifer, W. P., Cheng, B., Fang, Y., & Allen, R. (2007). Prenatal predictors of infant temperament. *Developmental Psychobiology, 49*(5), 474–484.

Willis, J. L. (1997). *Your guide to women's health. FDA consumer special report* (3rd ed.). Retrieved December 24, 1997, from http://www.fda.gov/oashi/aids/equal.html

Wilson, L. M., Reid, A. J., Midmer, D. K., Biringer, A., Carroll, J. C., & Stewart, D. E. (1996). Antenatal psychosocial risk factors associated with adverse postpartum family outcomes. *CMAJ, 154*(6), 785–799.

Wisner, K. L., Perel, J. M., & Wheeler, S. B. (1993). Tricyclic dose requirements across pregnancy. *American Journal of Psychiatry, 150*(10), 1541–1542.

14

Comorbid Presentations in Perinatal Mental Health: Dialectical Behavior Therapy as a Treatment Model

SUSAN DOWD STONE

When evaluating clients for the presence of perinatal mood disorders, it is critical to include a thorough multiaxial assessment to best formulate diagnosis and effective treatment planning. As pregnancy and childbirth require formidable personal resources across the biopsychosocial realm, lack of attention to any significant presentation along the axes could compromise treatment outcomes. While the distress of major mood disorders may be reliably captured by several evaluative rating systems (covered in chapter 5), further client exploration is then necessary to identify and target in treatment planning all contributing factors to ameliorate client distress and maximize treatment gains (Battle, Zlotnick, Miller, Pearlstein, & Howard, 2006; Conners, Grant, Crone, & Whiteside-Mansell, 2006).

Well covered elsewhere in this text (chapter 5) are basic assessment for perinatal mood disorders, associated risk factors, and medical conditions, which may prolong or worsen an affective episode. Also presented in this text are other social, alternative and psychological treatment resources for this population, such as peer support groups, psychodynamic approaches and interpersonal psychotherapy (chapters 6, 15, 16, and 18) some of which present empirical support for their consideration (Kopelman & Stuart, 2005; O'Hara, Gorman, Stuart, & Wenzel, 2000; Segre, Stuart, & O'Hara, 2004).

Less well researched and addressed, however, are studies focusing on treatments for perinatal clients who present with co-occurring disorders, that is, an affective disorder and the presence of comorbid eating disorders, substance abuse, personality disorders, or engagement in other behaviors such as smoking that compromise the pregnancy and the maternal/child outcomes. Despite acknowledgment of their frequent occurrence across the perinatal spectrum, such disorders often remain undiagnosed and untreated (Howard, Battle, Pearlstein, & Rosene-Montella, 2006). Exclusion of the multiaxial client in diagnostic focus and perinatal treatment research may partially explain noted disappointments in long-term treatment outcomes developed specifically for this population despite promising early relief from symptoms.

This chapter will focus on the identification of common perinatal comorbidities and offer an overview of a treatment design—Dialectical Behavior Therapy (DBT)—whose theory, design, and evidential findings for treatment of concurrent multiaxial disorders appear to align well with both the presumed etiology of perinatal mood disorders and management of complex cases. The model also offers guidance for clinicians in prioritizing complex treatment targets and ongoing consultative support.

While no large-scale studies applying DBT specifically to perinatal populations have been undertaken at press time, discussion of DBT's theoretical alignment with the recovery tasks in the perinatal period, qualitative elements similar to those in models effectively targeting perinatal depression, and a case study will be presented to demonstrate the model's application. Evidenced-based thinking will guide the model's suggested application in clinical settings until further research validates it as an evidence-based practice for this population (Center for Substance Abuse Treatment, 2007).

Comorbid presentations in the perinatal period are frequently referenced in perinatal literature calling for their evaluation, suggesting both their commonality and their association with depression and birth complications (Homish, Cornelius, Richardson, & Day, 2004; McMahon, Barnett, Kowalenko, & Tennant, 2004), yet current research on effective treatment protocols for this population tends to exclude research subjects presenting comorbid complexities, notably substance abuse, eating disorders, personality disorders, or suicidality (Reay, Fisher, Robertson, Adams, & Owen, 2006).

Statistics on the prevalence of perinatal mood disorders suggest that up to 22% of women experience diagnosable postpartum mood disorders (Ahokas, Kaukoranta, Wahlbeck, & Aito, 2001). Percentages of this group with comorbid or multiaxial diagnoses have been less quantified, but diagnostic information of participants in PPD treatment trials frequently reference comorbid conditions (James, 1998; Klier, Muzik, Rosenblum, & Lenz, 2001; Misri, Reebye, Corral, & Milis, 2004), including anxiety disorders, bipolar and adjustment disorders, eating disorders, PTSD, substance abuse, personality disorders, and additional psychosocial and medical stressors. A recent study by Battle et al. (2006) suggests that women seeking psychiatric services during the perinatal period are often more severely impaired and meet criteria for multiple comorbid conditions. These findings are unsurprising when considering that in women suffering from major depressive disorders (MDD) in the general population, up to 60% suffer from comorbid disorders (U.S. Department of Health and Human Services, 1999). The combination of rapid, extensive biological shifts emanating from pregnancy and birth, combined with profound psychosocial challenges requiring skillful management, strongly suggests that comorbid presentations which are known to be exacerbated by such stressors, could be even more likely along the perinatal spectrum.

The search for effective protocols responsive to these findings continues due to the paucity of studies—most of which are based on short-term treatment for postpartum depression only—involving significant numbers of women with co-occurring disorders, utilization of appropriate controls, and substantiation of gains through sufficient follow-up (Dennis, 2004). While the demonstrated effectiveness of current short-term treatment models in relieving symptoms of postpartum depression is not challenged here, it is suggested that untreated comorbid disorders may subvert retention of treatment gains in follow-up studies and may be a contributing factor in prolonging the primary affective episode.

Studies evaluating association between the duration and frequency of supportive psychotherapy, cognitive behavioral approaches, and psychopharmacological intervention and postpartum retention of gains (Hanusa, Perel, Sunder, & Wisner 2004; Huysman, 2003) appear to support the proposal that longer and more specifically focused treatment is needed to sustain postpartum recovery.

Additionally, the specific etiology and recovery tasks of postpartum spectrum disorders among multiaxial presentations infer that optimal treatment for high-risk clients might be best introduced when biological vulnerabilities first present and client motivation is high (pregnancy) and continue well into the postpartum period (Stone, 2006). Such focus would necessarily include comorbid disorders such as alcohol and substance abuse, eating disorders, personality disorders, suicidal ideation, smoking, and skills deficits impacting interpersonal transactions, and the medical outcome of the pregnancy.

COMMONLY OCCURING PERINATAL COMORBID DISORDERS

Alcohol Use

While the negative consequence of alcohol use before, during, and after pregnancy is well established and includes fetal alcohol syndrome, developmental problems, and behavioral issues, significant numbers of women will continue to drink alcohol during pregnancy (Chang et al., 1998). Despite the awareness of concurrent presentations of depression and alcohol abuse in the general population, there has been a lack of attention to this comorbid presentation in the perinatal period (Homish et al., 2004). One study determined that only 9% of pregnant alcohol users were identified by medical/obstetric staff during pregnancy (Chang et al., 1998). Yet, this population is excluded or underrepresented in treatment studies focusing on the perinatal period.

One recent study (Chang, McNamara, Wilkins-Haug, & Orav, 2007) found that less than 20% of women who tested positive for alcohol while pregnant ceased drinking during their first trimester, and only half were abstinent during the second half of their pregnancy. These studies suggest that the majority of alcohol use antenatally (including the period prior to realization of pregnancy), during, and after pregnancy continues to remain undetected and untreated! As some women will respond to pregnancy with attempts to alter patterns of use (Chang et al., 2007), evaluation for alcohol use and treatment supportive of maternal motivation for abstinence seems crucial early in the perinatal period. The T-ACE (tolerance, annoy, cut down, eye opener) evaluative tool administered early in pregnancy may help determine levels of drinking, or the presence of alcohol abuse, which is often underreported. The T-ACE was modified from the CAGE screening test and was designed to help identify alcohol use in obstetrical settings (Sokol, Martier, & Ager, 1989).

Substance Abuse

The use and abuse of substances during pregnancy also continues to be of major concern. Recent reports suggest that significant percentages of women (up to 4%) continue to use illicit drugs or binge drink during pregnancy (Conners et al., 2006). A study addressing the abuse of methamphetamine during pregnancy found it may be increasing (Derauf et al., 2007). Another study indicated ranges of from 1%–15% of pregnant women abusing substances into the third trimester of pregnancy, including ethanol (13%), cannabis (9.3%), cocaine (10%), and heroin (1%) (Chan, Klein, & Koren, 2003). Preterm birth rates of more than 16% have been found among women addicted to drugs compared with less than 10% among pregnant women who did not use drugs. Perinatal mortality rates as well as infant mortality rates were also much higher among women who used drugs during pregnancy (Dew, Guillory, Okah, Cai, & Hoff, 2006).

Such disorders affect the maternal child bond well beyond delivery as these impairments negatively impact physical caretaking of infants as well as the emotional quality of maternal–child interaction and can lead to long-term attachment difficulties. The damaging outcomes of unchecked maternal–child bond disruptions and their associated negative affective and behavioral outcomes are covered elsewhere in this text.

As substance abuse often co-occurs with depression and other affective disorders (Connors et al., 2006), this strong association again suggests the need for early evaluation specifically targeted for substance abuse in consideration of mental and physical health treatment planning throughout the pregnancy and postpartum. One tool that has been used in perinatal populations with good statistical validity and reliability is the DAST (Gavin, Ross, & Skinner, 1989; Svikis & Reid-Quinones, 2003).

Smoking

It is estimated that more than 30% of American women of childbearing age smoke cigarettes (Kuczkowski, 2005), and that preterm delivery of infants (up to 15%) and low birthweight (up to 30%) have been associated with smoking (Dew et al., 2006). In addition to the established health consequences to the mother and pregnancy, nicotine dependence has also been associated with depressive and affective disorders (Haas, Munoz, Humfleet, Reus, & Hall, 2004). While many new mothers may attempt to quit smoking upon discovery of pregnancy (Solomon et al., 2007), there is evidence that cessation of smoking itself can exacerbate an underlying mood disorder or relapse of previous depression (Haas et al., 2004).

Solomon et al. (2007) also found that women who stopped smoking prior to becoming pregnant had better long-term cessation outcomes than women who quit abruptly upon discovery of pregnancy. Depressed affect was one important factor found to increase the likelihood of smoking resumption in the postpartum among women who had quit upon learning of their pregnancy.

These studies again indicate the need for more proactive identification and treatment of mothers in three groups: those who smoke while pregnant (in order to prevent or reduce birth complications or preterm delivery and low birthweight), those who attempt smoking cessation at pregnancy and who may therefore be more susceptible to an affective episode or relapse, and those who are at high risk for smoking relapse postpartum, a health issue for both mother and the child who is then subjected to secondary exposure.

Eating Disorders

The incidence of women with eating disorders may peak during the childbearing years (Cohen, 2003) and has been identified in the perinatal period in ranges from 10%–12% (Franko et al., 2001). These reports seem reflective of statistics suggesting that from 10%–20% of women of childbearing age struggle with eating disorders, with the incidence among 18- to 24-year-olds double that of all other age groups (National Survey on Drug Use and Health, 2005). Reports evaluating the effects of eating disorders (anorexia nervosa or bulimia nervosa) on pregnancy complications have included failure to gain weight during pregnancy, hyperemesis gravidarum, higher incidence of miscarriage, cesarean section, and rates of depression approaching 34% (Franko et al. 2001; Franko & Spurrel, 2000; Morgan, Hubert, & Chung, 2006).

In addition, there are strong associations between maternal eating disorders and childhood feeding problems, as well as the possibility of a cross-generational component to the illness's transmission when such disorders escape detection and treatment (Cooper, Whelan, Woolgar, Morrell, & Murray, 2004). Of further interest were the findings that suggested specific kinds of obstetrical complications may be indicated in the etiology of eating disorders (Favaro, Tenconi, & Santonastaso, 2006).

While some studies have found a reduction in eating disorder symptoms during pregnancy, (Mazzeo et al., 2006), one study reported resumption of symptoms of bulimia nervosa by 9 months postpartum and anorexia nervosa symptoms at 6 months postpartum (Blais, 2000). As both illnesses are associated with higher rates of depression, this pattern appears to indicate the need for both early assessment and continuing evaluation well into the postpartum.

The identification of eating disorders can be difficult, but the introduction of the Eating Disorders Examination, an instrument of high reliability and validity (Peterson et al., 2007) at the prenatal interview may help identify the presence of the illness despite the client secrecy often associated with such disorders (Mitchell-Gieleghem, Mittelstaedt, & Bulik, 2002). Motivation to protect the unborn child, fear of obstetric complication and infertility bring some women to acknowledgment of their eating disorder. Others may pursue treatment for eating disorders upon consideration or discovery of pregnancy (Morgan et al., 2006), offering a therapeutic opportunity for remediation.

Personality Disorders

Screening for personality disorders during the prenatal interview is not common. Yet some findings suggest that including screening for personality disorders would additionally help identify women who might be at higher risk for depression (Denollet, Pop, Van Heck, Van Son, & Verkerk, 2005). The interpersonal problems often associated with personality disorders are of important clinical focus, as they may exacerbate symptoms of depression and anxiety on axis I; and anger, suicidality, or impulsive behavior on axis II (Morse & Pilkonis, 2007). In a recent study, women with avoidant, dependent, and obsessive-compulsive personality disorders experienced higher rates of new onset major depression in the postpartum period (Akman, Uguz, & Kaya, 2007). In addition, the risky behaviors, labile emotional states, and cognitive misinterpretations associated with borderline personality disorder can also be implicated in the etiology of depressive illness (Gratz & Gunderson, 2005). While response to medication can help reduce affective symptoms resulting from patterns of dysfunctional or impulsive behavior, without identification of the condition and responsive behavioral interventions, such disorders are likely to become chronic, resulting in repeated affective relapse.

Suicidality among depressed populations suffering from a comorbid personality disorder is another evaluative consideration for the prenatal assessment visit, yet presence of suicidality has been another excluding criteria in treatment studies for perinatal populations. One study (Lindhal, Pearson, & Colpe, 2005) found that while attempts and successful suicides are less frequent during pregnancy than in the general population of women, when death during the perinatal period does occur, suicide accounts for up to 20% of postpartum deaths. But the percentages of perinatal women who consider suicide or self-harm among those who are depressed have not been evaluated and remain unknown. The well-established association of depression co-occurring with personality disorders lends additional emphasis to the importance of early detection and responsive treatment.

Maternal interactions with children can suffer when patterns of thinking, reacting, and interacting are disrupted by cognitive distortions. For example, it has been found that maternal misinterpretations of infant eye contact avoidance can lead to erroneous conclusions of infant rejection, furthering possible withdrawal by the mother who feels her love is unreturned (Reck et al., 2004). Other damaging affects of perceptive disturbances in the maternal–child bond are covered elsewhere in this text and remain of primary concern.

Several themes emerge upon consideration of the preceding overview of the incidence and course of several perinatal comorbid conditions. First, they commonly co-occur with perinatal depression and can subvert treatment gains if not specifically addressed. Second, early detection and treatment in the prenatal or antennal period offers the greatest degree of protection from birth complications and negative maternal child outcomes and the best opportunity for retention of treatment gains. Third, pregnancy often motivates mothers contemplating pregnancy or who are pregnant to consider therapeutic intervention to long-standing issues, offering clinicians a window of opportunity to engage them in responsive treatments.

One model of care, which has been uniquely responsive to these conclusions, is the Day Hospital (Howard et al., 2006). The first of its kind in the country, The Day Hospital comprehensively evaluates, offers and/or arranges treatment for pregnant and postpartum women specific to their clinical presentations. After 5 years in existence, the model has presented encouraging results, receives community support from several stakeholders, and offers a realized vision of optimal care during the perinatal period. The didactic portion of the program includes many components of the model described below, which could work well in the context of centers offering comprehensive services to women across diagnostic ranges.

DIALECTICAL BEHAVIOR THERAPY

Dialectical Behavior Therapy may be an effective treatment choice when considering resources for the perinatal client with comorbid disorders as the model has been successfully applied to multiaxial presentations in nonprimiparious women. Its suggested method of prioritizing treatment targets according to those affecting life, interference with therapy and quality of life, (Linehan, 1993b), helps guide the clinical focus of complex cases while offering ongoing consultative support responsive to the heightened clinical effort required in management of such cases.

In addition, DBT includes many therapeutic features of models shown to be effective in the treatment of postpartum depression, such as task-oriented focus, psychoeducation, interpersonal skills, and efficacy in both group and individual formats. Uniquely emphasized in the model and of additional response to perinatal biopsychosocial issues may be DBT's nonshaming dialectic approach, therapist access via telephone support (which removes barriers of child care and transportation), and the health care provider collaboration integral to its delivery—a crucial treatment component during the perinatal period (Huysman, 2003).

DBT's underlying biosocial theory—that biology and environment are co-conspirators that can overwhelm coping systems in vulnerable individuals when perceived or actual invalidation produces sufficient tension (Dennis, 2004)—appears to offer unique alignment with the presumed etiology of postpartum mood and anxiety disorders (Glover & Kammerer, 2004; Miller, 1999; Parry, Piontek, & Wisner, 2002) as well as in the etiology of disorders associated with trauma (Van der Kolk, McFarlane, & Weisaeth, 1996) In addition, by encouraging client recovery responsibility, but not self-blame, the barrier of shame and society stigma so often noted in postpartum women (Bennett & Indman, 2003) can be addressed and reduced. Described in the *New York Times* science section as one of the "most popular new psychotherapies in a generation" (Carey, 2004), Dialectical Behavior Therapy extends its cognitive behavioral roots to include dialectic thinking as a powerful support to the change process.

Originally developed by Marsha Linehan for treatment of borderline personality disorder, Dialectical Behavior Therapy (Linehan, 1993a) demonstrated success in reducing self-harm, inpatient days, and treatment attrition in outpatient settings for this population (Dimeff, Koerner, & Linehan, 2001). As borderline personality disorder often presents with comorbid depression, suicidality, and substance abuse (American Psychiatric Association, 2000), these early gains led to program modifications for other populations in which behavioral containment or skills deficits in management of life tasks were prominent associated deficits with equally encouraging results (Wisniewski & Kelly, 2003). Findings have suggested that DBT may be successfully adapted for other disorders (such as eating disorders and substance abuse) in which dysfunctional behaviors serve to regulate emotions (Dimeff et al., 2001) or where skills deficits impede recovery.

In two full model studies for women with BPD comorbid with substance abuse referred to in Scheel (2000), reduction of substance abuse was superior to TAU (treatment as usual) in the first study and resulted in a lower percentage of opiate positive UAs in the second (Linehan, Schmidt, Dimeff, Craft, Kanter, & Comtois, 1999; Linehan, Dimeff, Reynolds, Comtois, Shaw, Welch, Heagerty & Kivlahan, 2002).

In another pre- and post test study of women diagnosed with binge eating disorder (Telch, Agras, & Linehan, 2001), participants attended the DBT skills group only but still achieved significant decreases in binge days and binge episodes that were maintained 6 months after treatment. Another study (Palmer et al., 2003), implemented an 18 month full DBT outpatient program for seven young women with a comorbid eating disorder and borderline personality disorder. At follow up, most patients were neither eating disordered nor self harming.

In an article considering adaptations of DBT for BPD or suicidal behavior, Robins and Chapman (2004) noted a study (Turner, 2000) that compared DBT to client-centered therapy in a community mental health setting over a period of 1 year for 24 clients. In this setting, the DBT skills training was incorporated into individual therapy in one group, but not the other. Results showed improvement in both groups, yet participants in the DBT-oriented individual therapy demonstrated greater improvement on variables such as reduction of suicide attempts, suicidal ideation, self-harm, anger, depression, impulsivity, and global mental health.

To practitioners utilizing cognitive behavior therapy in the treatment of emotion regulation disorders, DBT's attention to dichotomous thinking, assignment of client specific homework, and acknowledgment that analysis of deeply held schema cannot occur until skills acquisition takes place and a therapeutic relationship develops (Beck, Freeman, & Davis, 2004) seem to offer a natural theoretical extension. Levendusky (2000) notes that DBT may be the first cognitive behavioral therapy approach that is designed to treat complex and multifaceted clinical conditions.

And, current research in trauma that traces both the etiology of profound regulatory disorders and explains their impact on client's ability to correctly perceive and respond to environmental stimulants (Van der Kolk et al., 1996) also offers theoretical and practical support to the model by offering biological evidence (i.e., limbic system abnormalities found in brain images of clients suffering from PTSD) supporting DBT's mandate to first bolster client ability to manage increased arousal before initiating trauma-focused treatment (Becker & Zayfert, 2001).

Offering a full frontal attack on the constellation of symptoms associated with the dysregulatory process, Dialectical Behavior Therapy includes methods to alter client perceptions of precipitating events (dialectics), methods to dissipate a threatened escalation before chemical changes reinforce the intensity of the response or tolerate present affect (skills), and ways to empower clients to build skills outside the office (coaching calls, homework, focus on skills generalization). Finally methods to sustain and support the highly interactive therapist involvement are also a crucial model component (consultation team).

Dialectic Behavior Therapy appears to be imbued with principles ethically responsive to mental health treatment, including the need for practitioners to educate (skills training), advocate (insistence that change is possible), and intervene (active therapist involvement). Its dialectic view helps deepen clinicians' respect for the life that came before the current intervention and for client ingenuity in designing methods of survival. While validating the suffering that led to previous behavioral choices, DBT respectfully submits new options, helps clients locate and apply their own skills sets, offers new skills sets, and, most important, offers a new way of thinking about self and situations that can reduce anxiety and enhance problem solving.

Levendusky (2000) notes that DBT may be the first cognitive behavioral therapy approach designed to treat complex and multifaceted clinical conditions that may factor strongly in current global attempts to incorporate the model across treatment populations for which it was not originally designed. As clinicians struggle with limited treatment resources for complex cases with which they are increasingly charged, DBT is considered more and more as it appears to address and respond to the therapeutic dialectic that both acknowledges the etiology of emotion dysregulation disorders as biological—thereby removing client blame—while insisting that "patients may not have caused all of their own problems, but they have to solve them anyway" (Linehan, 1993a, p. 107). DBT's perspective that clients cannot fail, only treatment can, places the focus on therapist competency as well as client commitment. Its carefully measured and targeted treatment planning lends well to evaluative research and client reinforcement of progress.

The emerging data warrant consideration of DBT's inclusion for a variety of treatment populations when its guiding principles can be responsibly operationalized. Scheel (2000), after analysis of outcome studies offering full or partial model modifications, suggests that "if any partial incorporation of DBT concepts is made, adopting the empathic client conceptualization of DBT and providing therapist support would seem to be among those aspects that most safely and profitably could occur outside the standard DBT model" (p. 83).

While substantiation of DBT's application to the perinatal population is limited in this chapter to theory and case studies in group and individual settings, DBT's value as an effective model for treatment of multiaxial diagnoses has been well substantiated (Dimeff et al., 2001).

Following is a brief overview of DBT's components and tools (Stone, 2006). A thorough explanation of the model may be found in Linehan's text, *Cognitive Behavioral Treatment of Borderline Personality Disorder* (1993a) and the accompanying skills book *Skills Training Manual for Treating Borderline Personality Disorder* (1993b). DBT's cognitive behavioral rootedness may necessitate further formal study if there has not been prior clinical experience with CBT.

The DBT Skills Training Group delivers the didactic program components and meets weekly for up to 2 hours, gaining its structure and direction from the text's companion skills training manual. Modules include Core Mindfulness, Emotion Regulation, Interpersonal Effectiveness, and Distress Tolerance. This is not a psychotherapy group, but a forum for discussion of attempted skills generalization outside the group, continuously rewarding and reinforcing new behaviors through group acknowledgment. As the perinatal period may be one of imposed isolation for many women, the social support of the group format component may offer additional therapeutic benefits as peer support has been found to be of significant assistance in recovery from postpartum depression (Dennis, 2003).

Individual DBT Therapy supplements skills group training by offering personal attention to treatment goals (prioritized by those affecting life of mother and baby in this instance), therapy and quality of life, selection of target behaviors, and discussion of therapy-interfering behaviors. Individual comorbid presentations are addressed in this setting with focus on decreasing behaviors leading to interpersonal challenges, identifying behavioral precipitants, and increasing opportunities, activities and behaviors supportive of the change process, interpersonal effectiveness, and self respect.

Core Mindfulness introduces the dialectic thinking resulting in Wise Mind, in which practical and emotional needs negotiate a satisfactory solution to a problem. The dialectic view validates the emotional discomfort of changing behaviors while offering clear consequences to avoidance. The introduction of perspective that clients have choices and can even control their responses to environmental or internal stimulus is often a novel revelation for those who have felt helpless to control impulses. It offers new and often exhausted mothers an empowering option while attempting to skillfully manage the often overwhelming and multiple demands of motherhood.

Emotion Regulation offers skills to decrease suffering, reduce vulnerability, and understand emotional interplay with environment (Linehan, 1993b). Focus is on the value of client ability to independently return to and sustain emotional baseline prior to making behavioral choice or cognitive conclusions.

Interpersonal Effectiveness proposes methods of negotiating with self, situations, and others, challenging clients to tolerate the discomfort of difficult transactions while maintaining the self-respect of Wise Mind. A hierarchy for determining the value of keeping relationships and self-respect while achieving situational objectives is presented. The model focuses on current relational difficulties and includes role playing and formation of interpersonal boundaries where indicated.

Distress Tolerance helps clients develop an individualized "DBT toolbox" of skills, which may be resourced during emotional emergencies. Through personal experimentation and homework, clients develop immediate resources for the management of their emotions. They are taught that engagement in multisensory activities—those engaging sight, smell, taste, sound, and touch—can increase effectiveness of distractions meant to reduce emotional escalation.

Coaching Calls assists with skills generalization and offers additional therapist–client support between sessions. The call's purpose is to review the current issue, identify applicable skills, and construct a containment plan. In this way, therapist attention rewards attempts at adaptive behaviors, while discouraging the association between destructive behaviors and therapist response (Ben-Porath, 2004). It is easy to imagine the usefulness of this therapeutic resource in treatment of perinatal populations as it offers additional access to support when attempting skills generalization without the barriers of transportation or child care issues. Rarely abused when appropriately presented, the availability of this option is often of great reassurance in helping to elicit feelings of connectedness to the therapist and shoring up support for the change process.

ADAPTING DBT FOR POSTPARTUM DEPRESSION

Full implementation of DBT exacts a high commitment from clients and therapists alike, but it is currently often selected for multiaxial presentations. For the perinatal participant, it may be possible to integrate skills training with supportive individual therapy or introduce a homogenous group of postpartum women to DBT group skills training. Moderate stabilization of mood, absence of *active* suicidality and psychosis are important evaluative considerations prior to client initiation of DBT. Including the pediatrician, obstetrician, and other associated caregivers as part of the referent recovery team is crucial as observed interactions with the health care team provide useful feedback of client progress while helping to sustain theoretical treatment consistency. The pervasive philosophy embracing nonblaming dialectical perspective helps reduce client shame and often results in significant rates of client retention. One study that sought to evaluate the contributions of individual program components found that clients who perceived their DBT treatment to have been of value most emphasized the importance of the working client/therapist relationship, citing the nonjudgmental and validating qualities of their therapist as helping to create the environment for change (Araminta, 2000; Cunningham, Wolbert, & Lillie, 2004).

While attempts to analyze the efficacy of partialized DBT yield inconsistent results when modularized, more consistent findings emerge when key philosophies are implemented across treatment contexts. Scheel (2000) suggests that consideration of partialized DBT must include the responsible integration of its guiding principles and philosophy. And, Linehan (2000b) notes that the emphasis on balance and change can take many forms, limited perhaps only by the ingenuity and creativity of the therapeutic community.

CASE STUDY: INTRODUCTION OF DBT SKILLS IN A SUPPORT GROUP FOR POSTPARTUM DEPRESSION

The setting for this postpartum psychotherapy group of eight women was the outpatient program of a large regional hospital. The group was facilitated by a clinical social worker intensively trained in Dialectical Behavior Therapy and a member of a hospital-based interdisciplinary DBT consultation team. This group of eight women, five of whom were also treated with medication, met 90 minutes weekly and ranged from

6 weeks to 5 months postpartum. All eight women were receiving concurrent individual therapy on alternate weeks or PRN. Average session size was six women. Seven group members had been diagnosed with PPD; co-occurring disorders noted among five included bulimia, substance abuse (cannabis), and borderline personality disorder. After an overview of Dialectical Behavior Therapy, group members were asked for commitment to the demands of homework, diary cards, and consistent attendance. Consensus was unanimous and the dialectic nonblaming biosocial theory well appreciated.

Issues unique to the perinatal period included "finding myself again," "who am I now," and practical issues of parenthood requiring task-specific solutions such as time management, self-care, emotion regulation, remediation of dysfunctional family transactions, decision making, marital issues, assertiveness building, boundary setting, and reduction of shame and negative self-concepts. In addition, group members expressed a renewed motivation to confront long-standing dysregulatory and behavioral disorders in order to more effectively parent their child. Finally, the opportunity to relate their individual birth story to a compassionate group of peers was also a validating exercise in helping to achieve group cohesion and feelings of social support.

Individual sessions offered opportunities to designate and prioritize target behaviors unique to each participant's recovery plan. For example, the client recovering from cannabis abuse and bulimia focused on avoidance of cannabis, after identifying it as a precipitant to exacerbation of her bulimia and her affective recovery from depression. The client diagnosed with borderline personality disorder focused on reduction of impulsive responses, which brought regret and provoked suicidal ideation. The client consistently resourced distress tolerance skills, mindfulness, observation, and the empowering idea that she could *choose* not to respond to challenging situations until emotional baseline had been restored.

After 2 months, group members were able to begin sharing examples of skills application, which served as continuous group motivation. Each participant was encouraged to develop an individualized "toolbox" of DBT skills for distress tolerance, which usually included some skills and behaviors from all four DBT modules. These skills were resourced during client attempts to reduce or increase targeted behaviors.

Additional factors reported to be supportive of the DBT perspective included the nonjudgmental acceptance of group members, the consistency of the treatment, the quantity of the treatment (2 hours per week, including individual sessions and occasional coaching calls), the appeal of the treatment, and the psychoeducational component that helped postpartum women understand the complex interplay among the biological, psychological, and social stressors associated with the perinatal period. Clearly directed homework specifically tailored to accomplishment of new tasks and remediation of long-standing individual behavioral issues was also reported as highly supportive of treatment engagement.

The individual sessions and specifically the use of the diary card—a method for identifying and quantifying emotional and behavioral response—was described as highly useful. During the early weeks of recovery when gains seemed subtle or lacking, clients were able to compare weekly diary cards and notice improvements in mood and emotions from week to week.

The group continued to meet for several months with six members attending for 10 months. One moved out of the area and the eighth developed psychosis and was briefly hospitalized. The six who remained in treatment for the 10-month duration all reported substantial relief of symptoms. Three voluntarily maintained contact after discharge, reporting maintenance of skills and treatment gains at 4, 5, and 9 months posttreatment, respectively.

SUMMARY

The association of affective disorders with comorbid presentations in the perinatal period is well established. Common co-occurring disorders may include substance abuse, eating disorders, personality disorders, suicidality, and emotion dysregulation or skills deficits. In addition, the significant percentages of women experiencing antenatal depression may also be signaling the presence of subclinical or previously unaddressed disorders whose presence remained undiagnosed until the biopsychosocial stressors associated with pregnancy and motherhood exacerbated their presentation. There is substantial opportunity within the perinatal period to leverage the high motivation observed in many anticipating and expectant new mothers for treatment engagement. The possibility that therapeutic intervention could reduce or prevent generational passage of destructive behavioral patterns also offers inducement. Optimally, such interventions must be initiated prenatally or antenatally, extend well into the postpartum, and comprehensively offer specifically targeted focus for all clinical presentations.

Dialectic Behavior Therapy is a client-empowering form of treatment, which seeks to foster acceptance balanced with change and enhances the cognitive behavioral association of extensive empirical validation. Its Biosocial theory is uniquely compatible with the biopsychosocial factors thought to fuel perinatal spectrum disorders. Its efficacy as a treatment response to multiaxial presentations is strongly supported by research. DBT's modular multilayered approach allows concurrent targeting of Axis I and attendant Axis II diagnoses. DBT's nonblaming perspective helps reduce client shame, often a latent but profound barrier to successful treatment in this population, thereby increasing potential for the strong therapeutic alliance needed to affect change. Client retention for DBT participants tends to be high, and the model offers psychoeducation, didactic skills focus, and rigorous generalization of newly learned skills to environment.

While further studies of DBT's application to this population are encouraged to substantiate suggested theory, the model has been extensively validated as an efficacious treatment for multiaxial presentations (Robins & Chapman, 2004), including many of those outlined in this chapter. The reality of co-occurring disorders presenting during the perinatal period mandates specific attention and DBT attends to this process with a validating perspective, which could offer further encouragement to mothers contemplating treatment.

Dialectical Behavior Therapy could be an important component of a prenatal primary prevention program for women at high risk, as it offers a comprehensive response to the profound and inevitable biopsychosocial challenges accompanying motherhood. DBT's proposed length of treatment (1 year) may seem daunting but is responsive to findings that optimal perinatal treatment outcomes are more likely when interventions are introduced prenatally or antenatally and continued well into the postpartum period.

While the high level of commitment from therapist and client alike needed to optimize the model effectiveness may seem challenging, DBT's potential within this population to promote and sustain affective and behavioral recovery—as compared to the risks of no treatment or undertreatment—warrant its serious consideration. The new mother's often-intensified treatment motivation—fueled by her desire to more effectively parent her infant—will find ample opportunity within the DBT framework to repair many long-standing affective and behavioral issues. By helping women target the full spectrum of presenting conditions in the perinatal period and encouraging their early engagement in treatments powerfully responsive to all identified conditions, clinicians could increase positive outcomes, maternal empowerment, and optimal health for society's most critical dyad.

REFERENCES

Ahokas, A., Kaukoranta, J., Wahlbeck, K., & Aito, M. (2001). Estrogen deficiency in severe postpartum depression: Successful treatment with sublingual physiologic 17β-estradiol: A preliminary study. *Journal of Clinical Psychiatry, 62,* 332–336.

Akman, C., Uguz, F., & Kaya, N. (2007). Postpartum onset major depression is associated with personality disorders. *Comprehensive Psychiatry, 48,* 343–347.

American Psychiatric Association. (2000). *Diagnostic and statistical manual of mental disorders* (4h ed.). *Text Revision.* Washington, DC: Author.

Araminta, T. (2000). *Dialectical behavior therapy: A qualitative study of therapist and client experience.* Unpublished doctoral dissertation, California School of Professional Psychology, San Diego. (UMI No. 9958971)

Battle, C., Zlotnick, C., Miller, I. W., Pearlstein, T., & Howard, M. (2006). Clinical characteristics of perinatal psychiatric patients: A chart review study. *The Journal of Nervous and Mental Disorders, 194,* 369–377.

Beck, A. T., Freeman, A., & Davis, D. D. (2004). *Cognitive therapy of personality disorders.* New York: Guilford.

Becker, C. B., & Zayfert, C. (2001). Integrating DBT-based techniques and concepts to facilitate exposure treatment for PTSD. *Cognitive & Behavioral Practice, 8,* 107–122.

Bennett, S. S., & Indman, P. (2003). *Beyond the blues: A guide to understanding and treating prenatal and postpartum depression.* San Jose, CA: Moodswings Press.

Ben-Porath, D. D. (2004). Intersession telephone contact with individuals diagnosed with borderline personality disorder: Lessons from dialectical behavior therapy. *Cognitive & Behavioral Practice, 11,* 222–230.

Blais, M. A., Becker, A. E., Burwell, R. A., Flores, A. T., Nussbaum, K. M., Greenwood, D. N., Ekeblad, E. R., & Herzog, D. B. (2000). Pregnancy: Outcome and impact on symtomatology in a cohort of eating-disordered women. *International Journal of Eating Disorders, 27,* 140–149.

Carey, B. (2004, July 13). With toughness and caring, a novel therapy helps tortured souls. *The New York Times,* p. F1.

Center for Substance Abuse Treatment. (2007). *Understanding evidence-based practices for co-occurring disorders.* COCE Overview Paper 5. [DHHS Publication No. (SMA) 0704278]. Rockville, MD: Author.

Chan, D., Klein, J., & Koren, G. (2003). New methods for neonatal drug screening. *Neoreviews, 4,* e236.

Chang, G., McNamara, T. K., Wilkins-Haug, L., & Orav, E. J. (2007). Estimates of prenatal abstinence from alcohol: A matter of perspective. *Addictive Behaviors, 32,* 1593–1601.

Chang, G., Wilkins-Haug, L., Berman, S., Goetz, M. A., Behr, H., & Hiley, A. (1998). Alcohol use and pregnancy: Improving identification. *Obstetrics and Gynecology, 91,* 892–898.

Cohen, L. S. (2003). Eating Disorders. *OB-GYN News, 38,* 18.

Conners, N. A., Grant, A., Crone, C. C., & Whiteside-Mansell, L. (2006). Substance abuse treatment for mothers: Treatment outcomes and the impact of length of stay. *Journal of Substance Abuse Treatment, 31,* 447–456.

Cooper, P. J., Whelan, E., Woolgar, M., Morrell, J., & Murray, L. (2004). Association between childhood feeding problems and maternal eating disorder: Role of the family environment. *The British Journal of Psychiatry, 184,* 210–215.

Cunningham, K., Wolbert, R., & Lillie, B. (2004). It's about me solving my problems. *Cognitive & Behavioral Practice, 11,* 248–256.

Dennis, C. E. (2003). The effect of peer support on postpartum depression: A pilot random controlled trial. *Canadian Journal of Psychiatry, 48,* 115–124.

Dennis, C. E. (2004). Treatment of postpartum depression, part 2: A critical review of nonbiological interventions. *Journal of Clinical Psychiatry, 65,* 1252–1265.

Denollet, J., Pop, V., Van Heck, G. L., Van Son, M., & Verkerk, G. (2005). Personality factors as determinants of depression in postpartum women: A prospective 1 year follow-up study. *Psychosomatic Medicine, 67,* 632–637.

Derauf, C., LaGasse, L., Smith, L. M., Grant, P., Shah, R., Arria, A., Huestis, M., Haning, W., Strauss, A., Della Grotta, S., Liu, J., & Lester, B. M. (2007). Demographic and psychosocial characteristics of mothers using methamphetamine during pregnancy: Preliminary results of the infant development, environment and lifestyle study. *The American Journal of Drug and Alcohol Abuse, 3,* 281–289.

Dew, P. C., Guillory, V. J., Okah, F. A., Cai, J., & Hoff, G. L. (2006). The effect of health compromising behaviors on preterm births. *Maternal Child Health, 11,* 227–233.

Dimeff, L., Koerner, K., & Linehan, M. M. (2001). *Summary of research findings in DBT.* Retrieved October 2006, from www.behavioraltech.org

Favaro, A., Tenconi, E., & Santonastaso, P. (2006). Perinatal factors and the risk of developing anorexia nervosa and bulimia nervosa. *Archives of General Psychiatry, 63,* 82–88.

Franko, D. L., Blais, M. A., Becker, A. E., Delinsky, S. S., Greenwood, D. N., Flores, A. T., Ekeblad, E. R., Eddy, K. T., & Herzog, D. B. (2001). Pregnancy complications and neonatal outcomes in women with eating disorders. *American Journal of Psychiatry, 158,* 1461–1466.

Franko, D. L., & Spurrel, E. B. (2000). Detection and management of eating disorders during pregnancy. *Obstetrics and Gynecology, 95,* 942–946.

Gavin, D. R., Ross, H. E., & Skinner, H. A. (1989). Diagnostic validity of the drug abuse screening test in the assessment of DSM-III drug disorders. *British Journal of Addiction, 84,* 301–307.

Glover, V., & Kammerer, M. (2004). The biology and pathophysiology of peripartum psychiatric disorders. *Primary Psychiatry, 11,* 37–41.

Gratz, K. L., & Gunderson, J. G. (2005). Preliminary data on an acceptance-based emotion regulation group intervention for deliberate self-harm among women with borderline personality disorder. *Behavior Therapy, 37,* 25–35.

Haas, A. L., Munoz, R. F., Humfleet, G. L., Reus, V. I., & Hall, S. M. (2004). Influences of mood, depression history, and treatment modality on outcomes in smoking cessation. *Journal of Consulting and Clinical Psychology, 72,* 563–570.

Hanusa, B. H., Perel, J. M., Sunder, K. R., & Wisner, K. L. (2004). Postpartum depression, recurrence versus discontinuation syndrome: Observations from a randomized controlled trial. *Journal of Clinical Psychiatry, 65,* 1266–1268.

Homish, G. G., Cornelius, J. R., Richardson, G. A., & Day, N. L. (2004). Antenatal risk factors associated with postpartum comorbid alcohol use and depressive symptomatology. *Alcoholism: Clinical & Experimental Research, 28*(8), 1242–1248.

Howard, M., Battle, C. L., Pearlstein, T., & Rosene-Montella, K. (2006). A psychiatric mother-baby hospital for pregnant and postpartum women. *Archives of Women's Mental Health, 9,* 213–218.

Huysman, A. M. (2003). *The postpartum effect.* New York: Seven Stories Press.

James, K. (1998). *The depressed mother* (pp. 23–25, 123–139). London: Cassell Wellington House.

Klier, C. M., Muzik, M., Rosenblum, K. L., & Lenz, G. (2001). Interpersonal psychotherapy adapted for the group setting in the treatment of postpartum depression. *Journal of Psychotherapy Practice and Research, 10,* 124–131.

Kopelman, R., & Stuart, S. (2005). Psychological treatments for postpartum depression. *Psychiatric Annals, 35,* 556–566.

Kuczkowski, K. M. (2005). Drug addiction in pregnancy and pregnancy outcome: A call for global solutions [Letter to the editor]. *Substance Use and Misuse, 40,* 1749–1750.

Levendusky, P. G. (2000). Dialectical behavior therapy; so far so soon. *Clinical Psychology: Science and Practice, 7,* N1.

Lindahl, V., Peterson, J. L., & Colpe, L. (2005). Prevalence of suicidality during pregnancy and the postpartum. *Archives of Women's Mental Health, 8,* 77–87.

Linehan, M. M. (1993a). *Cognitive behavioral treatment of borderline personality disorder.* New York: Guilford Press.

Linehan, M. M. (1993b). *Skills training manual for treating borderline personality disorder.* New York: Guilford Press.

Linehan, M. M. (2000a). The empirical basis of dialectical behavior therapy: Development of new treatments versus evaluation of existing treatments. *Clinical Psychology: Science and Practice, 7,* 113–119.

Linehan, M. M. (2000b). Commentary on innovations in dialectical behavior therapy. *Cognitive & Behavioral Practice, 7,* 478–481.

Mazzeo, S. E., Slof-Op't Landt, M. C. T., Jones, I., Mitchell, K., Kendler, K. S., Neale, M. C., Aggen, S. H., & Bulik, C. M. (2006). Associations among postpartum depression, eating disorders, and perfectionism in a population-based sample of adult women. *International Journal of Eating Disorders, 39,* 202–211.

McMahon, C., Barnett, B., Kowalenko, N., & Tennant, C. (2004). Psychological factors associated with persistent postnatal depression: Past and current relationships, defence styles and the mediating role of insecure attachment style. *Journal of Affective Disorders, 84,* 15–24.

Miller, L. J. (1999). *Postpartum mood disorders.* Washington, DC: American Psychiatric Press.

Misri, S., Reebye, P., Corral, M., & Milis, L. (2004). The use of paroxetine and cognitive behavior therapy in postpartum depression and anxiety: A randomized controlled trial. *Journal of Clinical Psychiatry, 65,* 1236–1341.

Mitchell-Gieleghem, A., Mittelstaedt, M. E., & Bulik, C. M. (2002). Eating disorders and childbearing: Concealment and consequences. *Birth, 29,* 182–191.

Morgan, J. F., Hubert, L. J., & Chung, E. (2006). Risk of postnatal depression, miscarriage and preterm birth in bulimia nervosa: Retrospective controlled study. *Psychosomatic Medicine, 68,* 487–492.

Morse, J. Q., & Pilkonis, P. A. (2007). Screening for personality disorders. *Journal of Personality Disorders, 21,* 179–198.

National Survey on Drug Use and Health. (2005). *National mental health anti-stigma campaign.* U.S. Department of Health and Human Services, Substance Abuse and Mental Health Services Administration. Retrieved August 2007, from http://whatadifference.samhsa.gov/docs/SAMHSA_CDC_Report.pdf

O'Hara, M. W., Gorman, L. L., Stuart, C., & Wenzel, A. (2000). Efficacy of interpersonal psychotherapy for postpartum depression. *Archives of General Psychiatry, 57,* 1039–1045.

Palmer, R. L., Birchall, H., Damani, S., Gatward, N., McGrain, L., & Parker, L. (2003). A dialectical behavior therapy program for people with an eating disorder and borderline personality disorder—description and outcome. *International Journal of Eating Disorders, 33,* 281–286.

Parry, B. L., Piontek, C. M., & Wisner, K. L. (2002). Postpartum depression. *New England Journal of Medicine, 347,* 194–199.

Peterson, C. B., Crosby, R. D., Wonderlich, S. A., Joiner, T., Scrow, S. J., Mitchell, J. E., Bardone-Cone, A. M., Klein, M., & Le Grange, D. (2007). Psychometric properties of the eating disorder examination questionnaire: Factor structuring and internal consistency. *International Journal of Eating Disorders, 40,* 386–389.

Reay, R., Fisher, Y., Robertson, M., Adams, E., & Owen, C. (2006). Group interpersonal psychotherapy for postnatal depression: A pilot study. *Archives of Women's Mental Health, 9,* 31–39.

Reck, C., Hunt, A., Fuchs, T., Weiss, R., Noon, A., Moehler, E., Downing, G., Tronick, E. Z., & Mundt, C. (2004). Interactive regulation of affect in postpartum depressed mothers and their infants: An overview. *Psychopathology, 37,* 272–280.

Robins, C. J., & Chapman, A. L. (2004). Dialectical behavior therapy: Current status, recent developments and future directions. *Journal of Personality Disorders, 18(1),* 73–89.

Scheel, K. R. (2000). The empirical basis of dialectical behavior therapy: Summary, critique, and implications. *Clinical Psychology: Science and Practice, 7,* N1.

Segre, L. S., Stuart, S., & O'Hara, M. (2004). Interpersonal psychotherapy for antenatal and postpartum depression. *Primary Psychiatry, 11,* 52–56.

Sokol, R. J., Martier, S. S., & Ager, J. W. (1989). The T-ACE questions: Practical prenatal detection of risk drinking. *American Journal of Obstetrics and Gynecology, 160,* 863–870.

Solomon, L. J., Higgins, S. T., Heil, S. H., Badger, G. J., Thomas, C. S., & Bernstein, I. M. (2007). Predictors of postpartum relapse to smoking. *Drug and Alcohol Dependence, 90,* 224–227.

Stone, S. D. (2006). Using dialectical behavior therapy in clinical practice. In T. Ronen & A. Freeman (Eds.), *Cognitive behavior therapy in clinical social work practice* (pp. 147–166). New York: Springer Publishing.

Svikis, D. S., & Reid-Quinones, K. (2003). Screening and prevention of alcohol and drug use disorders in women. *Obstetrics and Gynecology Clinics of North America, 30,* 447–468.

Telch, C. F., Agras, W. S., & Linehan, M. M. (2001). Dialectical behavior therapy for binge eating disorder. *Journal of Consulting and Clinical Psychology, 69,* 1061–1065.

Turner, R. M. (2000). Naturalistic evaluation of dialectical behavior therapy-oriented treatment for borderline personality disorder. *Cognitive and Behavioral Practice, 7,* 468–477.

U.S. Department of Health and Human Services. (1999). *Mental health: A report of the Surgeon General—executive summary.* Rockville, MD: Author.

Van der Kolk, B. A., McFarlane, A. C., & Weisaeth, L. (1996). *Traumatic stress: The effects of overwhelming experience on mind, body and society.* New York: Guilford.

Wisniewski, L., & Kelly, E. (2003). The application of dialectical behavior therapy to the treatment of eating disorders. *Cognitive & Behavioral Practice, 10,* 131–138.

15

Treating Antepartum Depression: Interpersonal Psychotherapy

MARGARET SPINELLI

ANTEPARTUM DEPRESSION

The fact that 10%–13% of pregnant women experience depression dispels the myth of unconditional well-being during gestation (Gotlib, Whiffen, & Mount, 1989; Kumar and Robson, 1984; O'Hara, Zekoski, Philipps, & Wright, 1990). In a recent prospective longitudinal cohort study of 14,000 antepartum women, 13.5% scored above threshold for probable depression on the Edinburgh Postnatal Depression Scale (EPDS) at 32 weeks of pregnancy compared to 9.1% at 8 weeks postpartum. The prevalence is even greater in indigent populations (Evans, Heron, Francomb, Oke, & Golding, 2001).

Women with a history of depression are particularly vulnerable to pregnancy-associated recurrence (Frank, Kupfer, Jacob, Blumenthal, & Jarrett, 1987). The gonadal hormones once thought to be protective during pregnancy may provoke uncertain mood effects (Frank et al., 1987).

Supported by an NIMH Research Scientist Development Award for Clinicians (grant number MH-01276). This chapter has been adapted from M. Spinelli and J. Endicott (2003). Controlled clinical trial of interpersonal psychotherapy versus parenting education program for depressed pregnant women. *American Journal of Psychiatry, 160*, 555–562, with permission from the *American Journal of Psychiatry*.

Risk factors for depression (Graff, Dyck, & Schallow, 1991; Wisner and Stowe, 1997) during pregnancy include personal or family history of mood disorder; stressors such as marital dysfunction (Dimitrovsky, Perez-Hishberg, & Itskowitz, 1986); and demographic variables such as young age, minimal education, increased number of children, and a history of child abuse (Farber, Herbert, & Reviere, 1996).

Emphasis on puerperal depression has focused on the postpartum period. Many postpartum depressed women recall the onset of depressive symptoms during pregnancy.

When Hobfoll and colleagues (1995) evaluated 192 financially impoverished inner-city single women at two intervals during pregnancy, they found rates of depression at 27.5% and 24.5%. Seguin, Potvin, St. Denis, & Jacinthe (1995) found that 47% of women of low socioeconomic status and 20% of women with higher socioeconomic status scored >10 on the Beck Depression Inventory (BDI). Chronic stressors, financial and housing problems, negative life events, and inadequate social supports were all linked to high depressive symptomatology during pregnancy. Furthermore, that one-half of pregnant depressed women will have a postpartum depression (PPD) emphasizes the importance of prevention and early identification of risk (Dimitrovsky et al., 1986). These risks emphasize pregnancy as a paramount time for identification, treatment, and prevention of infant and family morbidity.

Timely and appropriate treatment is vital in order to avoid depression-associated appetite and weight loss. Pregnant depressed women are more vulnerable to nicotine, drug, and alcohol abuse, and failure to obtain adequate prenatal care (Zuckerman, Bauchner, Parker, & Cabral, 1990)—all factors that compromise fetal development. Maternal stress and depression during pregnancy are associated with lower birthweight and gestational age (Wadhwa, Sandman, Porto, Dunkel-Schetter, & Garite, 1993), delivery by cesarean section, and infants admitted to the neonatal care unit (Chung, Lau, Alexander, Chiu, & Lee, 2001).

INTERPERSONAL PSYCHOTHERAPY (IPT)

Interpersonal psychotherapy (IPT) (Klerman, Weissman, Rounsaville, & Chevron, 1984) was adapted from the school of interpersonal psychiatry based on the theories of Harry Stack Sullivan (Elkin et al., 1989). Sullivan emphasized the importance of social roles as they relate to family, friends, and community. The interpersonal psychotherapist is interested in the following data (Klerman et al., 1984): (1) the patient's current and past relationships; (2) the pattern of relationships; (3) beliefs, expectations, and role; and (4) associated affect and interpersonal experience.

Klerman and colleagues developed interpersonal psychotherapy for depression in 1984. It was designed to address symptoms of depression and subsequent interpersonal conflicts. While interpersonal issues may not cause depression, they frequently occur in the context of depression. The focus of treatment is depression as a biological illness (Klerman et al., 1984).

IPT is a 12–16 week treatment with a fixed endpoint created to treat nonpsychotic major depression (Klerman et al., 1984). The goals of IPT include decreased neurovegetative symptoms of depression, as well as resolution of interpersonal conflicts. Although emphasis is on the present, treatment may utilize the past as it relates to the present.

In the NIMH Treatment of Depression Collaborative Research Program (Weissman, Rounsaville, & Chevron, 1982), IPT was shown to significantly reduce depressive symptoms and improve function.

Several clinical trials have demonstrated the efficacy of IPT in the treatment of major depression (Elkin et al., 1989), postpartum depression (O'Hara, Stuart, Gorman, & Wenzel, 2000), depressed adolescents (Mufson, Weissman, Moreau, & Garfinkel, 1999), and maintenance treatment (Sloane, Staples, & Schneider, 1985; Weissman et al., 1979) of major depression. Furthermore, increased scientific evidence of the benefits of psychotherapy for depressed subjects treated with IPT compared to controls is associated with brain and physiological changes (Brody et al., 2001). To date, there has been one controlled clinical trial of individual psychotherapy for the depressed pregnant woman. IPT is a noninvasive treatment of proven efficacy that should be available in this underserved population.

IPT is a problem-focused psychotherapy. Klerman et al. (1984) have identified four problem areas to work from with the IPT patient. Because of the unique and developmental problems associated with gestation, an additional problem area addresses issues unique to pregnancy that cannot be covered using the original IPT problem set (Klerman et al., 1984) of grief, interpersonal role dispute, role transition, and interpersonal deficits. The fifth broad area, complicated pregnancy, addresses problems specific to gestation such as undesired pregnancy, medical problems associated with pregnancy itself, obstetrical complications, multiple births, and congenital anomalies.

PREGNANCY

While the journey from nonmotherhood to motherhood is essentially the same for all, each woman approaches it through her own perceptions and her own social and psychological experiences. Pregnancy has been described as a period of emotional crisis (Benedek, 1959). In fact, it is addressed more appropriately as a developmental period in which the mother-to-be transitions from independence to motherhood. This process may stir feelings about other relationships or other losses (St. Andre, 1993). The woman has increased dependency needs, and paradoxically fears both the loss of her identity as well as impending separation from the infant. If the woman has a history of complications such as stillbirth or spontaneous abortion, she may fear loss of the infant by death or illness.

The unique hormonal environment of pregnancy has significant physiological and psychological sequelae. Pregnant women experience a range of emotions from elation to fear to ambivalence. In addition, the woman must adjust to her own altered body image as well as the reactions of those around her. Normal pregnancy results in the recognition of conflicts. The developmental and psychological tasks of the woman with a medically complicated pregnancy are cumbersome. Women with psychosocial stressors, poor support systems, and lower SES have a more difficult time with the transition to motherhood. A high-risk pregnancy may result from complications, which include maternal disorders, obstetric difficulties, or fetal compromise. These complications may contribute to an already existing anxiety and make this an even more stressful time (Carr, 1993).

DEPRESSION DURING PREGNANCY

Serious sequelae of maternal mental illness are increased rates of accidental injury, child abuse, neglect (Scott, 1992), and, more seriously, infanticide. Furthermore, maternal–fetal attachment may be explored during gestation in order to facilitate resolution of conflicts or ambivalence before delivery (Robinson & Stewart, 1993).

Although selective serotonin reuptake inhibitors and some other antidepressant medications have demonstrated relative safety during gestation (Alwan, Reefhuis, Rasmussen, Olney, & Friedman, 2007; Chambers et al., 2006; Louik, Lin, Werler, Hernandez, & Mitchell, 2007; Wisner et al., 2000), absolute safety cannot be ensured. The infant's developing brain continues to be vulnerable to adverse events. Data remain limited by unknown long-term effects and have not been extrapolated to premature infants, multiple births, or infants with other birth complications.

Moreover, some women may not want to ingest medication and prefer nonpharmacological treatments. A recent pilot study by Oren and colleagues (2002) suggested that light therapy is beneficial for the treatment of antepartum depression. To date, this interpersonal psychotherapy study is the only randomized controlled clinical trial we know of that suggests an efficacious treatment for antepartum depression (see chapter 3 "Effects of Maternal Postpartum Depression on the Infant and Older Siblings").

The efficacy of interpersonal psychotherapy has been demonstrated in the treatment of postpartum depression (O'Hara et al., 2000). Furthermore, more scientific evidence for the benefits of psychotherapy for depressed subjects treated with interpersonal psychotherapy, compared to control subjects, is associated with brain and physiological change (Brody et al., 2001).

Since therapeutic guidelines dictate the use of a least invasive effective treatment to protect mother and fetus, the risk/benefit evaluation is the appropriate method for intervention. Decision analysis guides appropriate management. The initial step in the decision process is to determine the risk of untreated illnesses during pregnancy and consider factors that compromise fetal development.

The next step in the process is consideration of *treatment risk* such as medication. Psychotherapy provides an opportunity to explore conflicts and develop coping patterns for the changes and developmental tasks of pregnancy (St. Andre, 1993).

The application of IPT-P to the specific problems and needs of women with antepartum depression is manualized (Spinelli & Endicott, 2003), using guidelines and modifications around the issues of pregnancy. Unlike the above treatments, IPT-P addresses psychosocial concerns and stressors of parturition. IPT-P is a principal method of delivering care, and a first-line measure in the hierarchy of treatment guidelines.

GUIDELINES FOR INTERPERSONAL PSYCHOTHERAPY

The goals of IPT include (1) decreased neurovegetative symptoms of depression, and (2) resolution of interpersonal conflicts. IPT does not presume an interpersonal etiology of depression, but highlights the possibility that depression occurs in an interpersonal context.

In addition to biological change, pregnant women have significant stressors, that is, changing roles in society and family, concerns over obstetric difficulties, and acceptance of the parental role. IPT-P is designed to enable the patient to cope with interpersonal problems associated with symptom onset.

Klerman et al. (1984) described that strategies of IPT-P are separated into three phases of treatment. The initial phase comprises collecting an interpersonal inventory, psychoeducation, and selection of focal areas for treatment. The medical model is used and depression discussed as a biological illness. The major issues associated with depression are identified. A contract is then made with the patient to focus treatment in the selected problem area.

In the intermediate phase, the work of IPT-P addresses the identification of one or two of five problem areas associated with depression. The work of IPT-P begins with emphasis on the patient's particular problem as it is associated with depression. In the termination phase, feelings about termination, progress, and remaining work are considered.

Phases of IPT-P Treatment

IPT has been adapted to treat patients with depressive symptoms that occur during pregnancy. The patient cannot be actively suicidal, psychotic, or be using alcohol or drugs. During the initial phase of treatment, depressive symptoms are noted and monitored weekly. Psychoeducation is begun and an interpersonal inventory is collected. Identifying a problem area and the focus of treatment will be the substance of the treatment contract with the patient.

During the initial phase of treatment (weeks 1 to 4) the tasks of the therapist as described by Klerman et al. (1984) include (1) diagnose the depression, (2) assess suitability for treatment and feasibility of coming to sessions with some flexibility around childbirth issues, (3) conduct an inventory of significant others to determine the interaction between the patient and significant others, and feelings about pregnancy and the infant, (4) identify principal problem areas, (5) explain the rationale for interpersonal therapy, (6) make a treatment contract with the patient, (7) explain the patient's role in the treatment, and (8) begin treating symptoms.

This middle phase of IPT-P is the active phase of therapy. It is during the middle phase that important issues are explained and strategies for working through problems are discussed. While the initial phase has focused on assessment by the therapist, the middle sessions now shift responsibility from the therapist to the patient. The patient is encouraged to give up her "sick role" (Klerman et al., 1984) to actively bring the focus of the therapy into the sessions, and to be open to exploration. The therapist has several tasks: (1) monitor symptoms, (2) encourage the patient to discuss issues relevant to the identified problem area, and (3) identify feelings associated with the problem.

The termination of treatment for the pregnant mother can be complicated. If she has given birth before termination, she is accompanied by her baby in the final sessions. The task of termination is accomplished in the last four sessions (Klerman et al., 1984) and should include (1) explicitly discussing the end of treatment, (2) acknowledging this as a time of potential grieving, and (3) movement toward the recognition of the woman's independent competence.

PROBLEM AREAS FOR TREATMENT

Grief: If the patient associates depression with the death or loss of a loved one, then grief becomes the focus of treatment. The loss may not have a temporal relationship to the depression. Grief may have been postponed or the lost one inadequately mourned.

Pregnancy as a Role Transition: Parenthood and especially the period of pregnancy and motherhood is among the most common and complete transformations in human experience (Trad, 1990). The woman's self-concept is reorganized as she adapts to her new role as mother. The process is completed with the psychological separation from the child.

Interpersonal Deficits: If the patient is socially impoverished with few, if any, lasting relationships and has a history of extreme social isolation, personality deficits must be considered as treatment focus (Klerman et al., 1984). The relationship with the therapist, rather than significant others, will become the model for interaction.

Interpersonal Role Dispute: Klerman et al. (1984) define a role dispute as one in which two people have conflicting expectations in their relationship. An example is the pregnant woman who expects to stop work after her child is born and become a full-time mother, but because of a change in her husband's earnings, she must resume work.

Complicated Pregnancy: Pregnancy can be complicated by concurrent life events, such as a serious illness, obstetrical difficulties, death of a loved one, or a previous perinatal loss. The pregnancy may have been undesired as the result of rape. Other complications may be successful conception after a period of infertility or multiple gestations.

THE EFFICACY OF IPT-P

The use of IPT for antepartum depression was shown to be effective in the first NIMH study of pregnant women using the model of IPT adapted to pregnancy. The application of interpersonal psychotherapy to the specific problems and needs of women with antepartum depression is outlined in a manual (Spinelli & Endicott, 2003).

We report the results of a controlled clinical treatment trial of interpersonal psychotherapy (IPT-P) versus a Parenting Education Didactic (PEP-P). During the IPT-P or PEP, the participants met for 45-minute weekly sessions with therapists. Interpersonal psychotherapy was administered over 16 weeks, according to the manual by Klerman et al. (1984). The therapy was modified to antepartum depression according to the interpersonal psychotherapy manual (Spinelli & Endicott, 2003).

The parenting education program is a systematic didactic control condition of therapist-led weekly educational sessions. Patients were assigned a therapist and seen weekly for 45-minute sessions to discuss their symptoms and functioning. Similar to the interpersonal psychotherapy treatment, the parenting education control condition lasted for 16 weeks. During parenting education program sessions, the therapist emphasizes the developmental stages of pregnancy, delivery, parenting, and early childhood.

The parenting education control condition permits weekly evaluation of the patient's mood and control for contact with a professional as well as the nonspecific effects of repeated evaluations. In addition, the weekly contact with a therapist provides an ethical and reliable way of evaluating the patient's mood.

We report the results of a randomized controlled clinical treatment trial on the efficacy of 16 weeks of interpersonal psychotherapy compared to a parenting education control program.

Aims of the Study

The study consisted of a large sample of Dominican women in our catchment area at the New York State Psychiatric Institute at the College of Physicians and Surgeons of Columbia University. The aims of this study were to determine the efficacy of interpersonal psychotherapy versus a parenting education program for unipolar depressed nonpsychotic pregnant women and to test the feasibility of a placebo-controlled bilingual clinical treatment trial in an ethnically and economically diverse population of pregnant depressed women.

To our knowledge, this interpersonal psychotherapy treatment trial had the following three unique characteristics: (1) the first controlled clinical trial of individual psychotherapy for antepartum depression, (2) the first interpersonal psychotherapy study with a matched systematic nontherapeutic control group to assess the therapeutic benefits of interpersonal psychotherapy, and (3) the first reported bilingual interpersonal psychotherapy treatment in a population of socioeconomically deprived women.

Method

Training in Interpersonal Psychotherapy and Parenting Education

Two experienced therapists (with an MD and a CSW) received 1 year of interpersonal psychotherapy supervision. The interpersonal psychotherapy training program was modeled after that used in the National Institute of Mental Health (NIMH) collaborative study of treatment of depression (Elkin et al. 1989). A five-day didactic program described the clinical strategies of interpersonal psychotherapy in addition to the physical, psychological, and developmental phases of pregnancy.

The supervisor met with the therapists and provided written instruction, books on pregnancy, the postpartum, and early childhood as well as videotapes and visual aids that addressed the developmental stages of pregnancy, childbirth, and early parenting. There were few limitations on the content of instruction as long as the focus remained didactic. The therapists tailored the parenting education program sessions to the gestational age of the study participants.

Patients

The majority of women in our study group were immigrants from the Dominican Republic with few support systems and low socioeconomic status. Several factors increased the odds of depression in our group. There are conflicting data on the prevalence of depression among Hispanic immigrants (Hobfoll et al., 1995; Seguin et al., 1995). The ethnicity of our group must be seen against the backdrop of other circumstances such as poverty, isolation, chaos, pregnancy, immigrant status, and absence of the baby's father and other support systems. Studies of pregnant and postpartum women (Zuckerman et al., 1990) have addressed these variables.

More than 200 prospective research participants were recruited to the Maternal Mental Health Program from our outpatient clinics at the New York State Psychiatric Institute of Columbia University College of Physicians and Surgeons as well as other institutions in the New York metropolitan area. Professionals, community outreach programs, and former patients referred them.

A majority of Latina patients came from the social workers and midwives at our prenatal clinic in the Department of Obstetrics and Gynecology. Other subjects were self-referred, having heard about the Maternal Mental Health Program from newspapers, magazines, and radio announcements.

Fifty pregnant depressed women entered the study. Twenty-five were randomly assigned to the experimental treatment interpersonal psychotherapy group and 25 to the parenting education control program by using a table of random numbers. Thirty-eight women, who completed at least one interpersonal psychotherapy or parenting education program session, were included in the data analysis. English- and Spanish-speaking, physically healthy pregnant women between 6 and 36 weeks' gestation and 18 and 45 years of age were included in the study. Of the Latina women, 80% were Spanish-speaking. Consent forms were bilingual. All women understood the study and gave written informed consent to participate. Diagnostic inclusion criteria were based on *DSM–IV* criteria for major depressive disorder and a Hamilton Depression Rating Scale score = 12. Only pregnant women with major depression entered the study.

Patients were excluded if they had abused drugs or alcohol in the past 6 months, were acute risks for suicide, or had comorbid axis I disorders or medical conditions likely to interfere with participation in the study. Patients currently taking antidepressant medication were also excluded from the study.

Assessments of Change

After a baseline psychiatric evaluation, the Structured Clinical Interview for *DSM–IV* Axis I Disorders (First, Spitzer, Gibbon, & Williams, 1996) was administered to determine the presence of major depressive disorder and to rule out comorbid axis I diagnosis (American Psychiatric Association, 1994). All assessments were translated and back-translated to Spanish. The Hamilton Depression Scale (Hamilton, 1960) was the principal clinician-rated outcome measure. Because the discomforts of pregnancy may mimic somatic symptoms of depression (Klein & Essex, 1994), the patients were asked to evaluate whether symptoms such as appetite and weight change were likely due to pregnancy or depression.

The Beck Depression Inventory (Beck, 1985) is a self-rated measure of depressive symptoms in both the general and puerperal (O'Hara, Schlechte, Lewis, & Wright, 1991) populations. The cognitive-affective cluster of symptoms is the most sensitive to "true" depression during pregnancy (Huffman, Lamour, Bryan, & Pederson, 1990). Because the removal of the somatic cluster does not reduce the value of the Beck Depression Inventory, the somatic cluster was eliminated. The self-rated Edinburgh Postnatal Depression Scale (Harris, Huckle, Thomas, Johns, & Fung, 1989) emphasizes behavioral changes with no emphasis on somatic changes. Although primarily designed for postpartum mood states, it has been used as a sensitive measure in pregnancy (Murray & Cox, 1990) and translated into Spanish (Cox & Holden, 1994). The Edinburgh Postnatal Depression Scale is the only self-report mood scale validated for use during pregnancy and the postpartum period (sensitivity = 86%, specificity = 78%).

The Clinical Global Impression (CGI) scale (Petkova, Quitkin, McGrath, Stewart, & Klein, 2000) provides measures of severity and improvement of depressive symptoms.

Weekly assessments of mood change were administered before interpersonal psychotherapy or parenting education program sessions in order to avoid treatment effects. A modified version of the Maudsley Mother Infant Interaction Scale (Kumar & Hipwell, 1996) was used to measure mother-infant interaction in the postpartum period. A history of child abuse was reported by 47.0% of the women, sexual abuse by 28.0%, physical abuse by 25.0%, and both of the latter for 5.6%, while 73.0% reported a past history of major depression.

Results

There were no significant differences between the groups regarding race, marital status, gravity, education, employment status, income, or history of depression. The mean age of the interpersonal psychotherapy group was 28.3 years ($SD = 5.7$), and the mean age of the parenting education program control group was 29.3 years ($SD = 7.11$). Women entered the study at 21.5 weeks ($SD = 8.3$).

The efficacy of the two treatments was determined by comparing scores on measures of depressive symptoms (the Hamilton Depression Scale, the Beck Depression Inventory, the Edinburgh Postnatal Depression Scale) by using intent-to-treat analysis and the last phase as outcome, with the last score carried forward. A repeated analysis of variance model was used to compare outcome scores of the two groups at termination. Recovery status of the two groups was compared by using contingency-table chi-square tests and defined as a CGI score of 1 (very much improved) or 2 (much improved). Pearson's correlation coefficients were used to compare scores on the Maudsley Mother Infant Interaction Scale and the Hamilton Depression Scale. All statistical tests were two-tailed and used an alpha level of .05.

Interpersonal psychotherapy demonstrated significant advantage over parenting education for all mood scores, while both groups showed marked improvement over the course of treatment. The mood of the interpersonal psychotherapy treatment group improved significantly more than the parenting education program control group on scores on the Edinburgh Postnatal Depression Scale ($t = 2.99$, $df = 36$, $p = .005$).

The interpersonal psychotherapy treatment effect was significantly better than control effect on scores on the Hamilton Depression Scale ($t = 2.42$, $df = 36$, $p < .03$) and the Beck Depression Inventory ($t = 2.72$, $df = 31$, $p < .02$), respectively. The treatment group had a >50% improvement in mood symptoms on the Hamilton Depression Scale (52.4%) ($t = 8.85$, $df = 20$, $p = .001$) and the Beck Depression Inventory (52.4%) ($t = 5.35$, $df = 15$, $p = .001$), compared to the control subjects (29.4% and 23.5%; $t = 3.68$, $df = 16$, $p = .002$, and $t = 2.51$, $df = 16$, $p < .03$, respectively).

The difference in the recovery rate on the CGI was significant between the groups ($x^2 = 6.42$, $df = 1$, $p < .02$). The interpersonal psychotherapy group had a recovery rate of 60.0%, compared to the 15.4% rate of the parenting education control program.

There was a significant correlation ($r = .7$, $p < .05$) between the modified score (sum of five interactive items) on the Mother Infant Interaction Scale (Kumar & Hipwell, 1996) and the Hamilton Depression Scale in 11 patients at the first postpartum visit. The five interactive items of the Mother Infant Interaction Scale are (1) quality of emotional relationship with baby, (2) quality of interaction (i.e., responsiveness and sensitivity to baby by mother), (3) perceived risk to infant from mother, impulse, or rejection, (4) psychopathology incorporating baby, and (5) incident affecting baby.

DISCUSSION

Interpersonal psychotherapy resulted in a significant mood improvement relative to the parenting education program control condition based on all mood measures: the Hamilton Depression Scale, the Beck Depression Inventory, the Edinburgh Postnatal Depression Scale, and CGI symptom recovery. Most notable was the significant difference in the recovery rate between the treatment and control groups on the CGI.

The significance of the CGI recovery data is the absence of somatic symptoms. In addition, the clinician-derived measure has demonstrated minimum clinician bias, compared to outcome based on patient ratings (Petkova et al., 2000). A positive control effect on mood suggests that the control condition was therapeutic for some participants. Our Spanish-speaking therapist was uniquely sensitive to the cultural issues and language of this isolated group of young women, variables that likely contributed to a positive transference and therapeutic benefit. In addition, the control effects for our mood scales (the Edinburgh Postnatal Depression Scale: 11.8%, the Beck Depression Inventory: 23.5%, and the Hamilton Depression Scale = 29.4%) were similar to placebo responses in antidepressant medication studies (mean = 29.7%, *SD* = 8.3, range = 12.5–51.8) (Walsh, Seidman, Sysko, & Gould, 2002).

A central point of the study was the selection of a nontherapeutic systematized treatment control condition that enabled careful and sensitive detection of the benefits of interpersonal psychotherapy. Although interpersonal psychotherapy fared significantly better in some studies by use of a waiting-list control (Mufson et al., 1999), the specific benefit of psychotherapy remains undetermined because the condition did not permit examination or detection of the distinct efficacy of the interpersonal psychotherapy treatment itself. In contrast, the parenting education program controls for contact with a professional and duration of sessions as well as nonspecific effects of repeated evaluations, reassurance, and education (variables not controlled in the waiting-list control condition). Control for these measures and nonspecific therapeutic benefits enhanced our ability to assess the singular contribution of a focused interpersonal psychotherapy treatment and support our findings that the mood improvement in our group was attributable to the unique treatment effects of interpersonal psychotherapy.

The high attrition rate (32.0% for control subjects and 16.0% for treatment subjects) is attributed to several factors. First, three women left after delivery, and one left after a stillbirth. Second, child care and work demands were obstacles to care for sole-support mothers. The unpredictable nature of pregnancy and young motherhood demanded that the staff be sensitive to the unique needs of young and prospective mothers. Such complications as bed rest and delivery complications required flexible measures such as the use of telephone sessions and mechanisms for child care.

The study was composed of a predominantly fragile group of recent immigrants from the Dominican Republic. Homes were often transient and chaotic, with unpredictable and unstable support systems. For some, circumstances were even more tragic. Partners were involved in drug sales and street crime, and many were incarcerated. Two women left the study when they were reunited with incarcerated partners. Many women were lost to treatment and follow-up because of disconnected telephone numbers. In all the cases of women who were lost to follow-up, letters were sent with appropriate referrals. Our attrition rate suggests the need for more diligence in follow-up with mothers in less-permanent populations. An additional impediment to treatment may have been the duration of the treatment itself. Sixteen weeks required significant commitment and was a likely contributor to the attrition rate and our limited ability to collect postpartum information. Most interpersonal psychotherapy studies have successfully used treatment durations of 12 weeks (Mufson et al., 1999; O'Hara et al., 2000). Furthermore, mean depression scores improved by the seventh week of interpersonal psychotherapy and fluctuated slightly through week 12, indicating that a 12-week trial is probably sufficient.

One unexpected finding was the high incidence of reported child abuse (47.0%). Women with a history of childhood trauma are more likely to experience depression and suicidal ideation during pregnancy (Farber et al., 1996). Throughout normal pregnancy, the emotional attachment between mother and infant grows. The mother develops an elaborate internalized image of the fetus, a process conceptualized by Rubin (1984) as "binding in"; the fetus becomes part of the self. Consequently, the event of childbirth may exacerbate preexisting conflicts. Because parental and other early relationships may act as an imprint for future relationships, particularly with the infant, this signals the need for early identification of mothers at risk. A trusting relationship with a therapist may function as a protective factor, providing a high-risk mother with new ways of viewing herself and others.

Although this study was primarily about treatment success, limited information was available for postpartum follow-up. Seven of eight women treated with interpersonal psychotherapy had no postpartum depression, while one treated patient did. Of three available subjects in the control group, two had postpartum depression, and one did not. We can make few inferences from this limited data. However, this information emphasizes the importance of postpartum follow-up and the potential for prevention.

There was a significant correlation of the mother's improved mood with her ability to interact with the infant. Because this was illustrated at one time point in a small number of women ($N = 11$), the results are not generalizable. However, our findings support those of other researchers (Murray, 1992) and emphasize prevention. Depressed postpartum mothers are less sensitive to infant cues (Zuckerman et al., 1990) and are therefore less likely to soothe their infants, who tend to be withdrawn and inconsolable (Biringen & Robison, 1991; Zuckerman et al., 1990). Problems in behavior, cognition, and creativity often persist into early childhood and adulthood (Weissman et al., 1987). Poverty such as that described in our study group is also an important antecedent to postpartum depression (Hobfoll et al., 1995).

Halpern (1993) suggested that the presence of one or two difficult conditions, such as infant illness, poverty, and difficult personality, intensifies hostile feelings in the mother and emphasizes the vital need for psychiatric services. A striking finding was a history of depression in 73.0% of our group (Frank et al., 1987), data easily obtainable in antepartum clinics and obstetrician/midwife offices. Yet we frequently miss the opportunity for potential intervention and prevention in this accessible study group.

Another particular contribution of this study was the unique cross-section of an understudied population of socioeconomically deprived poorly educated immigrant women. Although immigrant women composed most of our group, African American, White, and Latina women of all socioeconomic backgrounds from the neighboring boroughs of Manhattan and the state of New Jersey were represented.

This study must be considered preliminary and the results considered in view of limitations such as the small group size and the large attrition rate. The benefit of treating mood disorders during pregnancy is far-reaching and extends to the nuclear family, the marital relationship, and parenting potential. Replication of this NIMH study with a larger, more diverse study group is currently underway and will provide generalizability and further information about the effects of ethnicity and socioeconomic status on the causes and treatment outcome of antepartum depression. Mechanisms for diligent follow-up are in place. Financial compensation for transportation and child care is provided to mothers in order to facilitate opportunities for treatment and provide greater study feasibility in this underserved population.

Since specific guidelines for effective, safe treatment of antepartum depression do not exist, interpersonal psychotherapy should be a first-line treatment in the hierarchy of treatment guidelines for depressed pregnant women.

REFERENCES

Alwan, S. A., Reefhuis, J., Rasmussen, S. A., Olney, R. S., & Friedman, J. M. (2007). The National Birth Defects Prevention Study: Use of selective serotonin-reuptake inhibitors in pregnancy and the risk of birth defects. *The New England Journal of Medicine, 356*(26), 2684–2692.

American Psychiatric Association. (1994). *Diagnostic and statistical manual of mental disorders* (4th ed.). Washington, DC: American Psychiatric Press Inc.

Beck, A. T. (1985). *Beck Depression Inventory.* In D. J. Deyser & R. C. Sweetland (Eds.), *Test critiques* (Vol. II, pp. 83–87). Kansas City, MO: Test Corporation of America.

Benedek, T. (1959). Parenthood as a developmental phase: A contribution to the libido theory. *Journal of American Psychoanalytic Association, 7,* 389–417.

Biringen, Z., & Robison, J. (1991). Emotional availability in mother-child interaction: A reconceptualization for research. *American Journal of Orthopsychiatry, 61,* 258–271.

Brody, A. L., Saxena, S., Stoessel, P., Gillies, L. A., Fairbanks, L. A., Alborzian, S., et al. (2001). Regional brain metabolic changes in patients with major depression treated with either paroxetine or interpersonal therapy. *Archives of General Psychiatry, 58,* 641–648.

Carr, M. L. (1993). *Normal and medically complicated pregnancies.* In D. E. Stewart & N. D. Stotland (Eds.), *Psychological aspects in women's health care: The interface between psychiatry and obstetrics and gynecology* (pp. 15–35). Washington, DC: American Psychiatric Press.

Chambers, C. D., Hernandez, S., Van Marter, L. J., Wesler, M. M., Louik, C., Jones, K. L., et al. (2006). Selective serotonin-reuptake inhibitors and risk of persistent pulmonary hypertension of the newborn. *The New England Journal of Medicine, 354*(6), 579–587.

Chung, T., Lau, T. K., Alexander, S. K., Chiu, H., & Lee, D. (2001). Antepartum depressive symptomatology is associated with adverse obstetric and neonatal outcomes. *Psychosomatic Medicine, 63,* 830–834.

Cox, J., & Holden, J. (1994). *Perinatal psychiatry: Use and misuse of the Edinburgh Postnatal Depression Scale.* London: Gaskell (Royal College of Psychiatrists).

Dimitrovsky, L., Perez-Hishberg, M., & Itskowitz, R. (1986). Depression during and following pregnancy: Quality of family relationships. *Journal of Psychology, 12,* 213–218.

Elkin, I., Shea, M. T., Watkins, J. T., Imber, S. D., Sotsky, S. M., Collins, J. F., et al. (1989). National Institute of Mental Health Treatment of Depression Collaborative Research Program: General effectiveness of treatments. *Archives of General Psychiatry, 46,* 971–982.

Evans, J., Heron, J., Francomb, H., Oke, S., & Golding, J. (2001). Cohort study of depressed mood during pregnancy and after childbirth. *BMJ, 323,* 257–260.

Farber, E. W., Herbert, S. E., & Reviere, S. L. (1996). Childhood abuse and suicidality in obstetrics patients in a hospital-based urban prenatal clinic. *General Hospital Psychiatry, 18,* 56–60.

First, M. B., Spitzer, R. L., Gibbon, M., & Williams, J. B. W. (1996). *Structured Clinical Interview for DSM–IV Axis I Disorders: Patient edition (SCID-P),* (Version 2). New York: New York State Psychiatric Institute, Biometrics Research.

Frank, E., Kupfer, D., Jacob, M., Blumenthal, S. J., & Jarrett, D. B. (1987). Pregnancy-related affective episodes among women with recurrent depression. *American Journal of Psychiatry, 144,* 288–292.

Gotlib, I. H., Whiffen, V. E., & Mount, J. H. (1989). Prevalence rates and demographic characteristics associated with depression in pregnancy and the post partum. *Journal of Consult Clin Psycho, 57,* 269–274.

Graff, L. A., Dyck, D. G., & Schallow, J. R. (1991). Predicting postpartum depressive symptoms and structural modeling analysis. *Perceptual and Motor Skills, 73,* 1137–1138.

Halpern, R. (1993). Poverty and infant development. In C. Zeanah (Ed.), *Handbook of infant mental health* (pp. 73–87). New York: Guilford.

Hamilton, M. (1960). A rating scale for depression. *Journal of Neurological and Neurosurgical Psychiatry, 23,* 56–62.

Harris, B., Huckle, P., Thomas, R., Johns, S., & Fung, H. (1989). The use of rating scales to identify postnatal depression. *The British Journal of Psychiatry, 154,* 813–817.

Hobfoll, S. E., Ritter, C., Lavin, J., Hulsizer, M. R., & Cameron, R. (1995). Depression prevalence and incidence among inner-city pregnant and postpartum women. *Journal of Consulting and Clinical Psychology, 63,* 445–453.

Huffman, L. C., Lamour, M., Bryan, Y. E., & Pederson, F. A. (1990). Depressive symptomatology during pregnancy and the postpartum period: Is the Beck Depression Inventory applicable? *Journal of Reproductive and Infant Psychology, 8,* 87–97.

Klein, M. H., & Essex, M. J. (1994). Pregnant or depressed? The effect of overlap between symptoms of depression and somatic complaints of pregnancy on rates of major depression in the second trimester. *Depression, 2,* 1994–1995.

Klerman, G. L., Weissman, M. M., Rounsaville, B. H., & Chevron, E. S. (1984). *Interpersonal psychotherapy in depression.* New York: Basic Books.

Kumar, R., & Hipwell, A. E. (1996). Development of a clinical rating scale to assess mother-infant interaction in a psychiatric mother and baby unit. *The British Journal of Psychiatry, 169,* 18–26.

Kumar, R., & Robson, K. M. (1984). A prospective study of emotional disorders in childbearing women. *The British Journal of Psychiatry, 144,* 35–47.

Louik, C., Lin, A. E., Werler, M. M., Hernandez, S., & Mitchell, A. A. (2007). First-trimester use of selective serotonin-reuptake inhibitors and the risk of birth defects. *The New England Journal of Medicine, 356*(26), 2675–2683.

Mufson, L., Weissman, M. M., Moreau, D., & Garfinkel, R. (1999). Efficacy of interpersonal psychotherapy for depressed adolescents. *Archives of General Psychiatry, 56,* 573–579.

Murray, D., & Cox, J. L. (1990). Screening for depression during pregnancy with the Edinburgh Depression Scale. *Journal of Reproductive and Infant Psychology, 8,* 99–107.

Murray, L. (1992). The impact of postnatal depression on infant development. *Journal of Child Psychology and Psychiatry, 35,* 343– 361.

O'Hara, M., Zekoski, E. M., Philipps, L. H., & Wright, E. J. (1990). Controlled prospective study of postpartum mood disorders: Comparison of childbearing and nonchildbearing women. *Journal of Abnormal Psychology, 99,* 3–15.

O'Hara, M. D., Schlechte, J. A., Lewis, D. A., & Wright, E. J. (1991). Prospective study of postpartum blues: Biologic and psychosocial factors. *Archives of General Psychiatry, 48,* 801–806.

O'Hara, M. W., Stuart, S., Gorman, L. L., & Wenzel, A. (2000). Efficacy of interpersonal psychotherapy for postpartum depression. *Archives of General Psychiatry, 57,* 1039–1045.

Oren, D. A., Wisner, K. L., Spinelli, M., Epperson, C. N., Peindl, K. S., Terman, J. S., et al. (2002). An open trial of morning light therapy for treatment of antepartum depression. *American Journal of Psychiatry, 159,* 666–669.

Petkova, E., Quitkin, F. M., McGrath, P. J., Stewart, J. W., & Klein, D. F. (2000). A method to quantify rater bias in antidepressant trials. *Neuropsychopharmacology, 22,* 559–565.

Robinson, G. E., & Stewart, D. E. (1993). Postpartum disorders in psychological aspects of women's health. In D. E. Stewart & N. L. Stotland (Eds.), *Psychological aspects in women's health care: The interface between psychiatry and obstetrics and gynecology* (pp. 115–138). Washington, DC: American Psychiatric Press.

Rubin, R. (1984). *Maternal identity and the maternal experience.* New York: Springer.

Scott, D. (1992). Early identification of maternal depression as a strategy in the prevention of child abuse. *Child Abuse Neglect, 16,* 345–358.

Seguin, L., Potvin, L., St. Denis, M., & Jacinthe, L. (1995). Chronic stressors, social support, and depression during pregnancy. *Obstetric Gynecol, 85,* 583–589.

Sloane, R. B., Staples, F. R., & Schneider, L. S. (1985). Interpersonal therapy versus nortriptyline for depression in the elderly. In G. D. Burrows, T. R. Norman, & L. Dennerstein (Eds.), *Clinical and Pharmacological Studies in Psychiatric Disorders: Biological Psychiatry.* (pp. 344–346). New Prospects. London: John Libbey.

Spinelli, M., & Endicott, J. (2003). Controlled clinical trial of interpersonal psychotherapy versus parenting education program for depressed pregnant women. *American Journal of Psychiatry, 160,* 555–562.

St. Andre, M. (1993). Psychotherapy during pregnancy: Opportunities and challenges. *American Journal of Psychotherapy, 47*(4), 572–590.

Trad, P. V. (1990). Emergence and resolution of ambivalence in expectant mothers. *American Journal of Psychotherapy, 44*(4), 577–589.

Wadhwa, P. D., Sandman, C. A., Porto, M., Dunkel-Schetter, C., & Garite, T. J. (1993). The association between prenatal stress and infant birth weight and gestational age at birth: A prospective investigation. *Am J Obstet Gynecol, 169,* 858–865.

Walsh, B. T., Seidman, S. N., Sysko, R., & Gould, M. (2002). Placebo response in studies of major depression: Variable, substantial and growing. *JAMA, 287,* 1840–1847.

Weissman, M. M., Prusoff, B. A., Dimascio, A., Neu, C., Goklaney, M., & Klerman, G. L. (1979). The efficacy of drugs and psychotherapy in the treatment of acute depressive episodes. *American Journal of Psychiatry, 136*(4B), 555–558.

Weissman, M. M., Rounsaville, B. J., & Chevron, E. (1982). Training psychotherapists to participate in psychotherapy outcome studies: Identifying and dealing with the research requirements. *American Journal of Psychiatry, 139,* 1442–1446.

Weissman, M. M., Gammon, G. D., John, K., Merikangas, K. R., Warner, V., Prusoff, B. A., et al. (1987). Children of depressed parents: Increased psychopathology and early onset of major depression. *Archives of General Psychiatry, 44,* 847–853.

Wisner, K. L., & Stowe, Z. N. (1997). Psychobiology of postpartum mood disorders. *Brain, Behavior and Reproductive Function, 15,* 77–90.

Wisner, K. L., Zarin, D., Holmboe, E., Appelbaum, P., Gelenberg, A. J., Leonard, H. L., & Frank, E. (2000). Risk-benefit decision making for treatment of depression during pregnancy. *American Journal of Psychiatry, 157,* 1933–1940.

Zuckerman, B., Bauchner, H., Parker, S., & Cabral, H. (1990). Maternal depressive symptoms during pregnancy and newborn irritability. *Journal of Developmental Behavior in Pediatrics, 114,* 190–194.

16

A Psychodynamic Approach to Treatment for Postpartum Depression

ALEXIS E. MENKEN

There is no shortage of literature about postpartum depression, but very little has been written about specific psychotherapeutic methods of treating the disorder (Brockington, 1992; Dunnewold, 1997). Within this narrow body of work, virtually nothing has been written about the psychodynamic approach (Blum, 2007). This is unfortunate because psychodynamic therapy, by its very nature, integrates a patient's unique history with the emotional challenges the person faces in the present. The current chapter argues that for women struggling with postpartum depression (PPD), this is exactly what needs to be examined: the experiences that have shaped their maternal identity as they've traveled from girlhood to womanhood.

The current chapter will outline and illustrate a psychodynamic approach to psychotherapy for PPD. It has been said that, "for therapy to be therapeutic, it is more important for the clinician to understand people than to master specific treatment techniques" (McWilliams, 1999, p. 9). On that note, this chapter doesn't offer specific techniques. Instead, it illustrates how psychodynamic therapy can be put into practice with patients who are struggling with PPD. Vignettes will help clarify how the treatment process works. This chapter will also explore how the patient–therapist relationship—replete with its dynamics of transference and countertransference—can be used to effect positive change. It is important to note that psychodynamic therapy requires a collaborative interplay between the therapist and the patient. Therefore, a patient must be able to address her conflicts, be capable of self-reflection, and not currently psychotic.

The psychodynamic theory that most informs this chapter hinges around the concept of Object Relations. Object relations, in its most basic sense, focuses on how early relationships and experiences influence the way we feel about ourselves and relate to others when we become adults. Within the realm of maternal mental health, early experiences that are internalized from girlhood lay the groundwork for the relationship a mother has with her child and with herself. This chapter begins with a focus on the nature and origins of maternal identity; it will then address the ways that women experience the unfolding of their maternal identity; finally, this chapter will concentrate on working with maternal identity from a psychodynamic perspective.

MATERNAL IDENTITY

What Is It and Where Does It Come From?

The moment a daughter is born, her maternal identity begins to develop. Her mother's loving touch, gentle voice, and the way she responds to subtle cues and meets her child's needs (or the lack thereof) all begin to lay the foundation for her daughter's relationship with the world around her. Mendell (1988) writes that the mother "becomes a lifelong model for her daughter to identify with, to differentiate herself from, and to bond with" (p. 22). Eventually, this mother–daughter template will greatly influence the daughter's feelings about and confidence in mothering her own child. Winnicott (1965) has explained that the degree to which one's mother has provided a "facilitating environment" (p. 239) will contribute to the development of mental health and may ultimately provide for a healthy sense of maternal identity. If a woman's early relationships are traumatic, she will have more difficulty developing secure bonds with others. At particular risk is the development of the woman's maternal identity and the relationship she will have with her child. It is beyond the scope of this chapter to address the potential role that nature plays in the development of maternal identity. We will, instead, focus on nurture and the enormous impact it has on a woman's subjective experience of being mothered and eventually mothering others.

Maternal identity is not only shaped by the relationship a woman has with her own mother. It is influenced by the relationship she has with her father, siblings, and/or significant relatives/caregivers. For example, based on this author's clinical experience, there seems to be a high degree of significant psychopathology in the fathers of women who suffer from postpartum depression. Pivotal life events, such as a woman's history of sexual experiences, abortions, and her feelings about her sexual partners also have a profound impact on maternal identity. Adoption; assisted reproductive technology; and feelings, thoughts, and fantasies about the meaning of infertility and about the possible donor sperm, ovum donor, and/or gestational carriers can also help shape a woman's view of herself as a mother.

How Does It Present Itself?

The first signs of a girl's nascent maternal identity can be detected as she plays. This is not limited to the prosaic cuddling or neglect of a doll or stuffed animal. It can be evident in the quality of the attachment she develops with objects and people around her. As a girl matures and becomes a young woman, her sense of herself as a mother becomes present in her thoughts, feelings, wishes, and dreams. Consciously or not, she begins to establish a relationship with her imagined child long before conception.

A woman's fantasies of herself as a mother usually begin to emerge more overtly during pregnancy. Researchers have demonstrated that when a pregnant woman's dominant thoughts concern fear about closeness and a lack of security, she will experience her pregnancy as largely stress-provoking (Monk, Leight, & Fang, 2007). If a woman has had fears about closeness and conflicted identification with her mother, these difficulties will often become prominent during pregnancy. For some women, the imagined experience of motherhood and the fantasy of the baby turn out to be concordant with their actual experience. For others, there is a great adjustment when reality arrives.

Maternal identity is fully expressed when a woman ultimately gives birth to her first child. The struggle to adjust to the realities of mothering and the capabilities a woman has or lacks can result in PPD. In one of the few articles written about the psychodynamics of women suffering from PPD, Blum (2007) argues that the disorder is characterized by three specific features: dependency conflicts, typically with a counterdependent adaptation (i.e., acting independent when in fact she feels completely needy and reliant on others); guilty inhibition of anger toward others; and conflicted identifications of the patient with her mother.

This last point—a woman's conflicted identification with her mother—is a major focus in the psychodynamic treatment of PPD. During therapy, a woman explores how she identifies (or not) with her mother and what kind of mother she herself wants to be.

For example, when Mary was pregnant for the first time, she described how her baby would fit seamlessly into her busy medical career. She anticipated that a full-time nanny would care for him, and she would not consider breastfeeding. She said, "My mother never breastfed and I was raised by a nanny so my mother could work. I would not consider doing this any other way." She overidentified with her own mother and could not imagine that she would feel differently about parenting than her mother had. When her baby arrived, the patient took off 6 weeks from work and discovered, much to her surprise, that she enjoyed breastfeeding and being at home with her child. Her mother pressured Mary to return to work, but Mary found herself torn between her mother's influence and her emerging maternal voice. Therapy helped Mary develop confidence in this voice and allow it to guide her on a maternal path that was separate from her mother's. During therapy, Mary became increasingly aware of the significance of her relationship with her grandmother, who had lived with her when she was a child. She recalled her grandmother as a very loving and "omnipresent" person in her life. She was able to relate her own feelings about mothering her baby to her feelings of being loved by her grandmother. Prior to giving birth, Mary's well-articulated concept of her own maternal identity was based on how she saw her own mother behave, but it was discordant with her actual experience of being a mother once the baby was in her arms.

In Mary's case, she was conflicted because she overly identified with her mother. A woman's overly dependent relationship with her mother is another common thread among women with PPD. Pines (1994) writes: "First pregnancy is an important developmental phase in a woman's lifelong task of separation-individuation from her own mother" (p. 114). When there is no such separation, it is very difficult for a new mother to find her own voice. For example, Jessica entered therapy when her daughter was 1 year old. She had begun to feel sad and weepy within the first few weeks of giving birth, but did not enter therapy until she became convinced that she was not merely struggling with "baby blues." Initially, Jessica described coming from a very close family. She reported that she spoke with her mother on the phone several times each day and sought parenting advice on a near-constant basis. Therapy, however, quickly revealed how helpless and overly dependent Jessica felt upon her mother—so much so that she felt she could not make any judgments or decisions relating to her child without asking for her mother's counsel. As she became more conscious of how intrusive and controlling her mother was, Jessica began to make small inroads into separating from her mother so she could determine how to function on her own.

To summarize, the experience of maternal identity presents itself in developmentally different ways throughout female development (e.g., through play, thoughts, fantasies, and wishes, and relationships). The development of this identity, while affected by many aspects of her life, is deeply affected by a woman's relationship with her mother. Maternal identity is, in part, related to how successfully a woman has separated from her own mother. Women with PPD often reflect a difficulty separating from their own mothers. The difficulty in separating from her own mother may present itself in terms of feeling needy, dependent, and inadequate, incapable of taking on the tasks of new motherhood. The difficulty in separating can also present itself with what Blum (2007) referred to as the counterdependent adaptation, in which case the woman may try to be overly independent to ward off her feelings of neediness. In either case, psychodynamic psychotherapy is a useful vehicle to help a new mother articulate these struggles and find her own voice.

How Do We Work With It?

Few experiences in life are more transformative than pregnancy, childbirth, and motherhood. Motherhood provokes major changes in a woman's body, marriage, identity, career, and interpersonal relationships. It is generally accepted that this cascade of biopsychosocial upheaval contributes greatly to PPD. But it cannot be overlooked that PPD is rooted not just in the present cascade of events, but also in a woman's history. McWilliams (1999) points out: "It is rare that someone comes to a therapist with a single, delimited difficulty" (p. 13). To wit, a woman seeking therapy because she is intensely anxious about Sudden Infant Death Syndrome is probably dealing with deeper issues, for example, perhaps her lifelong lack of self-confidence.

One of the greatest predictors of a postpartum depression is a prior history of depression, particularly depression during pregnancy. Therefore, pregnancy is an ideal time to address any concerns a woman might have about her own relationship with her mother and her own developing sense of maternal identity. Bergner, Monk, and Werner (in press) make a compelling argument for the role of psychotherapy during pregnancy. They write:

> Treatment allows for recognition, reclaiming and re-integrations of split off images and fantasies of self and other, particularly maternal representations, with which the woman becoming-mother and the fetus are for a time imbued. Such a process enlarges the psychic space within which the imagined baby can grow and become differentiated from problematic internal representations that are born of the mother's unsatisfying early primary relational experiences.

It is often difficult for women to admit to themselves and others that they are unhappy when they are pregnant, so the majority do not seek help at that time. This is unfortunate because an emotionally high-risk pregnancy merits the same degree of attention as what we commonly refer to as a physically high-risk pregnancy. When a postpartum patient finally makes it over the threshold of the therapist's door, it is, thus, crucial for the therapist to do a careful history to understand when the sadness actually began. The therapist should take a detailed history of the patient's emotional experiences during pregnancy: explore how the pregnancy was planned (or not); the woman's feelings about conception; and then her thoughts, feelings, memories, and wishes during the pregnancy.

Some women respond to the stress of new motherhood with a complete sense of disorganization and a breakdown in their own sense of identity. One of the goals of therapy is to help them tolerate this temporary destabilization and to view it as an opportunity for transformation in the service of growth. New mothers often come to therapy as a last resort, having tried many other things. Well-intended family members and sometimes even the obstetrician and/or pediatrician will tell a new mother that she just needs to get some rest. It is useful for a therapist to show the patient that he or she understands that she is not simply struggling with sleep deprivation. The therapist can explain to the patient that what she is experiencing is treatable and she will get better. The therapist should ask the patient if she could put her trust in the therapist's knowledge that she will improve, even if she herself doesn't feel that way.

It is also helpful to remind the depressed new mother that she must take care of herself before she can take care of her baby. It is useful to remind a new patient of how she is instructed to use the oxygen mask when flying on an aircraft. She must first put the oxygen on herself and then put it on her child. While this is counterintuitive, it is a concrete example of how the mother must take care of herself in order to take care of her child.

The first and foremost goal of psychodynamic psychotherapy for a woman with postpartum depression is to resolve her depressed mood so she has the fortitude to care for her baby. One way to achieve this goal is to help the new mother understand her maternal voice. What is her template for mothering? How did this form? Helping her to mother from a conscious place that is her own choice, not to repeat the way she was mothered, nor to mother in opposition to the way she was mothered, but rather to find her own authentic identity as a mother is the key.

It is helpful for the therapist to conduct a detailed inquiry of how the patient herself was mothered. Did she, for example, feel wanted, loved, safe, and nurtured? Or did she feel she was a bother or a burden to her mother? Exploring her own thoughts, fantasies, and feelings about her own sense of being mothered forms the groundwork for her own sense of who she is as a mother. As she can begin to articulate her own experience of being mothered, the patient will also begin to clarify how she herself is mothering, and, most important, how she would like to mother.

The therapeutic alliance—that is, the relationship that is built between the therapist and the patient—is the single most important healing factor in psychodynamic treatment. It gives patients an opportunity to resolve destructive patterns of relating through a collaborative relationship between the patient and therapist. It is the therapist's job to provide an empathic "holding environment," which Winnicott describes as "conveying in words at the appropriate moment something that shows that the analyst knows and understands the deepest anxiety that is being experienced, or that is waiting to be experienced" (Winnicott, 1965, p. 240). The therapist listens with concern, sustained attention, is nonjudgmental, and is therefore different from the woman's internalized objects from childhood (Pine, 1990). It is through this empathic environment that the patient is able to recognize her needs and find healthier ways of relating to others. This allows the patient to resolve her destructive object relations and to become more objective and autonomous so she has choices about how to relate in a genuine and spontaneous way. Behavior change is contingent upon the "provision of a new, corrective object relationship for the patient, one that can gradually enter into the world of internalized object relations" (Pine, 1990, p. 252).

In the object relations model, psychotherapy is inherently dyadic, that is, the therapy is co-created (Greenberg & Mitchell, 1983). Both therapist and patient enter the therapy relationship with transference and countertransference patterns. Transference is the patient's tendency to repeat old internalized object relations. Relational psychotherapy will enable the patient to develop an understanding of the distortions that she uses to maintain relationships. This pattern of relating reflects the patient's deeply ingrained set of object relations, therefore, it will emerge in all social interactions and the patient will elicit these distortions with everyone, including the therapist. Unlike Freudian psychoanalysis, relational psychotherapy does not require the therapist to work in a neutral or detached manner. Indeed, relational therapists believe neutrality cannot be obtained. Neutrality is defined by Greenberg as "the goal of establishing an optimal tension between the patient's tendency to see the analyst as an old object and his capacity to experience him as a new one" (Mitchel & Aron, 1999, p. 142). The therapist must use his or her own understanding of countertransference as a tool to learn about the inner world of the patient.

Transference and countertransference can take many forms. But when working with PPD, the patient often has the need that the therapist takes on a maternal transference with an empathic stance. Stern (1995) refers to this as the "good grandmother transference." When a new mother is having difficulty enjoying this new phase of her life, she wants nothing more than to be supported, valued, and encouraged to find the place within her that can blossom as a maternal figure. The power of the transference is not to be underestimated. This requires a more active and supportive role on the part of the therapist than one might traditionally strive for. Before the patient calls to schedule an appointment, she already has both conscious and unconscious thoughts about who she wants the therapist to be to her. Whether the patient is aware of her feelings toward the therapist, it is important to be immediately mindful of the developing transference. The transference to the therapist often involves conflicts regarding the patient's relationship with her own mother.

Stern argues that when working within the context of what he calls the *motherhood constellation,* the therapist must work within a therapeutic alliance that is different from that traditionally sought. The transference now focuses on themes related to mothering and being mothered. Specifically, Stern describes the work as involving three voices he terms the *motherhood trilogy.*

According to Stern, with the birth of a baby, the mother transitions into a new phase of life he terms the *motherhood constellation.* While this new phase is transient, it is also dominant and determines a new set of "action tendencies, sensibilities, fantasies, fears, and wishes" (Stern, 1995, p. 171). Stern defines the motherhood constellation in terms of the motherhood trilogy and four related themes. He describes the motherhood trilogy as the mother's major concern and areas that require the greatest work. These three areas are as follows: first, the mother's discourse with her own mother, especially her own mother as mother-to-her-as-a-child; second, the mother's discourse with herself, especially with herself-as-mother; and third, the mother's discourse with her own baby.

Stern also describes four themes and their related tasks that contribute to the motherhood constellation. His four themes are as follows:

- *First:* The life-growth theme (can she maintain the life and growth of the baby?).
- *Second:* Primary relatedness theme (can she emotionally engage with the baby in an authentic manner?).
- *Third:* Supporting matrix theme (will she know how to create the necessary support system?).
- *Fourth:* Identity reorganization theme (will she allow transformation of her own identity?).

During the course of therapy, it is useful to address the motherhood trilogy and its four related themes. However, it has been this author's experience that it is particularly useful to focus on the first part of Stern's trilogy, a woman's relationship with her own mother. In the words of Dinora Pines (1994), "Motherhood is a three-generation experience. Nevertheless, intrapsychically the problem is posed as to whether the pregnant woman is to identify herself with her introjected mother or to rival her and succeed in being a better mother than she was felt to have been" (p. 67). Thus, an important and central piece of work is to recognize the quality of a woman's identification with her own mother as mother-to-her. There has been much written on the new mother's transformation of her relationship with her own mother (Benedek, 1959). Exploring how she was mothered and focusing specifically on her definition of what it means to be a good mother are critical components to this work. The way the patient feels about how she was mothered forms the cornerstone of her own sense of maternal identity and thus her feelings about becoming a mother herself. A woman might try to be exactly as she imagined her mother was, or as illustrated in the following vignette, she might try to be quite the opposite.

Stephanie had an abusive, alcoholic, and punitive mother. She grew up with no sense of being mothered, nor was she made to feel safe in the world. Her father left when she was a toddler and she had no siblings. She became an excellent student and organized her identity around being the opposite of her mother. She became a high achiever, developed a successful corporate career, and married an equally successful businessman. When she gave birth, Stephanie read books, hired a 24-hour nurse for the first 3 months, and provided a very stable, organized home with strict schedules. She had two young children, and, although she worked full time, she attended to their entire needs: academic, social, physical, musical, etc. Stephanie sought psychotherapy while her children were in preschool for her own feelings of depression, intense sadness, and difficulty sleeping. In therapy, she worked on developing an awareness of how her sense of maternal identity had formed in reaction to her own mother. Initially, she spoke about her feeling of trying to care for her children "as if" she were their mother, taking cues from books, friends, and other experts. She did not feel genuinely connected to any internal authentic sense of herself as a mother. As she became increasingly aware of how her mothering was an attempt to be different from her own mother, she was eventually able to pay attention to her own inner experience when she was with her children. Over time, she began to figure out what kind of mother she herself wanted to be, not as the antithesis to her own mother, but to find her own sense of herself as a mother. In addition, she relied on the therapist as a maternal figure and was able to incorporate some of the positive feelings of being nurtured and cared for. She worked actively in the transference to express her feelings of fear about being cared for and exploring what it meant for her to learn how to feel safe in a nurturing environment.

Most mothers struggling with PPD are devastated by the thought that they are not good mothers. They also feel an intense societal pressure to be a good mother. It has been the experience of this author that when a patient is asked, "What is your definition of a good mother?" she will often become quite sad and tearful. Most women describe a supermother, the idealized perfect mother that is not based on any true experience of their own. Recognizing the destructiveness of this idealized image, Winnicott (1993) developed the concept of the "good-enough mother," in which he explains that mothers need not be spectacular, they need only be good enough (p. 123). The idealized image of the perfect superhero Mother may come from the media and/or from women's idealization of their own mothers.

For example, Katy came into therapy after the birth of her second child. Her marriage was in a crisis, and she felt she could barely manage her two young children without feeling completely overwhelmed. She reported feeling sad much of the day and described a crushing feeling of inadequacy. She described parenting her children with a feeling of intensity and a desire to enjoy every single moment, from putting on their socks in the morning to feeding them nutritious meals, to playing games after school. She was the eighth of nine children and felt that while her own mother always had a "handle on everything," she also felt that perhaps she was unwanted and her mother didn't enjoy parenting her because she had seven children before her. She began to view her intense efforts at superparenting as an attempt at reparation for the ways that her own mother was unavailable to her. A core piece of her own work was to find her own sense of herself as Winnicott's "good-enough mother," rather than comparing herself to her "amazing" and idealized mother whom she had both put on a pedestal and experienced as not fully present for her. A major goal of psychodynamic psychotherapy is to help each mother discover her own authentic voice, and to become the "good-enough" mother that she can be. In her book, *No Greater Love,* Mother Theresa (1989) captured the importance of accepting one's own capacity to love with the following words:

> Do not think that love, in order to be genuine, has to be extraordinary. What we need is to love without getting tired. How does a lamp burn? Through the continuous input of small drops of oil. What are these drops of oil in our lamps? They are the small things of daily life: faithfulness, small words of kindness, a thought for others, our way of being silent, of looking, of speaking, and of acting. (p. 22)

CONCLUSION

The psychodynamic approach to working with postpartum depression requires a focus on the development of maternal identity. It is through exploring a woman's past and her relationship with her own mother that the patient can become more aware of the templates she is working with as she strives to mother her baby. It is in the context of a nonjudgmental relationship with a therapist who provides a safe and nurturing environment that the patient can explore past patterns and work within the transference to become aware of her own patterns and opportunities for change. She can then find a way to love her baby without feeling like it is an exhausting effort, but rather an authentic way for her to be with her child. "Childbearing requires an exchange of a known self in a known world for an unknown self in an unknown world" (Rubin, 1984, p. 52). The goal of psychodynamic psychotherapy for postpartum depression is for the new mother to know and welcome her new self in her new world.

REFERENCES

Benedek, T. (1959). Parenthood as a developmental phase: A contribution to libido theory. *Journal of the American Psychoanalytic Association, 7*(3), 389–417.

Bergner, S., Monk, C., & Werner, E. A. (in press). Dyadic intervention during pregnancy? Treating pregnant women and possibly reaching the future baby. *Infant Mental Health Journal.*

Blum, L. D. (2007). Psychodynamics of postpartum depression. *Psychoanalytic Psychology, 24*(1), 45–62.

Brockington, I. F. (1992). Disorders specific to the puerperium. *International Journal of Mental Health, 21*(2), 41–52.

Dunnewold, A. L. (1997). *Evaluation and treatment of postpartum emotional disorders.* Sarasota, FL: Professional Resources Press.

Greenberg, J. R. (1999). Theoretical models and the analysts' neutrality. In S. A. Mitchel & L. Aron (Eds.), *Relational psychoanalysis: The emergence of a tradition* (pp. 131–152). Hillsdale, NJ: Analytic.

Greenberg, J., & Mitchell, S. (1983). *Object relations in psychoanalytic theory.* Cambridge, MA: Harvard University Press.

McWilliams, N. (1999). *Psychoanalytic case formulation.* New York: Guilford.

Mendell, D. (1988). Early female development: From birth through latency. In J. Offerman-Zuckerberg (Ed.), *Critical psychophysical passages in the life of a woman* (pp. 17–36). New York: Plenum.

Monk, C., Leight, K. L., & Fang, Y. (2007). *The relationships between women's attachment style and perinatal mood disturbance: Implications for screening and treatment.* Manuscript submitted for publication.

Pine, F. (1990). *Drive, ego, object & self.* New York: Basic Books.

Pines, D. (1994). *A woman's unconscious use of her body.* New Haven, CT: Yale University Press.

Rubin, R. (1984). *Maternal identity and the maternal experience.* New York: Springer.

Stern, D. N. (1995). *The motherhood constellation.* New York: Basic Books.

Teresa, Mother. (1989). *No greater love.* Novato, CA: New World Library.

Winnicott, D. W. (1965). *Maturational processes and the facilitating environment: Studies in the theory of emotional development.* Madison, CT: International Universities Press.

Winnicott, D. W. (1993). *Talking to parents.* Cambridge, MA: Addison-Wesley.

17

Health Literacy and Maternal Empowerment

LISA BERNSTEIN AND EVE WEISS

The What To Expect Foundation takes its name from the bestselling *What To Expect* series that has helped more than 27 million families from pregnancy through their child's toddler years. But, unfortunately, for as many families as those books have helped, they've missed the millions of families living in poverty who can neither afford, nor perhaps read, that book. With the United States' appallingly high infant mortality rate—28th in the world—and shockingly low literacy rate—approximately 36% of adult Americans have inadequate health literacy—clearly many families do not know what to expect during pregnancy and early parenting (I. Bennett, personal communication, December 5, 2007; National Assessment of Adult Literacy, 2003; Weiss, 2007). Thus the birth of The What To Expect Foundation, created by the series' author, Heidi Murkoff, and Lisa Bernstein, a former publishing executive and volunteer literacy tutor. The Foundation's Baby Basics Program provides comprehensive pregnancy and parenting information and health literacy support to underserved families, so they can become effective users of the health care system and empowered advocates for themselves and their family.

This chapter will review the common perinatal lived experiences of underserved expecting women in the public health system that inspired the creation of the Baby Basics Program. It will introduce the concepts of health literacy and research that shows how underserved families are affected by having "low health literacy." A case study of the Baby Basics Program illustrates how this program addresses these frustrations at the patient, provider, support staff, and community level. We will review the evidence of the relationship between literacy and health, and limited research on the link between health literacy and health status, and the proven correlation between maternal literacy and health outcomes. While there has been very little research on the linkage between health literacy, literacy, and depression—and even less on the linkage between a mother's literacy skills and her likelihood of developing perinatal depression—we hope this chapter illustrates and inspires all who work with this population to be sensitive to how the challenges and barriers inherent in the health care system, coupled with literacy concerns, could frustrate even the most healthy of pregnant women. These sensitivities will lead us to create a new paradigm to help providers and patients overcome the health literacy and mental health needs of vulnerable patients. We end with a list of specific health literacy and communication strategies that can be used right away with all patients.

PRENATAL CARE AND PUBLIC HEALTH EXPERIENCES

A low-income woman entering the prenatal center system may feel overwhelmed from the moment she places the first call for an appointment. Let's follow the experience from the patient's as well as the professional's perspective. First, a mom may have problems making an appointment and getting to her appointment on time. She must navigate a confusing phone system, perhaps sit on hold waiting to speak to a human, and then perhaps be unable to get an appointment before her first trimester. The moment she walks in the provider's door, a pregnant woman may be growled at by the clerical staff to take a seat. In many health centers, the clerical staff is overworked, and may feel underappreciated by the professional staff. Yet, a mother at her first appointment doesn't know that; to her, this receptionist is a major part of her health care experience.

Next come the health care forms, which a woman may not be able to read because of language or literacy barriers. (In fact, one mom told us that when she couldn't read or fill out the health forms, she felt "she had just flunked" the first test of motherhood.)

The waiting rooms of some prenatal care centers are beautiful, but others are dingy and poorly lit, with perhaps a TV blaring *Judge Judy* or some so-called educational program in the background. Written materials are rarely available in the waiting room to fill the time. Children's books or other educational or recreational materials are rarely available for bored children waiting with their mothers. Pregnant teens often stare at the squirming and screaming children in horror or fear. Mothers must frequently wait for 2 hours or longer before their names are called to see a doctor. Some programs will not give an exact appointment time—instead they instruct all mothers to show up at one time and then wait. And they must show up on time for this wait, or they will be cancelled for the day.

The providers at prenatal clinics often have at most 5 minutes to spend with a patient. This is not their fault, and it is an unfortunate reality of today's health care system. But from a patient's perspective, the doctors appear rushed, impersonal, and rude. (And, of course, with the level of overwork, the doctors may be feeling tired, anxious, and angry.) When doctors ask patients if they have any questions, we've noticed a curious disconnect. Mothers often shake their heads no, or cross their arms protectively and say "uh-uh." In focus groups, doctors said many of their moms have no questions—and surprisingly, some said it was because moms just didn't care. Moms, however, reported that they feared asking doctors questions for a variety of reasons: they didn't want to ask stupid questions; they weren't sure they knew the right medical words necessary to frame the question; the doctor had his hand on the door and his back to the patient before she could answer; or in the quick moments of the visit she had not summoned the courage to ask. Yet these moments are critical in ensuring adequate prenatal care. Research that has explored the reasons that women with low literacy give for obtaining prenatal care shows that women highly value the quality of communication with their prenatal providers, and, in fact, this is the most important factor in getting prenatal care (Bennett, Switzer, Aguirre, Evans, & Barg, 2006).

What have we learned? Clearly patient and provider perceive this moment very differently. Many mothers sit in the exam room feeling anxious instead of feeling cared for. Asking a question is a difficult skill for many patients. To ask a question at a prenatal or pediatric appointment, one needs to feel comfortable using health and body vocabulary; feel confident that it is a worthy question (after all, this is a busy, smart doctor); and have the assertiveness to pose that question. It is no wonder that many mothers shake their heads no.

These experiences may lead mothers to incorrectly perceive that the prenatal appointment is designed for the doctor's purposes, as a way to "check up on them." Not to care for them, but to inspect them to make sure they are properly taking care of their baby. Once they have their baby, they may face a similar experience with their pediatrician, a provider who is traditionally trained to care for and focus on the baby, not the parent. Among some underserved families and cultures, medical authorities are even perceived as suspect since they have the authority to report parents to child protective services.

While doctors are committed to patient well-being and care, they are rarely taught strategies or have tools that enable clear communication across literacy and cultural barriers. Even those with the best of intentions would be surprised by how often patients cannot correctly report back the most important topics discussed during their appointment. Unfortunately, little is written down to help patients remember, and the materials patients receive are rarely written to an appropriate reading level; they are often unattractive and condescending; and they are infrequently referred to during or following a visit.

Outside the exam room, the low-income prenatal patient must confront complex mental and physical navigation and negotiation in order to access and register for pregnancy Medicaid benefits. In states like Florida, prenatal care is free for anyone who cannot afford to pay, regardless of immigration status. Yet Floridian health departments have a difficult time reaching women to provide them with these services. In other states, those who do not qualify for prenatal care benefits due to their immigration status often are anxious when they do show up for appointments and are too frightened to give their real name or phone number to providers. Perhaps this is because they are unaware of laws forbidding health care providers to alert authorities or release information about undocumented patients.

A patient may also have trouble literally navigating the confusing corridors of large hospitals and reading the signs that will help her make it to her sonogram appointment on time—instead of arriving embarrassed and late. For some mothers, this is the first time they will have become entangled in this system. For others, it is just another "system" that leaves them confused or angry. Take these experiences and repeat them monthly, and we have a prescription for confusion, anger, hopelessness, and depression.

These insights, gleaned from our experiences working with these moms, contributed to the Baby Basics Program's organic evolution from book, to program, to philosophy of health care. In addition, these kinds of experiences—well-documented across the entire health care system—led the medical profession to more closely examine how literacy and cultural barriers affect health outcomes, and to create the term *health literacy*.

WHAT IS HEALTH LITERACY?

A 2003 study done by the U.S. Department of Education's National Assessment of Adult Literacy (NAAL) found that between 40% and 50% of American adults have only very basic or below basic literacy skills (this was a repeat of the initial NAAL 1993 study). These adults are from all backgrounds, races, and socioeconomic classes. Not surprisingly, low socioeconomic or immigrant status are often markers of lower literacy skills, and over a third of all mothers on Medicaid have limited literacy skills.

Leaders in the health care field began to note that some of the health care system's most seemingly intractable problems could be traced to the mismatch between the literacy demands of the health care delivery system and the literacy skills of its users (Rudd, Moeykens, & Colton, 1999). The term *health literacy* is commonly used to talk about this disconnect, and it is defined by the National Library of Medicine, the Institute of Medicine of the National Academy of Sciences, and Healthy People 2010 as "The degree to which individuals have the capacity to obtain, process and understand basic health information and services needed to make appropriate health decisions" (Nielsen-Bohlman, Panzer, & Kindig, 2004, p. 20).

Unlike the conventional definition of fundamental literacy—the ability to read and write—*health* literacy encompasses the skills required to understand complex medical information, communicate with providers, fill out health and insurance forms, and generally navigate a complex health care system (Allen & Horowitz, 2004).

The American Medical Association estimates that 90 million Americans—half of all adults—may struggle with low health literacy (American Medical Association Medical Student Section Community Service Committee, 2004). The report *Low Health Literacy: Implications for National Health Policy* states that the cost of low health literacy to the U.S. economy is in the range of $106 billion to $236 billion annually (Vernon, Trujillo, Rosenbaum, & DeBuono, 2007). According to the report, the savings that could be achieved by improving health literacy translates into enough funds to insure every one of the more than

47 million persons who lacked coverage in the United States in 2006, as well as reduce a tremendous cost burden for future generations.

Adults with low health literacy:

- Are often less likely to comply with prescribed treatment and self-care regimens
- Make more medication or treatment errors
- Fail to seek preventive care (Weiss, 1999)
- Are at a higher risk for hospitalization than people with adequate literacy skills (Baker, Parker, Williams, & Clark, 1998)
- Remain in hospital nearly 2 days longer (Kirsch, Jugebut, Jenkins, & Kolstad, 1993)
- Lack the skills needed to negotiate the health care system (Weiss, 1999)
- Have increased risk of depression symptomatology in pregnancy and in late life (Bennett, Culhane, & Elo, 2007)

Christina Zarcadoolas, PhD, Associate Professor, Department of Community and Preventive Medicine at the Mount Sinai School of Medicine, and lead author of *Advancing Health Literacy: A Framework for Understanding and Action* (Jossey-Bass, 2006) defines a health literate person as someone "able to use health concepts and information generatively—applying information to novel situations. Health literacy evolves over one's life and, like most complex human competencies, is impacted by health status as well as demographic, sociopolitical, psychosocial and cultural factors." In this more elaborated definition, health literacy is one of the many "literacies"; a wide "range of skills and competencies that people develop over their lifetime to seek out, comprehend, evaluate and use health information and concepts to make informed choices, reduce health risks and increase their quality of life" (C. Zarcadoolas, personal communication, November 15, 2007).

In fact, Zarcadoolas is exploring and defining a range of other "literacies" necessary to stay healthy and succeed in our complex society. She adds environmental literacy to the list—as in understanding and acting upon the evacuation plans for Hurricane Katrina, or the risk of toxic exposures—and she is also interested in "mental health literacy." Some cultures do not address, embrace, or even have the words for *mental health.* For example, some religions and cultures do not share the Western conception of free will and instead believe actions are divined or fated. Those born into generational or socially determined poverty and depression may believe "this is just the way life is." Just as a person with inadequate health literacy may not perceive the need to manage chronic conditions or practice preventative health behaviors, those with inadequate mental health literacy may not understand the nature of a psychological illness, let alone possible treatments. Without mental health literacy, a patient would not know or expect that there is an entire discipline of caring mental health professionals that can help them.

HEALTH LITERACY AND THE PERINATAL EXPERIENCE

A central question to explore is how does a woman's health literacy affect her pregnancy, her child's health, and her general sense of well-being during pregnancy and in the first years of motherhood? Studies have looked at how a mother's health literacy affects her access to prenatal care, her experience of care, and the health and well-being of her children.

Dr. Ian Bennett, Assistant Professor, Department of Family Medicine and Community Health, University of Pennsylvania School of Medicine, studied why women did not access prenatal services and how this was linked to their literacy skills. He found that "women with low literacy faced added hurdles to the navigation of the health care systems for themselves and their children. The stresses of poverty and an increased risk of depression further complicated the challenges of getting the services they need" (I. Bennett, personal communication, December 5, 2007). Immigrants face particularly high barriers to care. In a recent study among Latina prenatal care patients with limited English proficiency, Dr. Bennett found that participants commonly had inadequate literacy in Spanish. Among this group, Dr. Bennett identified a particularly high risk for maternal depressive symptomatology (Bennett et al., 2007).

"But ultimately, it is a matter of trust," Dr. Bennett continues. Patients need to feel safe and comfortable in order to access care. This is why he cautions against testing patients' literacy skills in a health care setting to determine their needs. Literacy tests can set up barriers to care and undermine the very feelings of trust that providers are trying to establish. Dr. Bennett has received an NIH grant to continue his studies on the associations between low literacy, the demands of the health care system, and perinatal depression, and is involved in a variety of interventions to change the experience for mothers.

Dr. Julie Gazmararian, a researcher at Emory University, stresses that mothers with low-health literacy tend to have feelings of shame and are eager to hide that they cannot read or cannot understand what their health care provider is explaining to them. They are unlikely to ask questions and are certainly unlikely to seek out further help. Studies have found that almost half of all patients with low functional literacy admitted feelings of shame; 67% had never told their spouses of their low literacy; and 53% had never told their children (Parikh, Parker, Nurss, Baker, & Williams, 1996; Wolf, Williams, Parker, Parikh, Nowlan, & Baker, 2007). Dr. Gazmararian wonders if the shame mothers feel admitting to limited literacy skills is similar to the shame felt by mothers suffering from perinatal depression. In both cases, we need to develop strategies to help mothers feel comfortable asking questions and empower women to admit they have a problem and to seek care and maintain treatment.

Dr. Lee Sanders, a practicing pediatrician and an Associate Professor of Pediatrics at the University of Miami Leonard M. Miller School of Medicine, cites estimates that between 31%–37% of adults of child-bearing age—his patients' parents—have limited health literacy skills (Committee on Health Literacy, 1999; Kutner, Greenburg, Jin, & Paulson, 2006). His studies and studies by other researchers suggest that a parent's literacy level has a more significant impact on their child's health than the family's socioeconomic status. He cites research in the United States that shows that mothers of lower literacy are less likely to have children who have a dedicated primary care provider and are more likely to have unmet health needs (Sanders, Thompson, & Wilkinson, 2007). Parent literacy skills also influence the developmental health of children. "On average, the poorer the parents' literacy skills," he says, "the fewer children's books they have in their home" (Sanders, Zacur, Haecker, & Klass, 2004, p. 424).

Dr. Sanders stresses the need for more research on the topic. "We know from international research that maternal literacy is very connected to birth outcomes, a higher likelihood that a child will be born prematurely, and a higher risk of infant mortality," he says (L. Sanders, personal communication, September 21, 2007).

As Dr. Perri Klass, a pediatrician, author, and the medical director of the pediatric literacy program Reach Out and Read, has observed, "a mother's reading skills often are fundamental to her family's prospects in life. Improved maternal literacy has a strong positive effect on child health, [because] as family literacy levels improve, parents become more effective users of the health care system" (Monsen, 2007). In one of the few studies to date that hones in on the relationship between literacy and depression, Barry D. Weiss et al. (2006) looked at whether improving literacy skills can lessen the severity of depression. The hypothesis was that "Individuals with limited literacy and those with depression share many characteristics, including low self-esteem, feelings of worthlessness, and shame" (Weiss, Francis, Senf, Heist, & Hargraves, 2006, p. 823). In a randomized clinical trial of 70 community health center patients who tested positive for both depression and limited literacy skill, he found that while patients under standard depression treatment showed some improvement, those who received both literacy education and treatment for their depression showed greater improvement. Though these patients are not suffering from perinatal depression, the report concludes that there may be a benefit to assessing the literacy skills of patients who are depressed and recommends that patients with both depression and limited literacy consider enrolling in adult education classes as an additional treatment for depression.

But a pregnant woman or new mother is unlikely to have the time, energy, or child care necessary to join an adult literacy class. As we've discussed, the very fabric of the prenatal health experience can cause feelings of helplessness and despair. Therefore, we must create a new paradigm that teaches providers how to better communicate with patients, advances their mental health and health literacy, and empowers patients to "obtain, process, and understand" health care.

THE BABY BASICS PROGRAM

> Often there was a wall between us and the people we were trying to serve. It was a wall of confusion and misunderstanding brought on by low functional literacy skills. And, unfortunately, it was sometimes shored up by our inability to recognize that our patients didn't understand the health information that we were trying to communicate. We must close the gap between what health care professionals know and what the rest of America understands about how to have a healthy pregnancy and a healthy baby. Not every American is a scientist or a health care professional, and we can't expect everyone to understand what it takes doctors, nurses, pharmacists and other health care professionals years of training to learn. That's why the Baby Basics Program is so important.
>
> —Former U.S. Surgeon General, VADM Richard Carmona, at the launch of the Houston Baby Basics Initiative (November 2, 2004)

Why We Created Baby Basics

Health literacy programs and research efforts typically focus on the patient's deficit rather than the flaws in the health care system. But the Baby Basics program tries to bridge the communication disconnect between providers and patients, providers and community-based organizations—and even the disconnect between the professional and support staff. The research discussed above, as well as close observation and our continuous best practices research, informed the creation and constant evolution of the Baby Basics Program. When we began to build the program in 2000, the term *health literacy* was not clearly defined, and research was just beginning to uncover women's unmet perinatal mental health needs. And though no one has yet directly studied the correlation between the two, as we built this program, we felt the connection was obvious.

We began with the understanding that a focus on women's health literacy and empowerment is essential; women organize their family's care and are central to the intergenerational transfer of learning and custom (C. Zarcadoolas, personal communication, November 15, 2007). For many at-risk women, pregnancy is their entry into our health system. It is a vulnerable time, but also an opportunity for positive intervention on many fronts. Pregnant women are especially receptive to tools, strategies, and supports that will help them do the best for their baby. Yet, most low-income women do not receive comprehensive, coordinated care, health literacy education, and the mental health services that would lead to healthier, happier pregnancies and would help moms build skills to advocate for their own and their family's health, education, and well-being. The Baby Basics program has four goals:

1. To provide prenatal and parenting materials to underserved families that are not only beautiful, comprehensive, and easy to read but also serve as a catalyst for learning and family literacy.
2. To empower, engage, and educate underserved parents so that they become effective users of the health care system and can advocate for themselves and their families.
3. To teach health care providers and educators how to use health literacy and cultural competency tools and strategies to improve patient communication and compliance.
4. To build community initiatives so that providers and educators are "all on the same page" and families receive integrated, coordinated prenatal and parenting messages.

The centerpiece of the Baby Basics program is *Baby Basics: Your Month by Month Guide to a Healthy Pregnancy,* a much-lauded, extensively researched, innovative prenatal guide/health literacy tool that is written to both a 3rd- and 5th-grade level. A publication of the What To Expect Foundation, the book addresses the medical, social, emotional, economic, cultural, and linguistic concerns of pregnant women (and men) living at or below the poverty level. Beneath its colorful cover, it is filled with illustrations, photographs, stories, and facts, and it is presented to mothers at their first appointment as a gift for them and their baby. For some mothers, this will be the first book they have ever owned. Before the creation of *Baby Basics,* mothers at most received poorly copied, unevenly stapled handouts that gave them a list of do's and don'ts. With *Baby Basics,* mothers have comprehensive, empowering information, presented with humor and respect.

The response to *Baby Basics* from health care providers, educators, and the mothers for whom it is meant has been overwhelmingly positive. In focus groups, we asked mothers for whom they thought this book was written. They all replied, "It was written for me." We also asked moms whom they would give their book to when their pregnancy was finished. Most moms said they would perhaps share the book, but they would want it back, because, they said, "it's mine."

How Baby Basics Works

Since the book's publication in 2002, close to 300,000 copies of *Baby Basics* have been provided to low-income pregnant women across the country. In 2004, *Baby Basics* was given an extensive cultural as well as linguistic translation into Spanish and renamed *Hola Bebe.* In 2007, *Baby Basics* was similarly translated into Chinese (*Xiao Bao Bao*) in partnership with the Charles B. Wang Community Health Care Center in New York City's Chinatown. More than 400 providers nationwide use and distribute the *Baby Basics* book, and 15 sites around the country have implemented a Baby Basics program, the most comprehensive of which are located in New York City.

The other tools used in a Baby Basics Program are the Baby Basics Planner and the Baby Basics Mom's Club Curriculum. The Planner acts as a portable, personal medical record for mothers and includes a place for moms to write down appointments and questions, a monthly list of commonly asked questions, and space for providers to write down page numbers to review and other recommendations. The planner has been translated into 14 languages. The Baby Basics Mom's Club Curriculum guides group educators, case managers, and home visitors with specific activities that teach prenatal education. These activities are infused with empowering health literacy skills, such as how to form a question and get a useful answer; how to navigate the health care system; and the critical medical terms in English that pregnant women should know to effectively ask questions and understand what is going on during labor and delivery.

Though there is a variety of Baby Basics models and programs across the country, we piloted our Baby Basics clinical model and evaluation at the Medical and Health Research Association of New York City, Inc.'s (MHRA) MIC Women's Health Services in Jamaica, Queens, from 2005 to 2007. At MIC, every mom receives a copy of the *Baby Basics* book and planner at her first appointment. By training the clerical staff and empowering them to develop a strategy and protocol for handing out the book, we help form human connections between the often-bored, snippy, or disassociated "lady behind the desk" and the often-frightened pregnant mom.

Mom is encouraged to attend drop-in Baby Basics Mom's Clubs in the education room (which has been painted to look like a *Baby Basics* book cover) instead of sitting in the waiting room for her appointment. Children's books are available for younger siblings. At the Mom's Club, health educators who have been trained in adult education and English-language education strategies run groups using the Baby Basics Mom's Club Curriculum. The group works together to look up topics in *Baby Basics*, provide support, validate mom's concerns, help her develop and role-play questions for the doctor, and make friends with other pregnant moms. When it's time for a mom's appointment, the nurse finds her in the Mom's Club and brings her to the exam room. The doctor or midwife, who also has been trained in Baby Basics strategies for communicating with patients, not only points to pictures in *Baby Basics* when talking to the mom, he or she also writes down key words and recommendations in her Baby Basics Planner and notes the page number so mom can look it up again when she gets home. Together, provider and patient review the monthly questions provided in the Planner or those mom has developed during the Mom's Club. Using the "teach-back method," the provider assesses mom's understanding by asking her how she will explain the specific topics they've just discussed to her friends or the baby's father. Of course, the doctor has also noted in the Planner which *Baby Basics* pages explain this information, as well as any other suggestions.

The Baby Basics Program has been adapted to work with the needs of staff at other settings. One hospital has trained volunteers, called BB Pregnancy Pals, to sit in the waiting room and ask moms if they've prepared questions for their doctor's appointment—"because this is *your* appointment and you have a right to have your questions answered." Together, mom and volunteer write down questions for the provider in the BB Planner and together look up information in the *Baby Basics* books. (Using an index to find information is just one of the skills this activity teaches.) The volunteer asks the mom to stop by after her appointment to ensure that she got answers to all of her questions. Another health care center did not have room for a Baby Basics Mom's Club onsite. Instead they have partnered with a nearby library and encourage moms to go there for a free, weekly BB Mom's Club run by a health educator (*and* they receive a library card!). The Baby Basics Program is also used by home visiting programs so that their education and care are coordinated with the provider's instructions and the entire health care community is on the same page.

MHRA conducted the evaluation of our Baby Basics pilot in Jamaica, New York. The evaluation was designed to measure program success by tracking process and outcome variables. Here are the findings:

1. After implementation of the Baby Basics Program at MIC Women's Health Center of Jamaica, the proportion of patients returning for postpartum care (n = 517) was significantly higher at the Baby Basics site, compared to the other MIC Women's Health sites that did not implement the Baby Basics Program (n = 2324); (chi square test p = .004).
2. Overall patient satisfaction increased over time at the intervention site, compared to all other centers.
3. The mean number of prenatal visits increased postintervention. This difference was statistically significant over time and comparing intervention to nonintervention sites.
4. Using more Baby Basics materials was not associated with increased visit duration, but using effective communication techniques was associated with increased visit duration.
5. Providers mentioned the *Baby Basics* book in every visit, but use of other Baby Basics materials during visits varied by provider.
6. Staff reported that the new strategies helped them communicate better without increasing the length of the visit, and that moms and dads were reading *Baby Basics* and not only learning, but enjoying what they learned.

We believe these findings show that empowering mothers, changing their prenatal experience, and giving them tools and strategies for truly engaging in their care encourage them to make better use of the services available. It also positively affects the provider's experience while not considerably extending the length of the visit. The finding that postpartum visits increased among Baby Basics participants felt particularly significant. Before our program was implemented, mothers rarely returned for their postpartum appointment. We posit that this was because they did not believe the appointment was for *them.* When participating in the Baby Basics Program, the entire prenatal care experience became positive and collaborative, rather than oppositional. Moms understood the reason for prenatal appointments. Thus, the last appointment had become a chance for them to get additional care and also to show off their new baby to their health care providers, their partners in health care.

Next Steps for Baby Basics

As a natural next step after the prenatal experience, in 2006 we began to research and develop the baby and family's "First Year Book." Working with cognitive behavioral therapists, literacy instructors, child development educators, pediatricians, and others concerned about the health of America's most vulnerable families, we are incorporating health literacy education, mental health support, and parenting advice in a new book and program that we hope will take the Baby Basics Program to new places for parents and providers. This program acknowledges that many of the new mothers we've observed, especially teens, appear "affectless." Are they overwhelmed and exhausted, or is there a generalized low-lying depression experienced by new mothers living in poverty? The curriculum will coordinate the stages of child development with reflective tools and exercises to help new parents discover personal behavioral strategies to help them to cope with the stresses of new parenthood and begin to overcome existing low self-esteem and depression issues.

Future Research

All of the researchers, providers, and educators who are cited in this study agree that we are just beginning to loosen the knot that intertwines the cycles of poverty, illiteracy, health literacy, perinatal depression, and even addiction. Many interesting paths and research were left out of this chapter due to space limitations, but we hope we've enticed you to do further reading and research on the topic. Can literacy instruction help alleviate symptoms of perinatal depression? What other interventions that are outside the norm for perinatal depression might work? How can literacy educators' understanding of the ways adults learn be integrated into cognitive behavioral therapy? And how can we measure a woman's feelings of satisfaction with her health care experience in a way that correlates with her feelings of self-efficacy during pregnancy, labor, and delivery, and motherhood? Medicine is just starting to discover that health is not all numbers, chemical indicators, prescriptions, and blood tests. We hope you'll want to help encourage that understanding.

Health Literacy Strategies

Now that you've learned about health literacy issues facing underserved women, there is a range of simple strategies for figuring out if a mother has literacy issues:

Let those with low literacy maintain their sense of dignity. Do not use literacy tests or screening tools as they are inappropriate in your setting. Instead you can do the following:

- When you hand a mother written material, do not ask her to read it to you. Instead you read aloud, and watch to see if her eyes track the material. Nonreaders cannot follow along—though it is a natural instinct for those who can.
- When you hand a mother written materials, hand it to her upside down. If she does not turn it right side up, it is possible that she cannot read it.
- Simply ask a mother how she likes to learn—by reading, listening to audiotapes, watching TV, or by doing. There are different types of learners, and many who cannot read or have reading disabilities prefer to learn in other ways. A mother with limited literacy skills may not be able to journal, but she can draw pictures, or cut out photographs that explore her feelings.

Regardless of a mother's literacy skills, there are some simple communication strategies for teaching that will help a mother retain the information you provide:

1. Speak simply, using plain language. One of the joys of getting an advanced degree is learning a whole new language. But the mothers you work with will not have received that degree. So speak simply and plainly, staying away from jargon.

2. Use the Teach-Back Method. Ask mom to restate back—or teach back to you—the messages that she heard. "What are you supposed to do when you go home?" "When you talk to the baby's dad or grandmother, how are you going to tell him or her what went on today?" This isn't a quiz, and you may want to preface these questions with a disclaimer—that she would be doing you a favor by helping *you* make sure *you* did a good job of explaining yourself.
3. Use excellent written materials—effectively. Avoid simply handing mothers written information at the end of a visit and telling them that the information you discussed is in this brochure. Instead, first read the brochure yourself and make sure it is written in clear, plain language and is easily understood. Familiarize yourself with the brochure and use its structure to structure your discussion. Open the brochure and point to each topic as you speak. Highlight or underline important words. Review the content and then mothers can go back to it later to review. A mother will be much more likely to look at the brochure again if you've used it with her.
4. Write things down. Pregnancy causes forgetfulness. New parenthood causes exhaustion—neither is conducive to memory. When you make a suggestion, or moms need to remember something, write it down—*neatly*, please! People with limited literacy skills will find someone who can read the information to them if necessary.
5. Make a drawing. No need for Picasso. Drawings engage parents, and it helps you think things through. Putting pen to paper will also slow you down, which will make it clearer.
6. Remember that you can have cultural differences with people who may have grown up in the same city as you, as well as people who grew up in distant lands. It's just more obvious that a woman who does not speak English cannot understand what you are saying.
7. Learn about the family literacy programs in your area and work out a referral protocol.
8. Find out more about Baby Basics by visiting www.whattoexpect.org

If you are providing perinatal counseling to a mother you suspect is having trouble communicating with her provider or understanding prescriptions, you can help her in these ways:

- If you suspect that a mom has trouble reading, ask her to bring in all of her medications. Then color-code each medicine (use different colored magic marker on each prescription pill bottle) and make her a simple chart to keep track of when and how often each "colored" pill is taken.
- If you are getting questions that are meant for the doctor, help mom write these questions down and encourage her to role-play, asking the doctor the question and imagining what kind of answer she needs.
- Offer to attend an appointment with her if this is practical, or help her enroll in a supportive home visiting program or other educational case management program.

REFERENCES

Allen, M., & Horowitz, A. (2004). *Understanding health literacy and its barriers.* Retrieved August 10, 2007, from www.nlm.nih.gov/pubs/cbm/healthliteracybarriers.html

American Medical Association Medical Student Section Community Service Committee. (2004). *Health Literacy.* Retrieved on August 10, 2007, from www.ama-assn.org

Baker, D. W, Parker, R. M., Williams, M. V., & Clark, W. S. (1998). Health literacy and the risk of hospital admission. *Journal of General Internal Medicine, 13,* 791–798.

Bennett, I., Culhane, J., & Elo, I. (2007). Literacy and depressive symptomatology among pregnant Latinas with limited English proficiency. *American Journal of Orthopsychiatry, 2,* 243–248.

Bennett, I., Switzer, J., Aguirre, A., Evans, K., & Barg, F. (2006). "Breaking it down": Patient-clinician communication and prenatal care among African American women of low and higher literacy. *Annals of Family Medicine, 4,* 334–340.

Committee on Health Literacy. (1999). Health literacy: Report of the Council on Scientific Affairs. Ad Hoc Committee on Health Literacy for the Council on Scientific Affairs, American Medical Association. *The Journal of the American Medical Association, 281,* 552–557.

Francis, L., Weiss, B. D., Senf, J., Heist, K., & Hargraves, R. (2007). Does literacy education improve symptoms of depression and self-efficacy in individuals with low literacy and depressive symptoms? A preliminary investigation. *The Journal of the American Board of Family Medicine, 20*(1), 23–27.

Kirsch, I. S, Jugebut, A., Jenkins, L., & Kolstad, A. (1993). *Adult literacy in America: A first look at the results of the National Adult Literacy Survey.* Washington, DC: Department of Education.

Kutner, M., Greenburg, E., Jin, Y., & Paulson, C. (2006). *The health literacy of America's adults: Results from the 2003 National Assessment of Adult Literacy (NCES 2006-483).* Washington, DC: National Center for Education Statistics, U.S. Department of Education.

Monsen, L. (2007). *Literacy initiatives boost maternal and child health, say experts.* Retrieved December 5, 2007, from www.usinfo.state.gov

National Assessment of Adult Literacy. (2003). *A nationally representative and continuing assessment of English language literary skills of American adults.* Retrieved December 12, 2007, from http://nces.ed.gov/naal/

Nielsen-Bohlman, L., Panzer, A., & Kindig, D. (Eds.). (2004). *Health literacy: A prescription to end confusion.* Institute of Medicine Report. Retrieved August 12, 2007, from www.nap.edu

Parikh, N., Parker, R., Nurss, J., Baker, D., & Williams, M. (1996). Shame and health literacy: The unspoken connection. *Patient Education Counseling, 27*(1), 33–39.

Rudd, R., Moeykens, B. A, & Colton, T. C. (1999). Health and literacy: A review of medical and public health literature. In J. Comings (Ed.), *Annual review of adult learning and literacy* (Vol. 1, chap. 5). New York: Jossey-Bass.

Sanders, L. M., Thompson, V. T., & Wilkinson, J. D. (2007). Caregiver health literacy and the use of child health services. *Pediatrics, 119,* 86–92.

Sanders, L. M., Zacur, G., Haecker, T., & Klass, P. (2004). Number of children's books in the home: An indicator of parent health literacy. *Ambulatory Pediatrics, 4,* 424–428.

Vernon, J., Trujillo, A., Rosenbaum, S., & DeBuono, B. (2007). *Case report: Low health literacy: Implications for national health policy.* Retrieved November 2007, from www.clearhealthcommunication.org

Weiss, B. (2007). *Assessing health literacy in clinical practice.* Retrieved on December 12, 2007, from www.medscape.com/viewarticle/566053

Weiss, B. D., Francis, L., Senf, J., Heist, K., & Hargraves, R. (2006). Literacy education as treatment for depression in patients with limited literacy and depression: A randomized controlled trial. *Journal of General Internal Medicine, 8,* 823–828. Retrieved December 14, 2007, from www.medscape.com/viewarticle/543730

Weiss, B. D. (1999). *20 common problems in primary care.* New York: McGraw-Hill.

Wolf, M., Williams, M., Parker, R., Parikh, N., Nowlan, A., & Baker, D. (2007). Patients' shame and attitudes toward discussing the results of literacy screening. *Journal of Health Communication, 12,* 721–732.

18

The Role of Social Support in the Prevention, Intervention, and Treatment of Perinatal Mood Disorders

JANE ISRAEL HONIKMAN

> The Support Groups represent the most significant and useful aspect of the renaissance in the recognition and treatment of postpartum illness.
>
> —James Alexander Hamilton, PhD, MD, August 30, 1988

This chapter will describe the history, principles, and types of social support. A specific and systematic social support approach will be detailed. Six stages will be recommended to organize a community-based social support network.

The role that social support plays in prevention, intervention, and treatment during pregnancy and the first postpartum year is based on research from cultural anthropology, psychology, sociology, nursing, and medicine. This research consistently has demonstrated that the lack of social support is an important modifiable risk factor for postpartum depression (Dennis & Letourneau, 2007). In general, parents with high levels of support are more satisfied with their babies, their roles, and with their lives overall and are less likely to develop postpartum depression (Kendall-Tackett, 1993). In addition to scientific research, there is a body of consumer-driven knowledge from the self-help movement. The progress of the perinatal social support movement has resulted from a convergence of knowledge and collaboration among all of these disciplines.

This chapter highlights the individuals whose research and writings led to the founding of Postpartum Support International. Their contributions laid the foundation of how pregnant and postpartum women, and their families, are acknowledged, supported, and treated today.

In a March 1984 letter to this chapter's author, James Alexander Hamilton, PhD, MD, a founder of the maternal mental health scientific organization, The Marcé Society, wrote, "Your organizations have enormous potential for helping people." He continues, "When I was most actively in practice I always had from 3 to 8 postpartum cases in the same ward. The first thing I did when a new case came in was to introduce her to a woman who was on the road to recovery. This is the best therapy possible. The woman with a postpartum illness is very dejected. She feels that she has failed, she has a character deficit. When she sees others with the same thing, in various stages of recovery, she knows that she is the victim of an illness, not a character failure. This is the most effective factor in recovery, in hospital patients, and it must be effective in lesser degrees of illness. I think that you could claim a lot of support and interest from feminist sources. I think that you could say, for the United States at least, that this field has been totally neglected by male-dominated medicine, which, with pitifully few exceptions, is totally ignorant of the kinds of stresses that are involved here."

Dr. Hamilton's words propelled self-help activists and health care professionals in their own communities into a global advocates' network for maternal mental health. He was a visionary whose first book, *Postpartum Psychiatric Problems*, was published in 1962. In his introduction he wrote, "Of all the ailments to which the human mind and body are vulnerable, none is more catastrophic than serious psychiatric illness following childbirth" (Hamilton, 1962). It was Dr. Hamilton who proposed using PPD as a "generic term to relate to all of the groups to a common cause" (Taylor, 1996, p. 132). Dr. Hamilton became the movement's mentor until his death in 1997 at age 90.

THE HISTORY OF SOCIAL SUPPORT: A CONVERGENCE OF SCIENCE AND SELF-HELP FOR PERINATAL FAMILIES

Harry Harlow, PhD, was one of the best-known psychologists of the 20th century. There is a link between what his research with primates demonstrated about affection and relationships and the field of perinatal social support. The Harlow legacy shows us that social isolation is devastating.

For more than a decade the research conducted at the Primate Laboratory at the University of Wisconsin, Madison, examined social support systems (Blum, 2002). His work and the research that followed his lead give us a view on love and the importance of social contact and support. Deborah Blum said, "The nature of love is about paying attention to the people who matter, about still giving when you are too tired to give. Be a mother who listens, a father who cuddles, a friend who calls back, a helping neighbor, a loving child" (Giberson, 2003, p. 25).

Harlow's findings have become incorporated into what is considered common sense childrearing practices today. He demonstrated the importance of mother, her role in providing constant comfort to her infant, as well as the significance of peer relationships and play. In 1975 he received a prestigious award, and his work was praised as being "of extreme significance for understanding those aspects of human behavior related to depression which originate in the formative years of mother-infant interactions" (LeRoy & Kimble, 2003, p. 296).

Dana Raphael focused on the link between successful breastfeeding and social support. She is a cultural anthropologist whose own experience led her to 15 years of intensive research on breastfeeding in animals. She then studied how mothers are treated in the United States, and more than 200 other cultures (Raphael, 1970, 1976, 1981). *Matrescence,* or the time of "mother-becoming," is the critical period when a girl becomes a woman (Raphael, 1975, 1988). This *rite de passage* is a process that includes, not only biological states of pregnancy and birth, but also her status, emotional state, identity, and relationships. Dr. Raphael introduced the word *doula* into our vocabulary as the person who assists the process of matrescence (Raphael, 1988).

Doulas of North America (DONA) wrote its position paper on the role of the postpartum doula in maternity care in 2002. "The doula's education, quiet support and guidance are a manifestation of the traditional postpartum support that our society is missing" (DONA, 2002, p. 1). In addition to practical help, the doula can offer new parents help with understanding the process of concrete problem solving. This extends to determining whether they have adequate social support (Kelleher, 2002).

There has been a significant contribution from British researchers and health care providers to the field of perinatal psychiatry. Among the scientific founders of the Marcé Society were Professors R. Kumar and I. F. Brockington. They edited two scholarly books on motherhood and mental illness during the 1980s. A growing body of research into psychopathology of reproduction demonstrated a vitality in the field (Brockington & Kumar, 1982). Of particular importance has been the development of the Edinburgh Postnatal Depression Scale (EPDS). John Cox and Jeni Holden edited a book in response to a conference held in 1991 to discuss the increasing use of the EPDS within the context of strategies for prevention (Cox & Holden, 1994).

An important contributor to the literature has been developmental psychologist Kathleen Kendall-Tackett. Her decision to write a book on postpartum depression for nurses came from her years as a child abuse researcher. She includes specific suggestions for interventions and referrals to appropriate community resources (Kendall-Tackett, 1993). A major researcher on postpartum mood disorders has been Michael O'Hara, PhD, at the Department of Psychology, University of Iowa. His work was supported by grants from the National Institute of Mental Health. All of the studies included the role of social support using tools such as the Childcare Stress Inventory, the Peripartum Events Scale, and the Social Support Interview (O'Hara, 1995).

M. Cynthia Logsdon, DNS, began her research interest in perinatal social support in the early 1980s. She became concerned with lack of support for new mothers and developed the Postpartum Support Questionnaire (PSQ) (Logsdon, Usui, Birkier, & McBride, 1996). It consists of 34 items and 4 Likert-type scales and is designed as either a self-report or by interview (Logsdon et al., 1996; Logsdon, 2003).

Cheryl Beck, DNSc, was the first to conduct a phenomenological study on postpartum depression. Prior to her research the science had been based upon quantitative designs using questionnaires. Dr. Beck's approach was to interview mothers who were suffering in order to describe the essential structure of the illness (Beck, 1992). Her research continued and by the end of the decade, Beck had developed a new screening scale. The Postpartum Depression Screening Scale (PDSS) improves detection through a 35-item Likert-type self-report instrument (Beck & Gable, 2000).

The role that culture plays in understanding postpartum mood disorders is described by Wile and Arechiga (1999). They recommend that research studies devoted to parenthood rites of passage must have the following guidelines: (1) provide accurate descriptions of the symptoms that mothers experience; (2) account for the cultural medium in which the behavior is expressed; and (3) include observations by individuals culturally immersed to translate customs and rituals describing a woman's pregnancy, birth, and postpartum experience.

Using data obtained from 26,877 women with newborns in the state of Iowa, race/ethnicity was found to be a risk factor for depressed mood in late pregnancy and the early postpartum period. Lower levels of social support emerged as a possible explanation for why African Americans reported more depression (Segre, Losch, & O'Hara, 2006). Another recent multiethnic study conducted at community health centers near Boston showed that having two or more friends or family members available for support lowered depressive symptoms in new mothers (Surkan, Peterson, Hughes, & Gottlieb, 2006).

THE SELF-HELP MOVEMENT

The concept of "helping one another" or "mutual aid" is the foundation of what evolved into "helping others help themselves," or self-help. The pioneers of the 19th century in the United States, fueled by waves of immigration, joined together in activities of mutual support. They formed agricultural cooperatives, provided end-of-life services, and financial assistance (Zola, 1979). These are early examples of tangible forms of environmental social support.

The evolution of providing emotional or psychological help is tied to how medical practices changed during the mid-20th century. Zola identified three basic barriers to the development of the self-help movement: (1) the nature of the groups' problems, (2) types of help to deal with the groups' problems, and (3) who would be appropriate for providing the help. His models focused on medical diseases considered to be "unacceptable." These included both physical and mental disabilities. He described a range of stigma of having a perceived deficit such as hearing or limb loss to extremely taboo behavioral disorders of mental illness. As medical advances were made in eradicating infectious diseases, sanitation practices more widely adhered to, and public health improved, there was a dramatic shift from curing patients to long-term care. This included the need for medical management, and it brought forth a change in patient–doctor relationships. An epidemiologist, John Cassel, used the term *social support* when describing the relationship between the vulnerability to disease and certain psychosocial processes (Logsdon, 2000). This shift opened an opportunity for patient involvement in illness treatment. It was the beginning of psychological self-help activities.

New social movements like the American self-help movement are the result of people wanting to meet and create places to come together.

Their tenacity to establish groups and networks provides a bridge between professionals and their own lived experiences (Taylor, 1996). In the early 1980s, Richard Marshall, MD, was one of the first medical professionals to acknowledge the importance of new parent support groups or parenting networks as substitutes for family and friends. He worked specifically with parents and families of premature and sick newborns at a neonatal intensive care unit (NICU). His perspective was based on observations that "a certain kind of concern and mutual support is available only from those peers in whom issues of authority and power are not important considerations" (Boukydis, 1986). Dr. Marshall recommended that professionals see parents as colleagues and members of the team to improve health outcomes for the infants. He continues that, "looking back, it seems obvious to ask consumers how we can better serve their needs, and yet in our professional training we are not taught to use such humility and common sense." The seventh edition of *The Self-Help Group Sourcebook: Your Guide to Community and Online Support Groups,* published in 2002 by the American Self-Help Group Clearinghouse, contained information on nearly 1,100 national and model one-of-a-kind groups, and international networks.

There are four common characteristics present in groups defined as self-help. First, they represent a dynamic process of mutual help in which knowledge is pooled, experiences are shared, hopes are reinforced, and efforts are joined. Second, they are composed of peers sharing a common problem or stressful life situation, providing the message that the participant is not alone. Third, groups are voluntary, charging no or minimal fee for help. Last, the locus of control is the group, rather than professionals. These factors promote true ownership, a sense of responsibility, and the feeling of being a community (Madara, 1990).

Sociologist Verta Taylor wrote extensively on the development of a formal postpartum social support structure in her 1996 book, *Rock-a-by-Baby.* While at Ohio State University, she theorized that today's social support movement was influenced by the larger women's movement that began in the 19th century. This is attributed to women continually searching for acknowledgment of their own experiences (Honikman, 1999). Verta Taylor describes a distinction that sets apart social support for new mothers from other forms of self-help as gender-specific. The feminine aspects of self-help include: (1) the concept that support groups promote the self-interest of each individual, and (2) caring for others is a route to individual empowerment (Taylor, 1996). British psychologist Jeni Holden describes *befriending* as an act that empowers a woman and helps her to gain a sense of her own competence. For example, one voluntary home visiting program, begun in 1992 throughout the United Kingdom, offers friendship, support, and practical help to young families (Cox & Holden, 1994).

THE EMERGENCE OF THE PERINATAL SOCIAL SUPPORT MOVEMENT

The first annual conference on Women's Mental Health Following Childbirth was convened by this chapter's author on June 28, 1987, in Santa Barbara, California. Among those attending this historic event were the founders of Postpartum Education for Parents (PEP) in Santa Barbara; Depression After Delivery (DAD) from the states of New Jersey, Washington, Ohio, Pennsylvania, and Utah; and the Pacific Post Partum Support Society (PPPSS) in Vancouver and Calgary, Canada (Honikman, 2000). Dr. James Hamilton gave the keynote address. He recommended that the participants form an organization and call it Postpartum Support International.

The mission of Postpartum Support International (PSI) is to promote awareness, prevention, and treatment of maternal mental health issues related to childbearing in every country worldwide. The nonprofit's members are the consumers, self-help groups, and professionals who lead the postpartum social support and mental health movement. PSI's infrastructure features a global social support network consisting of area coordinators who represent 50 states in the United States and 26 other countries. The PSI Office receives telephone calls and emails from women, their families in need of support and information, and professionals. When appropriate, these callers and emails are distributed to the area coordinators. The Web site at www.postpartum.net was established during the 1990s at Indiana University in Pennsylvania. PSI continues to sponsor an annual conference whose theme reflects the current trends in the scientific research and the role of support volunteers. The grassroots organization is a member of the National Institute of Mental Health's Outreach Partnership Program. On the global level, PSI is a member of the World Federation for Mental Health and has presented information about its worldwide network at its conferences on mental health promotion and prevention. Since the early 1980s, there has been an ongoing relationship with the Marcé Society, which promotes the international scientific research of perinatal mood disorders (Honikman, 2006). Central to the purpose of Postpartum Support International is the founder's vision to have a social support network in every community worldwide.

THE PRINCIPLES OF SOCIAL SUPPORT

The principles of social support are derived from evidenced-based research that has shown that: (1) empowerment, (2) ethnic minorities integration, (3) positive interpersonal interactions, (4) social participation, (5) social responsibility and tolerance, (6) social services, and (7) social support and community networks are the protective factors of good mental health (World Health Organization [WHO], 2004b, p. 21). Social support has both genetic and environmental variables. It is about who we are, how we interact with others, and external stressors. It includes accepting who we are, as well as giving, getting, and giving back again. It covers three domains: (1) the extent to which individuals are attached to others, (2) the individual's cognitive appraisal of the support, and (3) the response of others in the provision of support (WHO, 2004a, p. 33).

During the 1980s researchers from several disciplines noted the relationship between the importance of social support and the promotion of mental and physical health. Initial research in the 1970s investigated the "more is better" approach of whether support decreased stress directly, improved coping skills, or if it acted as a buffer to stress. It was found that support can be perceived as a burden if there was an expectation to give support back (Davis, Logsdon, & Birkmer, 1996). There were specific findings that new mothers were concerned about their need for emotional support and prolonged postpartum depression (Kruckman, 1996). Environmentally, there is a variety of social factors such as life stress, poverty, and child care that impact mothers and fathers. Research on postpartum depression concludes that a woman's level of social support is the most influential. This research has shown the relationship between levels of self-esteem, self-efficacy, lowered anxiety, and, therefore, the prevention of postpartum depression (Kendall-Tackett, 2005).

In all cultures and countries there is a universal message given to the women and their families who are experiencing pregnancy-related mood disorders. This is expressed in three simple phrases: (1) you are not alone (validation); (2) you are not to blame (reassurance); and (3) your experience is real, it is treatable, and you will be well (hope). This message reflects the dynamic process and principles of mutual help and social support (Honikman, 2002).

A recent Canadian study examined the influence of both global and relationship-specific perceptions of support in the first 8 postpartum weeks in a diverse sample of 594 mothers. It was found that relationship-specific (e.g., partner, mother, and other women with children) support was beneficial. Of significance was the issue of reliability and nurturance from her partner, as well as from other women with children. The conclusions suggested that strategies using relationship-specific interventions include positive alliances that provide opportunities for interaction with other mothers (Dennis & Letourneau, 2007).

THE TYPES OF SOCIAL SUPPORT

Social support has been classified into four types. These are: (1) material, (2) emotional, (3) informational, and (4) comparison. The first type of support is also called practical or instrumental help. Emotional support includes encouragement, affection, approval, and feelings of "togetherness." The definition of informational support includes sharing advice, answering questions, as well as facilitating active problem solving. Comparison support is derived when encouragement, advice, or information are shared between individuals with similar or the same situations (Davis, Logsdon, & Birkmer, 1996; Logsdon, 2003). Studies have shown that the predominant source of social support is provided to pregnant and new mothers by spouses (Logsdon, 2000).

A recent study of 1,216 families in 10 U.S. locations investigated the presence and patterns of social support and child care on the relationship between maternal depressive symptoms and child behavior problems at two developmental stages. The results showed that social support was a contributing factor. The conclusions suggest that health providers examine what social support is available to mothers, especially those not severely depressed. Further recommendations include providing child care so that mothers and their children can benefit from protective interactions with others (Lee, Halpern, Hertz-Picciotto, Martin, & Suchindran, 2006).

A Specific and Systematic Social Support Approach for Perinatal Families

After offering emotional telephone and peer group support for 20 years, this chapter's author wrote *I'm Listening: A Guide to Supporting*

Postpartum Families in 2002. The premise of the phase *mothering the mother* is the keystone of the message conveyed to perinatal families through a method of conversational, nonjudgmental emotional support. This approach believes that: (1) every mother needs a mother; (2) if a mother is not well, then her family is not well; and (3) mothers deserve care and are worthy of being the focus of society's attention. As previously stated, there is a universal message expressed throughout the perinatal social support movement. It has three simple components: (1) you are not alone; (2) you are not to blame; and (3) you will be well, your experience is real, and there is help available.

The author has written an outline called Steps to Wellness. This systematic approach is based upon Dr. George Albee's formula for reducing the incidence of mental disorders (Albee, 1982). This model is described by the formula:

$$\text{Incidence} = \frac{\text{Organic factors} + \text{stress}}{\text{Coping skills} + \text{self-esteem} + \text{support groups}}$$

The Step to Wellness outline is also based upon the experiences and recommendations of the British Health Visitors program implemented in the early 1990s. Their six key elements in the prevention of postpartum depression are: (1) continuity of care; (2) social support; (3) preparation for parenthood; (4) stress management, problem solving, and a plan of action; (5) referral to additional resources; and (6) education about emotional reactions to pregnancy, birth, and parenting (Gerrard, Elliott, & Holden, 1994).

The author's Steps to Wellness include the following nine steps: (1) Education, (2) Sleep, (3) Nutrition, (4) Exercise and Time for Myself, (5) Sharing With Nonjudgmental Listeners, (6) Emotional Support, (7) Practical Support, (8) Referrals to Professional, and (9) Plan of Action.

The First Step to being healthy is education because it confronts both denial of a problem and ignorance surrounding that problem. It also provides information and options for treatment. The expression *knowledge is power* is founded on the premise that without accurate information we become passive victims and fearful. If we can learn, then the fear is diminished. Reading accurate materials and listening to informed individuals is critical to maintaining and/or returning to good health.

Step Two is sleep. The body requires adequate and quality sleep to stay healthy and to heal. Pregnancy, labor, delivery, and the postpartum period interrupt the brain and body's ability to sleep. The key to healing is restorative or rejuvenating sleep; therefore, new parents must be given the opportunity to achieve this goal. The role of social support is crucial in determining if parents are receiving adequate and proper sleep, and, if not, to assist them. In extreme cases the brain will not "shut down or wake up" as it should, and medical intervention may be required. An excellent question to ask a new parent is, "Given the opportunity to sleep, can you sleep?"

The Third Step is nutrition. A majority of postpartum women may be eating poorly, some may be malnourished, and a few even starving themselves. The role that a social support person provides is asking the following important questions: (1) Do you have an appetite? (2) What are you eating? (3) What have you eaten today? and (4) What's there to eat in your kitchen? The appetite center in the brain is responsible for the feeling of hunger. The mother's (and sometimes the father's) inability to provide adequate nutrition may require medical intervention as well as psychologically emphasizing the important message that if the mother is not healthy, no one will thrive, including the baby.

Step Four is exercise and time for oneself. Social support networks are frequently found by getting outside and away from one's home. This is a double opportunity to be physically active to help the body return to a prepregnancy state, and to make new friends who are sharing this same experience of parenthood. It may also be a time to be away from one's baby. The message of this step is "You are worthy and deserving of being alone."

The Fifth Step is sharing with nonjudgmental listeners. Parents need to ask the question, "Who can I talk to about my feelings?" This is a risky proposition if one is surrounded by advice givers who may be well intentioned but uninformed and highly judgmental. The brain can also "shut down" and prevent verbalization. Social support networks surround mothers and fathers with validation and reassurance. The goal is to offer hope that, no matter what, it is okay to express negative emotions or experiences.

Step Six is the emotional support that is given back in response to Step Five. All new parents *need* and *deserve* emotional support from one's friends, family, faith community, professionals, and others in order to heal. There may be a range of reactions from the normal adjustment issues of parenthood to tremendous emotional turmoil, including mental illness. It takes time to listen well and it requires time. Anonymous volunteers may provide this step over a telephone, in a group setting, or between friends. Empathy is the foundation of this type of caring and concern.

Step Seven is practical support, sometimes called material help. Ideally, this step can be planned for in advance of the postpartum period. It may have already begun during pregnancy with help for household chores. If a social support network is established prior to parenthood, it eases the burdens, including financial and lack of time, of "normal" adjustment. When illness intervenes, a crisis can be avoided through the existence of individuals who can assist the family with cooking, cleaning, shopping, and child care.

The Eighth Step is offering referrals to professionals and other resources. This includes doctors, therapists, and social support networks. There is a general rule that applies to offering a referral to a paid professional. Three names should be given to someone seeking a referral. There is also the consideration of insurance. It can become a cycle of frustration to find a professional, but it is hoped that one's primary care doctor can work with new parents. In the perfect community, there is a social support network in place that can facilitate this process as well.

The final Ninth Step is called a Plan of Action because it takes the parent from being in a place of denial and/or ignorance to acknowledgment and self-advocacy. A parent can begin by self-evaluating the previous eight steps by asking, "What am I doing well, and what could I be doing better?" The outcome should then be "What can and should I do next?" The conversation has come full circle with the potential for a positive outcome.

The Six Stages to a Successful Social Support Network

The development of perinatal parent support networks in our own communities is needed in order to respond to the emotional needs of pregnant and postpartum families. These networks are the heart of social support. Their role is to link consumers with community resources. A review of research on social support in the early 1980s distinguished three areas of focus: (1) the potential or actual providers of support available to a person, (2) a person's internal appraisal of the availability and effectiveness of support, and (3) the activities involved in the provision of social support (Boukydis, 1986).

The oldest example of a continuously operating postpartum support organization in the United States is Postpartum Education for

Parents (PEP). This chapter's author and her own circle of social support established PEP in 1977 (Honikman, 1986). The experience of co-founding this all voluntary, community-based nonprofit is the basis of *Step by Step: A Guide to Organizing a Postpartum Parent Support Network in Your Community* (Honikman, 2000). It is a workbook designed in an outline format that has been divided into six stages. Some of the stages and steps can be done simultaneously.

> *Stage 1* asks you to visualize and start an organizational structure in which you will actualize your dream of a parent support network. It is imperative that you find others who share your vision and commitment to make this network real and viable.
>
> *Stage 2* requires you to research other parent support groups and networks that already exist in your community and beyond. The information and personal connections that you start to make in this stage will shape your decisions in the subsequent stages of this workbook.
>
> *Stage 3*, the Planning Stage, is the most time-consuming. It involves the "meat" of this work process. Starting with Step 1, you will begin to formulate your group's purpose, philosophy, goals, and objectives. In addition, you will make decisions regarding the services to provide and the group structure. There is a discussion of funding, along with volunteer and staff issues.
>
> *Stage 4* is about implementing the group's services. The contacts that you developed in previous stages will help you form an advisory board of professionals who serve your target population. The ideas that you and the core committee developed earlier will be turned into printed material and will represent your group. Through your group's outreach efforts, the general community starts to hear about what the new network will offer them. The last step is the implementation of service.
>
> *Stage 5* can feel both concrete and abstract. You deliver services; there's something to show for your hard work and vision. Yet it can feel anticlimatic when participant level starts low or drops off. If your group offers emotional support, the volunteers or service deliverers may not be able to measure the effects of their interventions/services. There are methods for evaluating a group's effectiveness, but this part of the process is often neglected. Without Stage 5, your group cannot endure.

Stage 6 encourages you to develop partnerships outside your group and to have a bearing on the services of other organizations in your local community. You'll learn how to set new goals and objectives to keep your group fresh and vital, and, should you care to, how to write your own account of starting the network.

SUMMARY

This chapter has reviewed the history, principles, types, and research of the role of social support in assisting perinatal families. There is a legacy left by decades of dedicated individuals and groups that indicate that mental and physical health require a holistic approach. An evolution of understanding indicates that emotional and practical support is a critical component of quality health care (Logsdon, McBride, & Birkimer, 1994). The biological and social scientists have combined their talents and resources to focus attention on the previously overlooked arena of maternal mental health. Postpartum Support International is the leader of the perinatal social support movement. The organization's goal and objectives are part of a transformation that is outlined by the President's New Freedom Commission of Mental Health. The goals include: (1) understanding that mental health is essential to overall health; (2) mental health care is consumer- and family-driven; (3) disparities in mental health services are eliminated; (4) early mental health screening, assessment, and referral to services are common practice; (5) excellent mental health care is delivered, and research is accelerated; and (6) technology is used to access mental health care and information (New Freedom Commission on Mental Health, 2003).

In response to the President's Commission, the Department of Health and Human Services (HRSA) wrote and published a booklet entitled *Depression During and After Pregnancy: A Resource for Women, Their Families, and Friends.* The recommendations listed are: (1) lean on family and friends; (2) talk to a health care professional; (3) find a support group; (4) talk to a mental health care professional; (5) focus on wellness; and (6) take medication as recommended by your health care provider (HRSA, 2006).

Author and clinical psychiatrist Valerie Davis Raskin, MD, captures the essence of this chapter in her latest book: "A common prescription I give: join a new-mother's group. Whether it's a support group for women with postpartum depression, a moms-newly-at-home group . . . , new mothers are often amazed at the confessions of other women, especially those who don't live in fear of being judged, for whom shame is not an ever-lurking shadow" (Raskin, 2007, p. 45).

REFERENCES

Albee, G. (1982). Preventing psychopathology and promoting human potential. *American Psychologist, 37,* 1043–1050.

Beck, C. T. (1992). The lived experience of postpartum depression: A phenomenological study. *Nursing Research, 41,* 166–170.

Beck, C. T., & Gable, R. (2000). Postpartum depression screening scale: Development and psychometric testing. *Nursing Research, 49*(5), 272–282.

Blum, D. (2002). *Love at Goon Park: Harry Harlow and the science of affection.* Cambridge, MA: Perseus.

Boukydis, C. F. Z. (1986). Support for early parenting: Research and theoretical perspectives. In C. F. Z. Boukydis (Ed.), *Support for parents and infants: A manual for parenting organizations and professionals* (pp. 11–37). New York: Routledge & Kegan Paul.

Brockington, I. F., & Kumar, R. (1982) *Motherhood and mental illness.* London: Academic.

Cox, J., & Holden, J. (1994). *Perinatal psychiatry: Use and misuse of the Edinburgh Postnatal Depression Scale.* London: Gaskell (Royal College of Psychiatrists).

Davis, D., Logsdon, M., & Birkmer, J. (1996). Types of support expected and received by mothers after their infants' discharge from the NICU. *Issues in Comprehensive Pediatric Nursing, 19,* 263–273.

Dennis, C. L., & Letourneau, N. (2007). Global and relationship-specific perceptions of support and the development of postpartum depressive symptomatology. *Social Psychiatry Psychiatric Epidemiology, 42*(5), 389–395.

Doulas of North America (DONA). (2002). *Position paper: The postpartum doula's role in maternity care.* Jasper, IN: Author.

Gerrard, J., Elliott, S., & Holden, J. (1994). The management of postnatal depression trainers manual. London: Sinsbury Centre for Mental Health.

Giberson, K. (2003). Learning about love the hard way. *Science & Spirit, 14*(2), 25–28.

Hamilton, J. A. (1962). *Postpartum psychiatric problems.* St. Louis: Mosby.

Health Resources & Services Administration (HRSA). (2006). *Depression during and after pregnancy: A resource for women, their families, and friends.* Rockville, MD: Author.

Honikman, J. I. (1986). How to start a parents' organization. In C. F. Z. Boukydis (Ed.), *Support for parents and infants: A manual for parenting organizations and professionals* (pp. 41–58). New York: Routledge & Kegan Paul.

Honikman, J. I. (1999). Role of self-help techniques for postpartum mood disorders. In L. J. Miller (Ed.), *Postpartum mood disorders.* Washington, DC: American Psychiatric Press.

Honikman, J. I. (2000). Step by step: A guide to organizing a postpartum parent support network in your community. Santa Barbara, CA: Author.

Honikman, J. I. (2002). I'm listening: A guide to supporting postpartum families. Santa Barbara, CA: Author.

Honikman, J. I. (2006). The role of Postpartum Support International in helping perinatal families. *Journal of Obstetric, Gynecologic, & Neonatal Nursing, 35*(5), 659–661.

Kelleher, J. (2002). *Nurturing the family: The guide for postpartum doulas.* Xlibris Corp. Retrieved March 16, 2008, from www.Xlibris.com

Kendall-Tackett, K. A. (1993). *Postpartum depression: A comprehensive approach for nurses.* Newbury Park, CA: Sage.

Kendall-Tackett, K. A. (2005). *Depression in new mothers: Causes, consequences, and treatment alternatives.* New York: Haworth Maltreatment and Trauma Press.

Kruckman, L. D. (1996). An anthropological view of postpartum depression: Disorders. In J. A. Hamilton & P. N. Haberger (Eds.), *Postpartum psychiatric illness: A picture puzzle* (pp. 137–148). Philadelphia: University of Pennsylvania Press.

Lee, L. C., Halpern, C. T., Hertz-Picciotto, I., Martin, S. L. & Suchindran, C. M. (2006). Child care and social support modify the association between maternal depressive symptoms and early childhood behavior problems: A U.S. national study. *Journal of Epidemiological Community Health, 60*(4), 305–310.

LeRoy, H. A., & Kimble, G. A. (2003). Harry Frederick Harlow: And one thing led to another . . . In G. Kimble & M. Wertheimer (Eds.), *Portraits of Pioneers in Psychology: Vol. V* (p. 296). Washington, DC: American Psychological Association.

Logsdon, M. C. (2000). *Social support for pregnant and postpartum women.* Washington, DC: Association of Women's Health, Obstetric and Neonatal Nurses.

Logsdon, M. C. (2003). The postpartum support questionnaire. In O. L. Strickland & C. DiIorio (Eds.), *Measurement of nursing outcomes: Vol. 3. Self-care and coping* (2nd ed., pp. 129–141). New York: Springer Publishing.

Logsdon, M. C., McBride, A. B., & Birkimer, J. C. (1994). Social support and postpartum depression. *Research in Nursing & Health, 17,* 449–457.

Logsdon, M., Usui, W., Birkmer, J., McBride, A. (1996). The postpartum support questionnaire: Reliability and validity. *Journal of Nursing Measurement, 14*(2). 129–141.

Madara, E. J. (1990). Maximizing the potential for community self-help through clearinghouse approaches. *Prevention in Human Services, 7,* 109–138.

New Freedom Commission on Mental Health. (2003). *Achieving the promise: Transforming mental health care in America. Executive summary.* DHHS Pub. No. SMA-03-3831. Rockville, MD.

O'Hara, M. (1995). *Postpartum depression: Causes and consequences.* New York. Springer Publishing.

Raphael, D. (1970, February 8). When mothers need mothering. *The New York Times Magazine,* 67–69.

Raphael, D. (1975). Matrescence, becoming a mother: A "new/old" rite de passage. In D. Raphael (Ed.), *Being female: Reproduction, power and change* (pp. 65–71). Chicago: Aldine.

Raphael, D. (1976). *The tender gift, breastfeeding: Mothering the mother—the way to successful breastfeeding.* New York: Schocken Books.

Raphael, D. (1981). Why supportive behavior in human and other mammals? *American Anthropologist, 83,* 634–638.

Raphael, D. (1988). New patterns in doula client relations. *Midwife Health Visitor & Community Nurse, 24,* 376–379.
Raskin, V. D. (2007). *The making of a mother: Overcoming the nine key challenges from crib to empty nest.* New York: Ballantine Books.
Segre, L. S., Losch, M. E., & O'Hara, M. (2006). Race/ethnicity and perinatal depressed mood. *Journal of Reproductive and Infant Psychology, 24*(2), 99–106.
Surkan, P. J., Peterson, K. E., Hughes, M. D., & Gottlieb B. R. (2006). The role of social networks and support in postpartum women's depression: A multiethnic urban sample. *Maternal Child Health Journal, 10*(4), 375–383.
Taylor, V. (1996). *Rock-a-by-baby: Feminism, self-help, and postpartum depression.* New York: Routledge.
Wile, J., & Arechiga, M. (1999). Sociocultural aspects of postpartum depression. In L. J. Miller (Ed.), *Postpartum mood disorders* (pp. 83–98). Washington, DC: American Psychiatric Press.
World Health Organization. (2004a). *Promoting mental health concepts: Emerging evidence, practice. Summary Report.* H. Herrman, S. Saxena, & R. Moodie (Eds.). Geneva: Author.
World Health Organization. (2004b). *Prevention of mental disorders: Effective interventions and policy options. Summary Report.* C. Hosman, E. Jané-Llopis, & S. Saxena (Eds.). Geneva: Author.
Zola, I. K. (1979). Helping one another: A speculative history of the self-help movement. *Archives of Physical Medicine and Rehabilitation, 60,* 452–456.

Resource List

This is not an exhaustive list, but offers a starting point for further information/services.

American Psychiatric Association—Postpartum depression website
www.healthyminds.org/postpartumdepression.cfm

ASRM (American Society For Reproductive Medicine)
www.asrm.org

AWHONN—Provides professional resources and support empowering nurses to provide superior evidence-based care to newborns and to women throughout the lifespan.
www.awhonn.org/awhonn/

The Emory Women's Mental Health Program—Established in 1991, primarily focuses on the evaluation and treatment of emotional disorders during pregnancy and the postpartum period.
www.emorywomensprogram.org/

Massachusetts General Hospital Women's Mental Health Program—Provides a range of current information, including discussion of new research findings in women's mental health and how such investigations inform day-to-day clinical practice.
www.cwmh.wordpress.com/about/

MediSpin—NIMH-funded website offering information for consumers and mental health practitioners on perinatal mood disorders. The site also offers CME provider courses for those interested in developing this practice specialty. Most information offered in English and Spanish.
www.mededppd.org

NASPOG (The North American Society for Psychosocial Obstetrics and Gynecology)—A society of researchers, clinicians, educators and scientists involved in women's mental health and healthcare. Formed in the 1960s as a collaboration among Obstetrician Gynecologists, Psychiatrists and Psychologists, the Society's aim is to foster scholarly scientific and clinical study of the biopsychosocial aspects of obstetric and gynecologic medicine.
www.naspog.org/

National Association of Social Workers with Perinatal Practice Specialty
www.socialworkers.org

New Jersey Department of Health and Senior Services—A website for consumers and healthcare professionals available in English and Spanish, developed by the first state in the union to pass PPD legislation.
www.state.nj.us/health/fhs/ppd/index.shtml

Postpartum Progress—Nation's most widely read blog on PPD issues, by Katherine Stone, offering current information, stories from survivors, news items and books.
www.postpartumprogress.typepad.com

Postpartum Support International—World's largest non-profit organization offering information, annual educational conference and other services for women, their families suffering from perinatal mood disorders, and the health care professionals who serve them, including free live session with perinatal mental health experts via 800 bridgeline. With coordinators in most United States and 26 countries around the world, PSI's network helps connect women and families with the services they need in their area. The website also offers links to many other national and international programs/services including websites for families, fathers and other information. PSI also offers a nationally recognized certificate training program for those interested in forming or facilitating support groups in a professional or lay capacity. Coordinators warm line and website information offered in English and Spanish.
www.postpartum.net
1-800-944-4773

RESOLVE—The National Infertility Association
www.resolve.org

Index

O

P

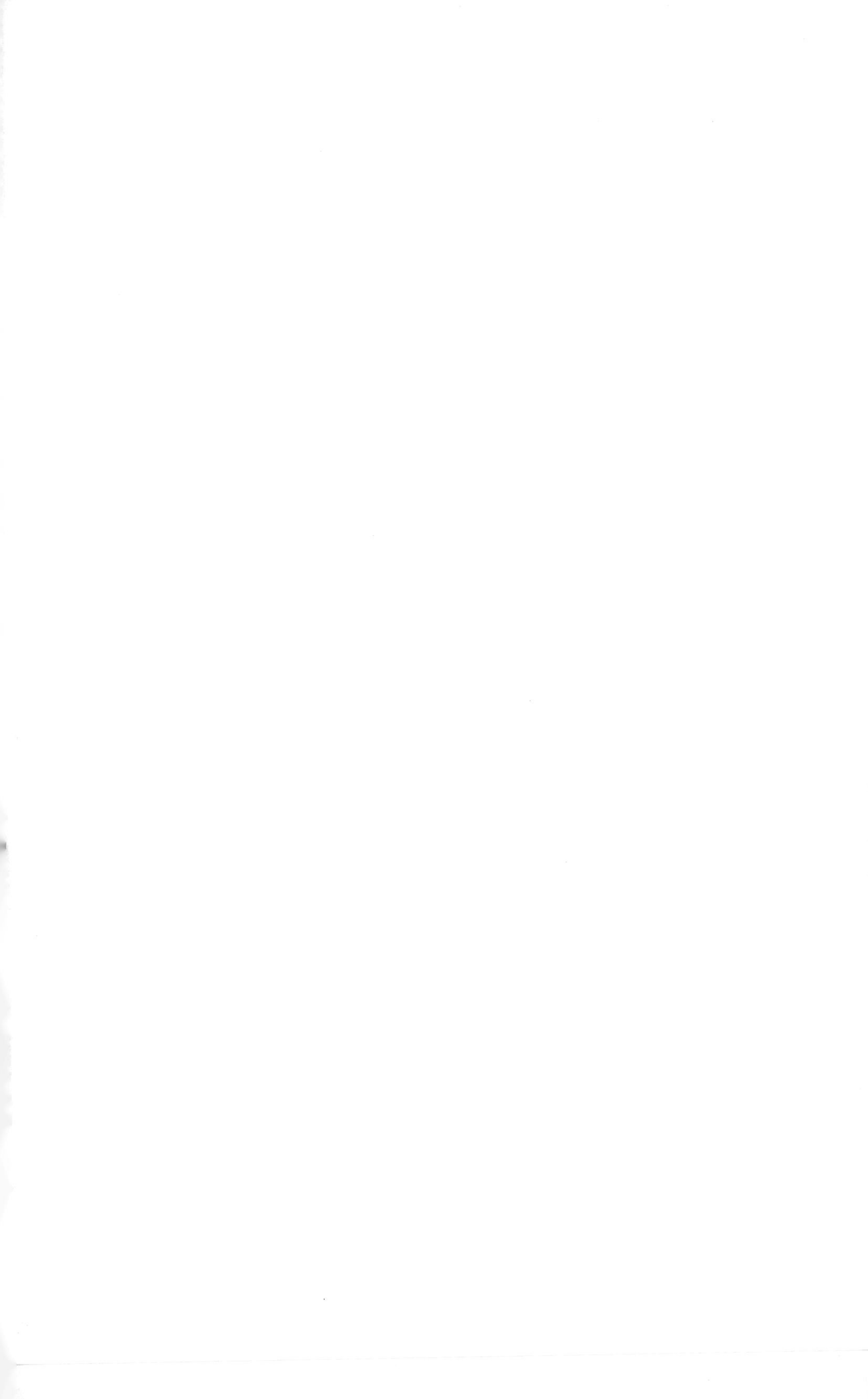